Modern Management of Testicular Cancer

Editor

SIAMAK DANESHMAND

UROLOGIC CLINICS
OF NORTH AMERICA

www.urologic.theclinics.com

Consulting Editor
SAMIR S. TANEJA

August 2019 • Volume 46 • Number 3

ELSEVIER

1600 John F. Kennedy Boulevard ● Suite 1800 ● Philadelphia, Pennsylvania, 19103-2899

http://www.theclinics.com

UROLOGIC CLINICS OF NORTH AMERICA Volume 46, Number 3
August 2019 ISSN 0094-0143, ISBN-13: 978-0-323-68234-3

Editor: Kerry Holland
Developmental Editor: Laura Kavanaugh

Urologic Clinics of North America (ISSN 0094-0143) is published quarterly by Elsevier Inc., 360 Park Avenue South, New York, NY 10010-1710. Months of issue are February, May, August, and November. Business and Editorial Offices: 1600 John F. Kennedy Blvd., Suite 1800, Philadelphia, PA 19103-2899. Periodicals postage paid at New York, NY and additional mailing offices. Subscription prices are $387.00 per year (US individuals), $757.00 per year (US institutions), $100.00 per year (US students and residents), $450.00 per year (Canadian individuals), $946.00 per year (Canadian institutions), $520.00 per year (foreign individuals), $946.00 per year (foreign institutions), and $240.00 per year (Canadian and foreign students/residents). Foreign air speed delivery is included in all *Clinics* subscription prices. All prices are subject to change without notice. **POSTMASTER:** Send address changes to *Urologic Clinics of North America*, Elsevier Health Sciences Division, Subscription Customer Service, 3251 Riverport Lane, Maryland Heights, MO 63043. **Customer Service: 1-800-654-2452 (US). From outside the United States, call 1-314-447-8871. Fax: 1-314-447-8029. E-mail: JournalsCustomerServiceusa@elsevier.com (for print support)** and **JournalsOnlineSupport-usa@elsevier.com (for online support).**

Reprints. For copies of 100 or more, of articles in this publication, please contact the Commercial Reprints Department, Elsevier Inc., 360 Park Avenue South, New York, New York 10010-1710. Tel.: 212-633-3874; Fax: 212-633-3820; E-mail: reprints@elsevier.com.

Urologic Clinics of North America is covered in MEDLINE/PubMed (*Index Medicus*), *Excerpta Medica, Current Contents/Clinical Medicine, Science Citation Index,* and *ISI/BIOMED.*

Contributors

CONSULTING EDITOR

SAMIR S. TANEJA, MD
The James M. Neissa and Janet Riha Neissa
Professor of Urologic Oncology, Professor of
Urology and Radiology, Director, Division of
Urologic Oncology, Vice Chair, Department of
Urology, NYU Langone Medical Center, New
York, New York, USA

EDITOR

SIAMAK DANESHMAND, MD
Associate Professor of Urology (Clinical
Scholar), Director of Urologic Oncology,
Director of Clinical Research, Urologic
Oncology Fellowship Director, USC
Norris Comprehensive Cancer Center, USC
Institute of Urology, Los Angeles, California,
USA

AUTHORS

RAFAT ABONOUR, MD
Division of Hematology and Medical Oncology,
Melvin & Bren Simon Cancer Center, Indiana
University School of Medicine, Indianapolis,
Indiana, USA

NABIL ADRA, MD, MSc
Division of Hematology and Medical Oncology,
Melvin & Bren Simon Cancer Center, Indiana
University School of Medicine, Indianapolis,
Indiana, USA

PETER ALBERS, MD
Professor, Department of Urology,
University of Duesseldorf, Medical Faculty,
Heinrich-Heine-University, Duesseldorf,
Germany

ADITYA BAGRODIA, MD
Assistant Professor, Department of
Urology, The University of Texas
Southwestern Medical Center, Dallas,
Texas, USA

MICHAEL JANNEY BILES, MD
Department of Urology, The James Buchanan
Brady Urological Institute, Johns Hopkins,
Baltimore, Maryland, USA

MICHAEL A. BROOKS, MD
Fellow in Urologic Oncology, Urology
Department, Glickman Urologic and Kidney
Institute, Cleveland Clinic, Cleveland, Ohio,
USA

CLINT CARY, MD, MPH
Associate Professor, Department of Urology,
Indiana University School of Medicine,
Indianapolis, Indiana, USA

SIAMAK DANESHMAND, MD
Associate Professor of Urology (Clinical
Scholar), Director of Urologic Oncology,
Director of Clinical Research, Urologic
Oncology Fellowship Director, USC Norris
Comprehensive Cancer Center, USC Institute
of Urology, Los Angeles, California, USA

HOOMAN DJALADAT, MD, MS
Associate Professor of Clinical Urology,
Institute of Urology, USC Norris
Comprehensive Cancer Center, University of
Southern California, Los Angeles, California,
USA

RICHARD S. FOSTER, MD
Professor, Department of Urology, Indiana
University School of Medicine, Indianapolis,
Indiana, USA

RASHED A. GHANDOUR, MD
Urologic Oncology Fellow, Department
of Urology, The University of Texas
Southwestern Medical Center, Dallas, Texas,
USA

SAUM GHODOUSSIPOUR, MD
Urologic Oncology Fellow, USC Norris
Comprehensive Cancer Center, USC
Institute of Urology, Los Angeles, California,
USA

ALIREZA GHOREIFI, MD
Research Fellow of Urologic Oncology,
Institute of Urology, USC Norris
Comprehensive Cancer Center, University of
Southern California, Los Angeles, California,
USA

ROBERT J. HAMILTON, MD, MPH, FRCSC
Division of Urology, University Health Network,
Princess Margaret Cancer Centre, Toronto,
Ontario, Canada

ANDREAS HIESTER, MD
Department of Urology, University
of Duesseldorf, Medical Faculty,
Heinrich-Heine-University, Duesseldorf,
Germany

ZACHARY KLAASSEN, MD, MSc
Division of Urology, Medical College
of Georgia, Augusta University, Georgia
Cancer Center, Augusta, Georgia,
USA

**CHRISTIAN K. KOLLMANNSBERGER, MD,
FRCPC**
Clinical Professor, Department of Medicine,
Division of Medical Oncology, BC Cancer -
Vancouver Cancer Center, University of British
Columbia, Vancouver, British Columbia,
Canada

JEAN-MICHEL LAVOIE, MD, FRCPC
Fellow, Genitourinary Service, Division of
Medical Oncology, Department of Medicine,
BC Cancer - Vancouver Cancer Center,
University of British Columbia, Vancouver,
British Columbia, Canada

ACHIM LUSCH, MD
Department of Urology, University of
Duesseldorf, Medical Faculty, Heinrich-Heine-
University, Duesseldorf, Germany

TIMOTHY A. MASTERSON, MD
Associate Professor, Department of Urology,
Indiana University School of Medicine,
Indianapolis, Indiana, USA

AKANKSHA MEHTA, MD, MS
Department of Urology, Emory University
School of Medicine, Atlanta, Georgia, USA

LUCIA NAPPI, MD, PhD
Department of Medicine, Medical Oncology
Division, BC Cancer Agency, Department of
Urologic Sciences, Vancouver Prostate Centre,
University of British Columbia, Vancouver,
British Columbia, Canada

DANIEL NETTERSHEIM, PhD
Professor, Department of Urology, Urological
Research Lab, Translational Urooncology,
University of Duesseldorf, Medical Faculty,
Heinrich-Heine-University, Duesseldorf,
Germany

CRAIG NICHOLS, MD
Testicular Cancer Commons, Vancouver,
Washington, USA; SWOG Group Chairs Office,
Portland, Oregon, USA

ALESSANDRO NINI, MD
Department of Urology, University of
Duesseldorf, Medical Faculty, Heinrich-Heine-
University, Duesseldorf, Germany

PHILLIP MARTIN PIERORAZIO, MD
Associate Professor, Urology and Oncology,
Department of Urology, The James Buchanan
Brady Urological Institute, Johns Hopkins,
Baltimore, Maryland, USA

BRUCE J. ROTH, MD
Professor, Department of Medicine, Division of
Oncology/BMT, Washington University in St.
Louis, St Louis, Missouri, USA

ROBERT CRAIG SINEATH, MPH
Department of Urology, Emory University
School of Medicine, Atlanta, Georgia,
USA

NIRMISH SINGLA, MD
Urologic Oncology Fellow, Department
of Urology, The University of Texas
Southwestern Medical Center, Dallas, Texas,
USA

ANDREW J. STEPHENSON, MD
Professor, Urology Department, Glickman
Urologic and Kidney Institute, Director, Center
for Urologic Oncology, Cleveland Clinic,
Cleveland, Ohio, USA

LEWIS J. THOMAS, MD
Fellow in Urologic Oncology, Urology
Department, Glickman Urologic and Kidney
Institute, Cleveland Clinic, Cleveland, Ohio,
USA

Contents

The Role of Imaging in the Diagnosis, Staging, Response to Treatment, and Surveillance of Patients with Germ Cell Tumors of the Testis   315

Lewis J. Thomas, Michael A. Brooks, and Andrew J. Stephenson

> Germ cell tumors (GCTs) of the testis are cured with the successful integration of surgery, chemotherapy, and/or radiation therapy in most cases. The favorable results are a consequence of improved risk stratification, risk-adapted chemotherapy, reduced morbidity of treatment, and appropriate integration of multimodal therapy. The success of these approaches depends on accurate staging with imaging studies of the testis, retroperitoneum, and thorax. This article reviews the indications for imaging and performance characteristics of modalities in the diagnosis, staging, surveillance, and follow-up of patients with GCTs. We also highlight the current guideline recommendations for imaging in treatment of patients with GCTs.

Management of Primary Testicular Tumor   333

Alireza Ghoreifi and Hooman Djaladat

> In any man with a solid testicular mass, cancer should be considered until proven otherwise. Radical inguinal orchiectomy is the treatment of choice in patients with testis mass. Placement of a testicular prosthesis is safe with a very low complication rate and should be offered to all patients undergoing radical orchiectomy. In patients with widespread or life-threatening advanced disease, delayed orchiectomy following chemotherapy is recommended. Testis-sparing surgery can be performed in highly selected patients with solitary testicle mass, bilateral testicular tumors, or strong suspicion of a benign lesion.

Preservation of Fertility in Testis Cancer Management   341

Robert Craig Sineath and Akanksha Mehta

> The presence of cancer in the testis, as well as the therapies used to treat testis cancer, can impair fertility potential for affected men. Fertility preservation is an important aspect of survivorship care and should be offered to all patients before initiating treatment. The only established means of fertility preservation in men is cryopreservation of sperm. Methods for fertility preservation in prepubertal boys are still experimental. Physicians treating men with testicular cancer should be familiar with the available options. This article outlines testicular cancer and its treatment's effects on fertility, fertility preservation options, and barriers to accessing this specialized care.

Management of Clinical Stage I Germ Cell Tumors   353

Bruce J. Roth

> Experience demonstrates multiple paths to cure for patients with clinical stage I testicular cancer. Because all options should provide a long-term disease-free rate near 100%, overall survival is no longer relevant in decision making, allowing practitioners to factor in quality of life, toxicity, cost, and impact on compliance.

Surveillance for clinical stage I seminoma and clinical stage I nonseminoma has become the preferred option. The contrarian view is that a risk-adapted approach should persist, with surveillance for low-risk individuals and active therapy high-risk individuals. However, results obtained in unselected patients provide a strong argument against the need for such an approach.

Management of Stage II Germ Cell Tumors   363

Rashed A. Ghandour, Nirmish Singla, and Aditya Bagrodia

There are several treatment approaches for stage II germ cell tumors (GCTs), and a thorough understanding of the staging classification and histologic differences in tumor biology and therapeutic responsiveness is critical to determine an effective, multimodal management strategy that involves urologists, medical oncologists, and radiation oncologists. This article discusses contemporary management strategies for stage II GCTs, including chemotherapy, radiotherapy, retroperitoneal lymph node dissection (RPLND), and surveillance. Patient selection, histology, and extent of lymphadenopathy drive management, and, as both treatment and detection strategies continue to emerge and be refined, the management of patients with stage II GCT continues to evolve.

Current Management of Disseminated Germ Cell Tumors   377

Jean-Michel Lavoie and Christian K. Kollmannsberger

The modern treatment of disseminated germ cell tumors (GCT) relies largely on cisplatin-based regimens, particularly combination chemotherapy with bleomycin, etoposide, and cisplatin. This article reviews the evidence supporting its use as well as common alterations based on prognostic grouping or contraindications to bleomycin. Special topics around the management of intermediate/poor prognosis choriocarcinoma and brain metastases are included. The management of residual masses for both seminoma and nonseminoma is discussed as well as long-term follow-up care of patients. Finally, the management of relapsed disseminated GCT is addressed.

Postchemotherapy Resection of Residual Mass in Nonseminomatous Germ Cell Tumor   389

Saum Ghodoussipour and Siamak Daneshmand

The introduction of cisplatin-based chemotherapy has revolutionized the care of patients with disseminated testicular germ cell tumors. Although a majority are cured with chemotherapy alone, surgical resection continues to play a role because one-third will have residual mass after chemotherapy. In this article, we review the current indications for postchemotherapy resection in nonseminomatous germ cell tumors, including masses greater than 1 cm, resection after salvage chemotherapy, with elevated markers, after late relapse, and for growing teratoma syndrome. We also highlight technical considerations of this often-challenging surgery, including the need for adjunctive procedures, extraretroperitoneal resections, and modern techniques to minimize morbidity.

Indications for Surgery in Disseminated Seminoma   399

Phillip Martin Pierorazio and Michael Janney Biles

Seminoma is commonly diagnosed in young men, and it has therefore become a disease of long-term survivors. As the late toxic effects of radiation and chemotherapy are better understood, it is becoming imperative to focus management advance-ments on reducing exposure to toxic agents. Retroperitoneal lymph node dissection (RPLND) currently is indicated as a salvage procedure in postchemotherapy patients with residual masses. Primary RPLND currently is being further explored in patients with clinical stage IA and clinical stage IB disease in 2 prospective studies.

Retroperitoneal lymph node dissection (RPLND) is complex; however, recent ad-vances in technology have allowed adoption of the robotic platform for highly select cases. Initial case series have shown improved cosmesis, less blood loss, and decreased length of stay compared with open RPLND. Our preference for perform-ing robotic RPLND is via a transperitoneal approach with the patient in the supine position, thus facilitating a bilateral template dissection identical to that used in all our open procedures. Robotic RPLND should mimic the open approach with regard to oncologic principles and should only be performed by clinicians well versed in open RPLND.

Growing teratoma syndrome (GTS) is a rare clinical phenomenon in patients with nonseminomatous germ cell cancer defined by growing metastatic mass during ongoing or directly after completed chemotherapy with timely decreasing tumor markers and postpubertal teratoma exclusively after resection. GTS was first described in 1982, and few reports have been published. The limited number of studies and the resulting lack of exact knowledge about development, differentia-tion, and treatment of GTS leaves several clinical problems regarding treatment and follow-up unsolved. This review provides an overview of clinical diagnosis and disease management and an approach to explain the molecular development of GTS.

Retroperitoneal lymph node dissection is an integral part of the management of testicular cancer. Surgical approach and outcomes have improved over the past de-cades. Several factors influence the complexity of the operation, including numerous patient characteristics and disease-related characteristics. An important consideration lies in the fact that this is largely a vascular operation, and techniques of vascular control should be comfortable for the urologic surgeon performing the procedure. This article discusses the known surgical complications related to this operation and their relative incidence reported throughout the literature.

Germ cell tumors (GCT) are the most common cancer in men between 15 and 35 years of age and the incidence has increased during the past several decades. This article reviews the current knowledge on high-dose chemotherapy (HDCT) and stem cell transplant for salvage treatment of patients with relapsed metastatic GCT. Furthermore, the authors attempt to dissect the controversy of using standard-dose versus high-dose therapy as initial salvage and identify patients who are most likely to benefit from HDCT and peripheral blood stem cell transplant.

Two clusters of microRNAs have been discovered highly expressed by seminoma and nonseminoma germ cell tumors. They are secreted in blood of patients with testicular germ cell tumors and can be extracted from the serum or plasma and quantified by real-time–polymerase chain reaction. Results have confirmed the feasibility of the technique and demonstrated that sensitivity and specificity of those microRNAs in detecting viable germ cell tumors are higher than with current methods. If operation characteristics are confirmed in larger studies, those micro-RNAs will be valuable to manage equivocal clinical scenarios characterized by high uncertainty and high risk of over-treatment or under-treatment.

UROLOGIC CLINICS OF NORTH AMERICA

Preface

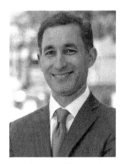

Siamak Daneshmand, MD
Editor

At first glance, it may appear that we have compiled another round of redundant articles on a topic that has for the most part been rather stagnant over the past 2 decades. The pioneering work of investigators and institutions in the 1970s and 1980s led the path to what we now enjoy as an era of very high cure rates in testicular cancers. The last decade has seen a reduction in adjuvant therapies in stage I disease and a shift toward patient-centered management with resultant decrease in the burden of treatment. Many opportunities for improved delivery of care however still remain. In this issue, we have broadly covered the main areas of modern testicular cancer management, from imaging and management of the primary testicular tumor, to stage-specific treatment and a detailed description of microRNA (miRNA) as a novel biomarker. The emerging theme within management of germ cell tumors is meaningful population-based reduction in imaging intensity, adjuvant therapy, and overall use of chemotherapy, while maintaining excellent cure rates. While we no longer routinely advocate surgery for low-risk stage I nonseminoma and in patients who achieve a complete response following chemotherapy, we are exploring the therapeutic value of retroperitoneal lymph node dissection (RPLND) for early-stage seminoma and miRNA-positive nonseminoma in novel clinical trials. No matter what the approach, we have seen a significant decrease in the morbidity of surgery while maintaining the principles of anatomic dissection set forth decades ago. There is now a marked focus on fertility preservation with nerve-sparing surgical techniques and widespread availability of sperm banking. All of these topics are discussed in the various articles in this issue.

I am enormously thankful to the expert authors who have contributed the outstanding articles within this issue. They are each drivers of innovation and practice the art of medicine with passion and precision. This issue serves not only as a modern reference but also as a guide for optimal management of germ cell cancers around the world. There are more novel molecular-based discoveries on the horizon, which will undoubtedly lead to a paradigm shift in recommendations for surgery and systemic therapy in the very near future, and we look forward to being on the forefront of these breakthroughs.

Siamak Daneshmand, MD
USC/Norris Comprehensive Cancer Center
Institute of Urology
1441 Eastlake Avenue, Suite 7416
Los Angeles, CA 90089, USA

E-mail address:
daneshma@med.usc.edu

Urol Clin N Am 46 (2019) xiii
https://doi.org/10.1016/j.ucl.2019.05.002
0094-0143/19/© 2019 Published by Elsevier Inc.

urologic.theclinics.com

The Role of Imaging in the Diagnosis, Staging, Response to Treatment, and Surveillance of Patients with Germ Cell Tumors of the Testis

Lewis J. Thomas, MD[a], Michael A. Brooks, MD[a], Andrew J. Stephenson, MD[a,b,*]

KEYWORDS

- Testicular neoplasms • Neoplasm staging • Retroperitoneal space • Radiation therapy • Risk

KEY POINTS

- Imaging is critical for the diagnosis, staging, surveillance, and follow-up of patients with testicular cancer.
- Ultrasound and MRI are the main modalities for imaging of the testis. Computed tomography (CT) and MRI are used for imaging of the retroperitoneum. CT, MRI, and chest radiographs are used for imaging of the chest.
- Fluorodeoxyglucose-PET is useful in imaging of post-chemotherapy seminoma patients with residual masses, but has limited utility otherwise.
- Regimens for surveillance and follow-up are based on the risk, timing, and location of potential relapses.
- Although imaging is critical for rapidly diagnosing relapses; serum tumor markers, symptoms, and physical examination also play important roles.

INTRODUCTION

Germ cell tumor (GCT) of the testis is the model of a solid-organ malignancy that can be cured with multimodal therapy, even in advanced stages. Selection of appropriate therapies for patients with GCT is based on numerous variables including histopathologic assessment, serum tumor marker levels (STM), imaging findings, and patient preference. Current imaging modalities used in the staging, follow-up, and surveillance of GCT include plain radiographs (chest, [CXR]), ultrasound (US), computed tomography (CT), MRI, and fluorodeoxyglucose (FDG)-PET. These tests have different indications, costs, radiation exposures, and availabilities. The selection and timing of appropriate imaging studies is paramount in the accurate diagnosis, staging, response to treatment, and posttreatment surveillance of patients to optimize outcomes.

Imaging guidelines for GCT are rarely based on level 1 evidence and few head-to-head studies comparing different modalities have been performed. Recommendations instead rely on retrospective data describing patterns, risks, and locations of relapses in different disease states.

Disclosure Statement: No disclosures.
a Urology Department, Glickman Urologic and Kidney Institute, Cleveland Clinic, Glickman Tower, Q10. 9500 Euclid Avenue, Cleveland, OH 44108, USA; b Center for Urologic Oncology, Cleveland Clinic, Cleveland, OH 44195, USA
* Corresponding author. Center for Urologic Oncology, Cleveland Clinic, Cleveland, OH 44195.
E-mail address: ajs213@case.edu

Urol Clin N Am 46 (2019) 315–331
https://doi.org/10.1016/j.ucl.2019.05.001
0094-0143/19/© 2019 Published by Elsevier Inc.

urologic.theclinics.com

In addition, specific targeted imaging techniques have not been developed for testis cancer. Despite these issues, oncologic outcomes for patients with GCT are quite good; however, further research into imaging offers the hope of reducing the burden of surveillance/follow-up regimens or of improving on the ability to stratify early-stage patients and reduction of overtreatment.

This review summarizes key imaging tests and regimens used in the management of patients with GCT. Key guidelines are described, as well as the evidence underpinning those guidelines. Finally, areas of uncertainty are discussed, and we describe our approach to imaging in patients with GCT, particularly where it deviates from the recommended regimens.

The imaging regimens described in the figures are common regimens that the authors use in surveillance of patients with testis cancer. They are not in complete concordance with either European Association of Urology (EAU) or National Comprehensive Cancer Network (NCCN) guidelines, although they are based off interpretations of much the same evidence. In addition, although imaging is critical to testis cancer surveillance, other factors including history/physical examination, STMs, and patient preference all play a role in developing appropriate follow-up regimens.

DIAGNOSIS
Imaging of a Testicular Mass

Ultrasound
Trans-scrotal ultrasound with color Doppler (ultrasound) is the primary modality for imaging of testicular masses. Ultrasound is a widely available, nontoxic, low-cost technique, and has high sensitivity for GCTs (100% in some series).[1] Studies of ultrasound typically include color-Doppler imaging, which characterizes the vascularity of a lesion and can aid in distinguishing benign from malignant findings. Current guidelines, including the NCCN and the EAU, both recommend ultrasound for evaluation of any patient with a suspected testis mass.[2,3] However, performing a confirmatory ultrasound should not delay referral of a patient with suspected testis cancer for definitive management.

Imaging of the contralateral testis for germ cell neoplasia in situ or synchronous primary tumor
Bilateral GCT occurs in approximately 2% to 3% of patients, although presentation is usually metachronous. An asymptomatic, nonpalpable synchronous primary tumor in the contralateral testis is rare. Nevertheless, the contralateral unaffected testis should be evaluated by ultrasound to rule

out other testicular pathology that may influence the decision to perform orchiectomy or perform ancillary tests (eg, atrophic testis and need for sperm-banking pre-orchiectomy). Germ cell neoplasia in situ (GCNIS) is the premalignant lesion associated with the development of invasive GCT and is associated with 80% to 90% of invasive GCT and is present in the contralateral testis in 5% to 8% of patients with GCT.[4] Approximately 50% of patients with GCNIS will develop invasive GCT within 5 years.[5] Abnormal ultrasound echotexture of the testis is a common but nonspecific finding associated with contralateral GCNIS, although diagnosis is dependent on pathologic assessment.[6] There are no guideline recommendations for ultrasound follow-up of the contralateral testis.

Benign testicular masses
Although most intratesticular masses are malignant, there are benign intratesticular findings that providers should be aware of. This includes cysts, infection, infarction, hemorrhage, scar/fibrosis, tubular ectasia, intratesticular varicocele or spermatocele, Leydig cell hyperplasia, adrenal rest, sarcoidosis, and lipoma. Occasionally these benign etiologies can be diagnosed by ultrasound, history, and examination, although often they are diagnosed by orchiectomy pathology. In particular, practitioners should be wary of cystic lesions, as teratoma can often present as a cystic mass on ultrasound. Some of the relevant examination and imaging findings of these lesions are noted in **Table 1**.

MRI for testis masses
MRI can often be used to aid in the diagnosis of equivocal testicular lesions. MRI has a high sensitivity for testicular malignancies and a reasonable ability to discriminate benign from malignant lesions. Tsili and colleagues[10] reported on 33 patients with ultrasound-diagnosed testicular masses and compared the MRI findings with the eventual pathologic diagnosis. MRI had a sensitivity of 100% for testicular malignancies, and a specificity of 87.5%. Malignant lesions were noted to be isointense on T1 imaging, with variable characteristics on T2 imaging, and heterogeneous enhancement with contrast (gadolinium) administration. The false-positive result was granulomatous orchitis, which had heterogeneous enhancement on contrast administration similar to a malignant lesion. Benign diagnoses that were correctly identified by MRI included tubular ectasia of the rete testis, hemorrhagic necrosis, and fibrosis/scar.

Table 1
Common benign intratesticular findings that may be mistaken for germ cell tumor on scrotal ultrasound or examination

Pathology	Examination	Imaging
Epididymoorchitis	Firm and tender testis and cord, possible constitutional or lower urinary tract symptoms.	Ultrasound: hyperemic testis/cord on Doppler imaging, enlarged testis/cord. MRI: T1 hyperintense, T2 hypointense. Preservation of testicular septations.
Infarct	Acute pain/swelling, chronic findings may vary. Associated history of sickle-cell disease, epididymoorchitis, or inguinal surgery.	Ultrasound: hypoechoic region with diminished flow on color Doppler, may be wedge shaped. MRI: Isointense or heterogeneous on T1, hypointense on T2. Nonenhancing or rim-enhancing on contrast images. MRI can better demonstrate the "wedge shape" and mediastinal orientation.
Intratesticular hematoma	Soft on examination. Occasionally tender or with trauma history although can be spontaneous.	Ultrasound: Acute lesions may be hyperechoic, resolving lesions typically hypoechoic/cystic. Evolve over time. MRI: hyperintense on T1, varying T2 appearance (may have dark rim of hemosiderin). No contrast enhancement.
Simple cyst	Often nonpalpable on examination, if palpable should be soft. Larger cysts or those with complex features may be teratoma.	Ultrasound: smooth thin wall, anechoic, no shadowing. MRI: fluid signal characteristics. No contrast enhancement.
Epidermoid cyst	Firm intratesticular lesion, nontender.	Ultrasound: "onion-skinning" appearance, negative color-Doppler. MRI: T2 hypointense rim with sharp margins. Heterogeneous, occasionally with "target" appearance. No contrast enhancement (avascular).
Tunica albuginea cyst	Typically, older patients. Often located at the upper-anterior or lateral aspect of testis. Can be nonpalpable.	Ultrasound: similar to simple cyst. MRI: similar to simple cyst.
Scar/Fibrosis	Often nonpalpable, or feels like a solid mass. Typically asymptomatic.	Ultrasound: hypoechoic, often with poorly defined borders. Occasional associated calcifications. MRI: low intensity on T1/T2, no contrast enhancement.
Tubular ectasia/ Dilated rete testis	Typically asymptomatic and nonpalpable.	Ultrasound: Multiple small cystic/tubular areas near the mediastinum of the testis. MRI: High signal intensity on T2, isolated to mediastinum testis.

(continued on next page)

Table 1
(continued)

Pathology	Examination	Imaging
Spermatocele (intratesticular)	Soft intratesticular mass.	Cystic appearing lesion on ultrasound, can displace the testicular parenchyma. MRI with noninvasive well-demarcated cystic lesion.
Varicocele (intratesticular)	Often with associated extratesticular varicocele. Testicular pain occasionally present.	Ultrasound with dilated veins and high color Doppler flow. MRI: T1/T2 hypointense, tubular structure. Early enhancement with contrast (vascular).
Leydig cell hyperplasia	Small often nonpalpable nodules on examination. Associated with early puberty/virilization in children or adolescents. Often asymptomatic in adults, can have infertility/gynecomastia.	Ultrasound: hypo or hyperechoic nodule with normal margins. Typically small (<10 mm). Can be multifocal/bilateral. MRI: Isointense on T1, hypointense on T2. Enhance with contrast.
Lipoma	Often a soft or nonpalpable lesion. Diffuse testicular lipomatosis is a common finding of Cowden syndrome.	Ultrasound: hyperechoic lesions without internal flow. MRI: T1 and T2 hyperintense.
Microlithiasis	Found in multiple clinical scenarios, often benign, controversial association with germ cell neoplasia in situ.	Ultrasound: multiple punctate hyperechoic regions, with or without shadowing. MRI: not visible.

Data from Refs.[7–9]

Cramer and colleagues[11] reported on a similar cohort and found that preoperative MRI correlated with pathologic diagnosis in 100% of cases. The most common benign diagnosis thought to be a malignancy based on ultrasound/examination was orchitis (15/20 benign cases). In patients with equivocal clinical and ultrasound examinations, Serra and colleagues[12] reported that MRI was able to correctly diagnose 91% of patients, whereas ultrasound was correct only 29% of the time. Sensitivity for malignancy was 83%, with 1 patient with a small seminoma misidentified on MRI. An associated cost analysis demonstrated that MRI could be cost-saving in equivocal cases. Similar to the Cramer cohort, orchitis was the most misdiagnosed by ultrasound/examination.

Finally, Muglia and colleagues[13] reported on a cohort of patients with equivocal ultrasound findings who underwent MRI. They found that MRI provided "additional correct information" in 82% of cases, and was incorrect in only 7%. The study also reviewed all patients referred for ultrasound, and found that only 3.6% were then referred for MRI, implying that history, examination, and ultrasound evaluation provided sufficient diagnostic information in the vast majority of cases.[14]

Ultrasound is the primary modality for workup of the patient with a suspected testis cancer and should be done in every case. Ultrasound is both sensitive and specific for GCTs, and provides a definitive diagnosis in most cases. Ultrasound can help identify contralateral testis abnormalities, but is nonspecific for pathology, and is not recommended during follow-up. MRI is useful in situations when the initial examination and ultrasound findings are equivocal, and has a reasonable ability to discriminate benign from malignant findings.

Key Points

- Ultrasound is highly sensitive for testicular malignancies.
- MRI is useful in equivocal situations and is excellent at distinguishing benign from malignant pathologies.
- MRI imaging should include T1 and T2 sequences, as well as a contrast-enhanced sequence.
- The most common confounding diagnosis is orchitis.
- Ultrasound of the contralateral testis is used primarily to rule out a synchronous primary

tumor or other intratesticular pathology. Otherwise, it should not be used in the surveillance of patients with testis cancer.

STAGING
Retroperitoneum

GCT follows a predictable pattern of spread from the testis via the lymphatics to the retroperitoneal lymph nodes in the vast majority of cases. Nonseminomatous GCTs (NSGCT) have a higher probability of systemic spread via hematogenous route as compared with seminoma. The frequency of clinical metastases at diagnosis is 20% and 60% to 70% in patients with seminoma and NSGCT, respectively.[15] Cross-sectional imaging of the abdomen and pelvis is recommended by both the NCCN and EAU for initial staging.[2,3] In addition, both groups note that either CT abdomen/pelvis (CT-AP) or MRI with contrast can be performed, citing data that describe similar sensitivity and specificity for diagnosing nodal disease for the two modalities.[16,17] Generally, CT is used for staging unless contraindications to intravenous contrast exist. However, groups such as the Swedish-Norwegian Testicular Cancer group, have used MRI routinely for staging/surveillance.[18,19] If using MRI for staging, then MRI should be used during surveillance/follow-up to allow comparison.

Size of positive lymph nodes

One of the controversies surrounding staging of the retroperitoneum is determination of the appropriate lymph node size cutoff to distinguish positive from negative nodes. Traditionally, a 10-mm cutoff has been used to define retroperitoneal adenopathy. However, this is based off older studies using early forms of CT or lymphangiography.[20] More recent evaluations have reported the 95th percentile of maximum short-axis diameter of nodes on CT and MRI systems to be 3 to 5 mm.[21] In studies of patients undergoing primary retroperitoneal lymph node dissection (RPLND), positive subcentimeter nodes are frequently found. Hilton and colleagues[22] reported on a cohort of patients with NSGCT undergoing primary RPLND, and found that using a 10-mm cutoff yielded a sensitivity of 37% with specificity of 100%, an unacceptably high rate of false-negative findings. Conversely, a size criteria of 4 mm had sensitivity of 93%, but specificity of 58%, meaning that nearly half the patients with nodes >4 mm in size obtained no oncologic benefit from RPLND. Leibovitch and colleagues[23] similarly reported on a cohort of 143 patients with NSGCT undergoing primary RPLND, but included landing zone as a variable in their assessment. They found that a cutoff of 10 mm yielded a sensitivity of 59% and specificity of 97%. However, a 3-mm cutoff in the primary landing zone (right interaortocaval, left pre- and para-aortic) as well as a 10-mm cutoff outside the primary landing zone increased the sensitivity to 91% but dropped the specificity to 52%. This trade-off in sensitivity for specificity in patients with retroperitoneal adenopathy up to 10 mm in size drives the controversy over the optimal management of patients with stage I NSGCT disease.

Fluorodeoxyglucose-PET

Better imaging tools could help stratify which patients can be observed versus treated. To that end, the Medical Research Council (MRC) group examined the role of FDG-PET in patients with high-risk clinical stage I NSGCT. The trial was stopped early because of a high rate of relapse among those with negative PET scans (63% at 1 year). Thus, at least currently, PET has no role in the staging of patients with NSGCT.[24] One area of potential interest is the use of FDG-PET in the staging of seminoma patients with small or equivocal nodes. Ambrosini and colleagues[25] reported on a diverse cohort of seminoma patients, and noted a sensitivity of 92% for FDG-PET lesion detection. Such high sensitivity could help with staging, and some high-volume centers are now using FDG-PET to try to delineate stage I from stage IIa seminoma; however, this strategy has not been validated at this time and is not guideline recommended.

In summary, cross-sectional imaging of the retroperitoneum with CT-AP should be performed at the time of diagnosis. This may be performed once the orchiectomy pathology is known and should be done within 4 weeks of diagnosis. The primary landing zone for right and left-sided GCTs should be heavily scrutinized. Visible nodes (particularly 6–10 mm in size) should be regarded with a moderate degree of suspicion for metastases, especially if high-risk primary tumor features (lymphovascular invasion) are present. In the presence of equivocal cases, the clinician may consider short-term imaging follow-up (4–8 weeks) before finalizing treatment plans. A 10-mm cutoff is used to identify suspicious nodes outside the primary landing zones. In general, pelvic lymph node metastases are rare in the absence of extensive retroperitoneal lymph node involvement.

Chest

Seminoma

NCCN and EAU guidelines recommend chest imaging as part of the workup for newly diagnosed seminoma and NSGCT. For patients with pure seminoma, the NCCN recommendation is to perform a CXR and CT-AP first, with CT-chest performed only if abnormalities are noted.[3] This practice is backed by data reported by Horan and colleagues,[26] who reviewed the staging chest CT from 182 seminoma patients. Among those with negative CT-AP, intrathoracic metastases were diagnosed in 1 patient who was identified with CXR as well as chest CT. Thirteen additional patients had abnormal chest CTs despite a negative CT-AP, but were found to have benign findings. This high false-positive rate and poor positive predictive value can lead to significant patient anxiety and unnecessary further testing. In addition, in the 13% of the cohort with positive retroperitoneal imaging, lung metastases were still fairly rare (2 of 24 cases, 8%). CT was able to identify both cases, but found an additional 5 cases with concerning findings that ended up being benign. Therefore, practitioners should be aware that even in patients with retroperitoneal adenopathy, pure seminoma lung metastases are rare, and CT-chest has a low positive predictive value (29%). This allows for appropriate patient counseling and hopefully a reduction in test-associated anxiety (**Fig. 1**).

Contrary to the NCCN approach for seminoma patients, EAU guidelines recommend chest CT in the staging of all patients with testicular cancer. This recommendation is based on evidence from See and Hoxie,[27] who examined a cohort of patients with both seminoma and NSGCT, and noted that CXR failed to identify lesions eventually proven to be metastatic disease in 22% of cases (4 of 18). However, no patients would have been missed if the NCCN chest imaging strategy had been used. Thus, and in particular for seminoma patients, we favor using CT-AP and CXR first, and performing CT-chest only if abnormalities are noted.

Nonseminomatous germ cell tumor

For NSGCT, both NCCN and EAU recommend CT-chest in the staging evaluation. Although the cohort described by See and Hoxie[27] included patients with NSGCT, it represented a small number of patients. A larger review by White and colleagues[28] examined both staging and surveillance chest CTs in patients with NSGCT and compared findings with clinical follow-up and CXR results. CXR identified only 35% of intrathoracic metastases noted by CT. In addition, 7% of patients with intrathoracic metastases had a concurrent negative CT-AP examination. However, the article notes that isolated chest metastases in otherwise clinical stage I patients were never identified.[28] Thus, it may be reasonable to use CXR, CT-AP, and STM to screen for those who require a staging chest CT, although this is not guideline recommended.

In summary, all patients should undergo chest imaging in the initial staging of GCT to rule out intrathoracic metastases. CXR is an appropriate test for patients with negative CT-AP imaging. CT-chest is not recommended in the initial

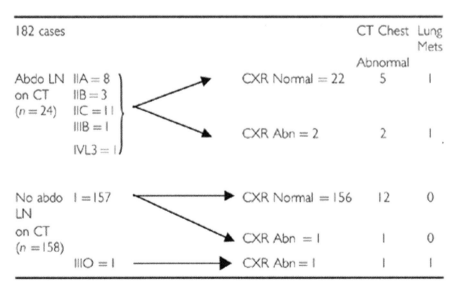

Fig. 1. Results of CXR and CT imaging for staging of seminoma. For patients with no retroperitoneal adenopathy, lung metastases were rare and identified by CXR. Abnormalities identified in seminoma patients undergoing chest CT are commonly benign (even in stage II disease). (*From* Horan G, Rafique A, Robson J, Dixon AK, Williams M V. CT of the chest can hinder the management of seminoma of the testis; it detects irrelevant abnormalities. Br J Cancer. 2007;96(6):882-885; with permission.)

staging of patients with seminoma because of high false-positive rates. CT-chest may be considered for patients with NSGCT, even for those without findings on CT-AP imaging, especially if factors associated with a risk of hematogenous spread exist (eg, lymphovascular invasion, choriocarcinoma) or when retroperitoneal lymph node dissection is planned. All patients with evidence of retroperitoneal lymph node metastases on CT-AP imaging or evidence of rising post-orchiectomy STMs should undergo CT-chest imaging before definitive treatment plans are made.

Brain/Bone Imaging

Imaging of the bone and brain is rarely indicated in the initial staging of patients with GCT. NCCN and EAU guidelines both recommend brain imaging in symptomatic patients or those with high-risk features. High-risk features include beta-HCG greater than 5000, AFP greater than 10,000, nonpulmonary visceral metastases (NPVM), extensive lung metastases, or primary choriocarcinoma. A review of patients presenting with brain metastases noted that very high beta-HCG levels were common (53% with beta-HCG >100K), almost all patients had concomitant lung metastases (94%), many had NPVM (46% with bone/liver metastases), and most were NSGCT (95%). Of note, only 53% presented with neurologic symptoms.[29]

Bone imaging is rarely used in testis cancer, and is only recommended for symptomatic patients. Similar to brain metastases, isolated bone metastases are exceedingly rare. As targeted bone therapy in the absence of symptoms is rare, the value of detecting the occasional asymptomatic bone metastasis seems limited.

Summary

Staging of patients with testis cancer primarily focuses on the retroperitoneal lymph nodes and intrathoracic metastases. Imaging of the retroperitoneal nodes is done with CT-AP, or MRI if contraindications to contrast exist. Subcentimeter but visible lymph nodes in the primary landing zones are concerning for metastases and can be considered for treatment or followed very closely. In seminoma patients, CXR may be used for initial staging if the CT-AP is negative for disease. In NSGCT, CT-chest is currently recommended for staging, although CXR may be just as accurate in otherwise stage I patients. Bone imaging is reserved for high-risk patients with symptoms, whereas brain imaging can be useful in specific asymptomatic high-risk situations.

Key Points

- CT-AP is used for staging of retroperitoneal nodes, MRI if contrast contraindications exist.
- Chest CT may be avoided in seminoma patients with a negative CT-AP and negative CXR.
- CXR or CT-chest can be used to stage NSGCT, although current guidelines recommend CT.
- Visible retroperitoneal nodes (even if <1 cm) in the primary landing zones commonly harbor disease.
- Nodes >1 cm outside the primary landing zone are considered positive.
- Bone imaging should be done only in symptomatic patients with known advanced (stage III) disease.
- Brain imaging should be done only in symptomatic patients with known advanced disease or asymptomatic patients with advanced disease and high-risk features.

IMAGING AFTER TREATMENT
Seminoma

Post-adjuvant stage I treatment
Patients with clinical stage I seminoma who undergo adjuvant radiation therapy or carboplatin chemotherapy are at very low risk of relapse. Imaging regimens are thus fairly low intensity and short duration (**Fig. 2**). Seminoma does have potential for later relapse, particularly in patients receiving chemotherapy (median relapse of 25 months), so many recommended regimens do extend out to 3 years. Relapse more than 3 years post-adjuvant treatment is rare (0.2%) and the value of further surveillance is uncertain. In addition, outcomes of late-relapse patients are favorable. However, current EAU guidelines do recommend a late CT at 60 months, presumably to catch such asymptomatic late-relapse patients. Of note, the location of relapse differs substantially between patients undergoing different adjuvant treatments. For those with dog-leg radiation, most relapses are in mediastinal or neck lymph nodes (65%). For those with isolated para-aortic radiation, pelvic relapses make-up 37%, whereas neck/mediastinal were 26%. Finally, for those undergoing chemotherapy, most relapses (67%) were retroperitoneal.[30] Thus, for patients undergoing radiation, pelvic imaging may be important if a para-aortic field is used and may be unnecessary if a dog-leg is used. Similarly, in patients who undergo any radiation therapy, a high degree of suspicion should be applied to any chest/pulmonary symptoms during follow-up, and chest CT should be strongly considered for such patients.

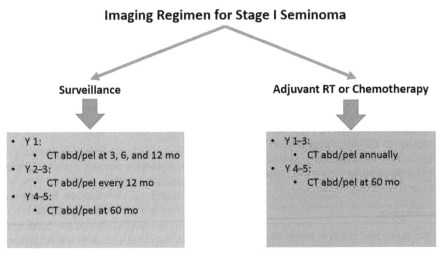

Fig. 2. Common regimens used by the authors for follow-up of stage 1 seminoma patients.

Post-radiation treatment

For seminoma patients with clinical stage IIa or nonbulky IIb disease, radiation therapy is a potential treatment option (as is chemotherapy). Such patients should rarely have a large residual mass after therapy, so surveillance is reliant on CT-AP and CXR (**Fig. 3**). Similar to surveillance after treatment of stage I disease, relapse is uncommon and is typically within the first 3 years. Post-radiation relapses also have a favorable prognosis with chemotherapy, reducing the value of aggressive imaging follow-up. A current frontier in the treatment of nonbulky stage II seminoma patients is the use of primary RPLND. Although small cohorts have been reported, there is currently not enough data on this technique to define the patterns/timing of relapse and thus dictate the appropriate post-therapy imaging regimen. As such, we use the same imaging protocol for RPLND patients as for post–radiation therapy patients.[31]

After chemotherapy

For seminoma patients with CS II/III who undergo chemotherapy, residual mass size plays a critical role in prognosis. Series of post-chemotherapy seminoma patients have established a 3-cm cutoff as a significant risk for residual disease versus fibrosis. Herr and colleagues[32] reported on a series of 55 seminoma patients who underwent post-chemotherapy RPLND. They noted that 30% of patients with residual masses >3 cm had disease present, whereas 0% of those with masses <3 cm had disease present. Results of the SEMPET trial (discussed in the next section) agree, with only 9% of patients with masses <3 cm having residual disease, whereas 50% of

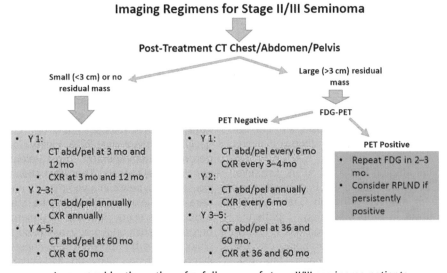

Fig. 3. Common regimens used by the authors for follow-up of stage II/III seminoma patients.

those with masses >3 cm had residual disease.[33] These findings allowed providers to observe seminoma patients with <3 cm post-chemotherapy masses. However, a substantial portion of patients with larger residual masses were still being unnecessarily exposed to additional therapy (typically surgery). Thus, additional tools were needed to help assess risk in seminoma patients with >3 cm post-chemotherapy masses.

Fluorodeoxyglucose-PET

FDG-PET helps in stratifying seminoma patients with post-chemotherapy masses >3 cm. Although early reports on FDG-PET were underwhelming, the modality gained traction from the dramatic results of the SEMPET trial. SEMPET was a prospective evaluation of 33 patients with residual retroperitoneal masses >1 cm in size following chemotherapy for seminoma. The trial reported results stratified by size of the residual mass, and correlated PET results to clinical or histologic outcomes. FDG-PET was able to predict disease presence in both small and large residual mass groups with a high degree of accuracy (specificity of 100%, sensitivity of 89%).[33]

Further follow-up of the cohort has yielded similar results. A 2005 update included 54 patients with 74 residual masses. FDG-PET correctly identified residual disease in all patients with residual masses >3 cm, but only 1 of 4 masses <3 cm in size. No false-positive results were noted.[34] These findings reinforced that FDG avid masses >3 cm in size are highly concerning for malignancy, and can serve as a strong indication for RPLND. However, FDG-PET was an insufficient tool for ruling out residual disease in patients with small residual masses.

Although the results of the SEMPET study have made FDG-PET important in stratifying post-chemotherapy seminoma patients, further studies have not demonstrated the same accuracy, with some reporting appreciable false-positive rates (15%–75%) whereas false negatives in >3 cm residual masses remained rare.[35–38] This is in line with our clinical experience. We have seen several false-positive FDG-PET studies, including some with persistently positive FDG-PET scans even on imaging several months after completion of chemotherapy (**Fig. 4**) The reasons for false-positive examinations are varied and include

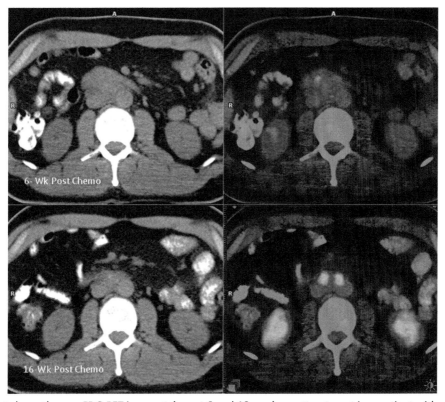

Fig. 4. Post-chemotherapy FDG-PET images taken at 6 and 16 weeks posttreatment in a patient with pure seminoma. RPLND was performed after the 16-week positive scan and pathology demonstrated fibrosis/scar. Patient has subsequently been free of relapse.

residual inflammation, fibrotic tissue, or confounding benign etiologies (such as sarcoidosis).[39]

Current guidelines

Both EAU and NCCN recommend FDG-PET for the stratification of seminoma patients with post-chemotherapy masses >3 cm in size. The recommendation is to perform the imaging at least 6 weeks after completion of chemotherapy, as earlier FDG-PET is thought to lead to false-positive results. NCCN guidelines do allow for surveillance of patients with residual masses >3 cm who do not have access to FDG-PET; however, the recommended regimen is very intense. A negative FDG-PET results in a less intense surveillance regimen (see **Fig. 3**). EAU guidelines do not specify a regimen for patients managed without FDG-PET, and recommend the standard follow-up regimen that can be used for all patients with remission (defined as mass <3 cm or >3 cm and FDG-negative) after therapy.

Our approach is to perform an initial post-chemotherapy CT-chest/abdomen/pelvis at approximately 4 to 6 weeks. If this demonstrates a residual mass >3 cm we then perform an FDG-PET at 2 to 3 months post-chemotherapy. If the FDG-PET is positive, we typically repeat FDG-PET several months later to confirm the findings. For those with masses <3 cm in size or with a negative FDG-PET, observation is recommended due to the high rate of fibrosis (see **Fig. 4**).

Nonseminomatous Germ Cell Tumor

Post-adjuvant stage I treatment

Following adjuvant treatment of stage I NSGCT, relapse is uncommon (9% for RPLND, 1% for chemotherapy), and typically occurs within 2 years.[40] As such, imaging regimens are of low intensity and of short duration (**Fig. 5**). For those with pathologic stage II disease following RPLND, follow-up is based on the receipt of adjuvant chemotherapy (**Fig. 6**). If adjuvant therapy is given, then the risk of relapse is very low (1%), and a short low-intensity follow-up regimen can be used.[41] If no adjuvant therapy is given, then the risk of relapse is substantially higher (>40%), and a more aggressive regimen is recommended. Most relapses in this cohort occur rapidly, and many are detected by elevated STM.[42]

Post-chemotherapy

For patients with disseminated disease (clinical stage II/III) primary chemotherapy is the mainstay of treatment. However, post-chemotherapy consolidative surgery may be needed. Accurate imaging assessment is critical to differentiate patients who require surgery from those that do not.

Size of residual mass

Post-chemotherapy RPLND (PC-RPLND) is recommended for patients with normalization of STMs and a residual retroperitoneal mass. Studies have demonstrated that either persistent GCT or teratoma may be present in more than 50% of patients on RPLND pathology.[14,43,44] Multiple studies have looked at using imaging to try to predict post-chemotherapy residual pathology. Steyerberg and colleagues[14] reported on a multi-institutional cohort of PC-RPLND patients and noted rates of residual disease (teratoma or GCT) in 28% of patients with residual masses 1 to 10 mm in size, and 26% in those with residual masses that shrank by more than 70%. A follow-

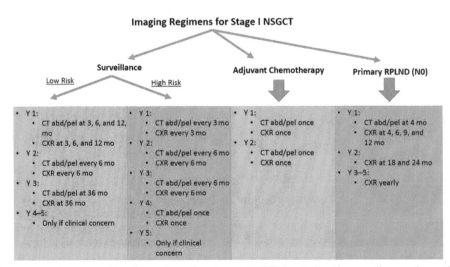

Fig. 5. Common regimens used by the authors for stage I NSGCT treated with surveillance, chemotherapy, or RPLND (with negative pathology).

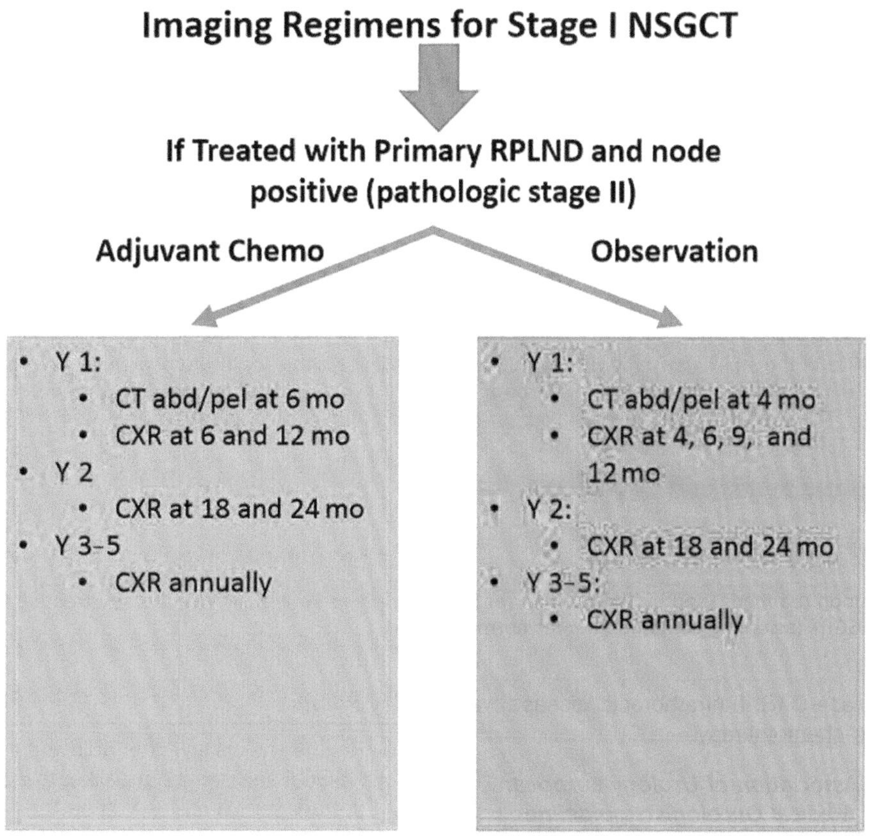

Imaging Regimens for Stage I NSGCT

If Treated with Primary RPLND and node positive (pathologic stage II)

Adjuvant Chemo

- Y 1:
  - CT abd/pel at 6 mo
  - CXR at 6 and 12 mo
- Y 2
  - CXR at 18 and 24 mo
- Y 3-5
  - CXR annually

Observation

- Y 1:
  - CT abd/pel at 4 mo
  - CXR at 4, 6, 9, and 12 mo
- Y 2:
  - CXR at 18 and 24 mo
- Y 3-5:
  - CXR annually

Fig. 6. Common regimens used by the authors for patients (typically stage I/IIa) found to be pathologic stage II after RPLND.

up paper looking at decision analysis for PC-RPLND additionally reported residual disease in 27% of patients with masses 1 to 10 mm that shrank more than 70%, and 22% for patients with masses 1 to 10 mm with no teratoma in the orchiectomy specimen.[45] Even series reporting on complete radiographic responses (no visible nodes), have noted retroperitoneal relapse rates of ∼7%.[46] There is a consensus that patients with residual masses >10 mm should undergo post-chemotherapy surgical resection if markers are negative. The management of patients with visible masses less than 10 mm in size is controversial. Some investigators have advocated for observation, whereas others favor surgical resection. Although the pathologic data described previously suggest risk with observation, long-term follow-up series have demonstrated low rates of relapse and mortality.

MRI and fluorodeoxyglucose-PET
Evaluation of the retroperitoneum in the post-chemotherapy setting has also been investigated using MRI and FDG-PET. Similar to staging, MRI is equivocal to CT for identifying retroperitoneal

lymphadenopathy.[17] However, it also has poor ability to discriminate fibrosis from residual disease.[16] FDG-PET is hampered because teratoma is not FDG avid. In addition, residual retroperitoneal inflammation/fibrosis can uptake FDG, leading to false-positive results. A multicenter cohort trial by Oechsle and colleagues[47] using FDG-PET in a post-chemotherapy NSGCT cohort with residual masses >1 cm noted a positive predictive value of just 59% and a poor negative predictive value of 50%, as compared with PC-RPLND pathology. As such, there is no role for FDG-PET imaging for patients with NSGCT after chemotherapy.

Regimens
Frequency of abdominopelvic imaging after chemotherapy depends on if PC-RPLND is performed, and then based on the pathology of the RPLND specimen (**Fig. 7**). For patients with fibrosis, relapse rates are typically 10% or less, with most occurring early. As such, a short low-intensity regimen is recommended. For those with residual teratoma/GCT or who are observed post-chemotherapy a more intensive and longer regimen is recommended. For both, chest CT

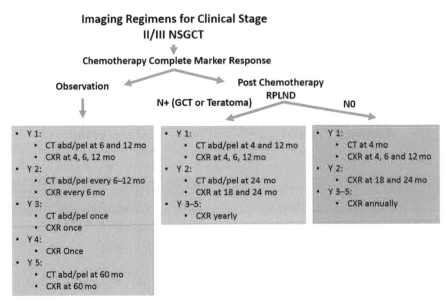

Fig. 7. Common regimens used by the authors for imaging follow-up after chemotherapy treatment of clinical stage II/III NSGCT (assuming complete marker normalization).

should replace CXR if intrathoracic disease was present pre-chemotherapy.

European Association of Urology/European Society of Medical Oncologists guidelines

Of note, both the European Society of Medical Oncologists and the EAU recommend a simplified regimen for all patients who receive treatment. Although this regimen is overall very reasonable, it groups together a wide array of patients with very different relapse risk profiles. As such, our typical regimens are more reflective of NCCN recommendations, which appropriately reduce the imaging and follow-up burden for those with lower risk of relapse.

Chest imaging

Some researchers have called into question the value of routine CXR in patients with disseminated NSGCT who undergo chemotherapy. Gietema and colleagues[48] described a series of 290 such patients with complete responses following chemotherapy. Relapse occurred in 11.4% of patients, with most identified by a rise in STM or symptoms. For the cohort, they identified more than 10,000 CXRs performed, with no relapses identified. Although this is a remarkable number of negative scans, this cohort was primarily treated before the generation of current guidelines (on average, each patient received >30 CXR examinations). Current guidelines (and our regimens) continue to recommend CXR during follow-up, with chest CT used in those with a history of intrathoracic disease or symptoms.

Key Points

- Relapse risk is low after adjuvant treatment of NSGCT and seminoma alike, thus the follow-up regimens are of low intensity.
- Seminoma has a longer median time to relapse, leading to longer imaging follow-up.
- Post-chemotherapy node size in NSGCT is an insensitive predictor of residual disease (especially chemo-resistant teratoma).
- FDG-PET does not help in identifying residual disease after chemotherapy in patients with NSGCT.
- Post-chemotherapy node size less than 3 cm has a low risk of relapse in seminoma patients.
- Nodes >3 cm in post-chemotherapy seminoma patients have a high rate of residual disease.
- FDG-PET can help identify residual disease in post-chemotherapy seminoma patients with nodes >3 cm in size.
- Chest radiographs may be of limited value in post-chemotherapy surveillance but are still recommended in follow-up of NSGCT.

IMAGING FOR SURVEILLANCE OF CLINICAL STAGE I DISEASE
Abdominal Imaging

A downside of surveillance for patients with NSGCT is the need for frequent imaging. Current NCCN guidelines for patients with CS1 disease recommend 4 to 9 CT-AP examinations over the first 5 years of observation. The intense but short nature of the regimen is because most relapses will occur within 3 years (median time to relapse of 6 months, 1% after 3 years).[49] EAU guidelines are similar and recommend retroperitoneal imaging twice during year 1, once at 24 months, once at 36 months, and once at 60 months. An additional scan at 18 months can be done for lymphovascular invasion (LVI)-positive patients. A common regimen that we use is described in **Fig. 6**.

Radiation exposure

A theoretic and controversial concern with surveillance regimens is the burden of medical radiation, which may increase the risk of developing a secondary malignancy. There is no definitive evidence that surveillance imaging increases the risk of secondary cancers, although observational studies support a possible association. Van Walraven and colleagues[50] analyzed a cohort of 2569 Canadian men with testis cancer who underwent an average of 10 abdominal/CT scans (110 mSv exposure) during their follow-up. Patients undergoing radiotherapy were excluded, and many patients underwent no therapy at all (69%). The cohort was followed for a median of 11.2 years. Fourteen patients developed secondary abdominopelvic malignancies. However, the investigators observed no association between amount of radiation exposure and risk of developing a malignancy. Other studies of radiation risk have used attributable risk based on models generated by the biologic effects of ionizing radiation VIII (BEIR VII) report.[50] Such studies have demonstrated a 0.5% to 2% lifetime attributable risk of secondary malignancy attributed to medical imaging during surveillance for testis cancer. The difference in results may be from using a lifetime-risk endpoint versus the intermediate term cohort follow-up of 11 years, or from the use of a model-based estimate instead of actual outcomes data.

Low frequency and low-dose CT regimens

Regardless of the radiation risk controversy, there remains interest in trying to determine the optimal frequency of imaging. Rustin and colleagues[51] performed a randomized-controlled trial (MRC TE08) comparing CT scans (chest/abdomen, no pelvis) at 3 and 12 months versus 3, 6, 9, 12, and 24 months in a surveillance NSGCT population. There was no significant difference in the relapse characteristics between the groups, with similar rates of intermediate-risk disease, STM levels, and node size. However, the surveillance protocol included aggressive STM measurements and CXR follow-up (monthly × 1 year, every 2 months × 1 year, every 3 months × 1 year, and so on). In addition, the study enrolled only a small number of higher-risk patients (LVI). However, the study demonstrates that for patients with NSGCT, frequent STM measurements can effectively diagnose many relapses and possibly avoid the burden of CT imaging.

Another route to reduce the burden of medical radiation is to use low-dose CT protocols. Chung and colleagues[52] reported on a series of patients with stage I testicular cancer on surveillance who were followed with noncontrasted low-dose CT scans. They noted that only 1 of 255 patients had low-dose scans of poor diagnostic quality. In addition, they noted no false-positive low-dose scans, and minimal difference in lymph node size between the low and standard dose scans at time of relapse (<1 mm). Using the low-dose protocol reduced radiation exposure by 55%. This single-center experience warrants replication, as it could reduce the contrast and radiation that patients with testis cancer are exposed to.

Seminoma

Seminoma surveillance patients have a low rate of relapse, but longer median relapse time (14 months, 9% with relapse after 3 years).[49] Thus, longer imaging follow-up must be done (see **Fig. 2**) particularly given the limited value of STM in diagnosing relapse. EAU guidelines are similar, with retroperitoneal imaging recommended twice during both year 1 and year 2, once at 36 months, and once at 60 months.

The use of MRI versus CT for surveillance is suspected of being equivocal. Currently, the MRC group is performing a trial of MRI in staging/surveillance of patients with clinical stage I seminoma (Trial of imaging and schedule in seminoma testis [TRISST]). This trial (which has completed accrual) will compare 4 arms, 2 with CT and 2 with MRI. The CT and MRI arms will be split into regimens with imaging at 6, 18, and 36 months (3 scan) versus imaging at 6, 12, 18, 24, 36, 48, and 60 months (7 scan).[53] Hopefully this trial will settle questions regarding CT versus MRI for retroperitoneal imaging, and also clarify the value (or lack thereof) of frequent retroperitoneal imaging for surveillance seminoma patients.

Chest imaging for nonseminomatous germ cell tumor and seminoma surveillance

The value of chest imaging in patients with stage I seminoma or NSGCT on a surveillance regimen is unclear, as isolated chest relapse without retroperitoneal disease is rare. Kollmannsberger and colleagues[49] have nicely summarized the patterns of relapse and methods of detection in a multicenter cohort of both NSGCT and seminoma patients being managed with surveillance. For patients with NSGCT, relapse was first diagnosed by CT-AP or STM in most patients, with only 2 of 213 relapses detected by CXR initially. For seminoma patients, no relapses were detected by CXR. A similar cohort of patients with NSGCT described by La Pena and colleagues[54] identified only one relapse by CXR (<1%). However, Rustin and colleagues[51] reported diagnosing 5 relapses purely by CXR in MRC TE08 (described previously), although it should again be emphasized that their CXR protocol was notably more aggressive than anything currently recommended by guidelines.

Guidelines

Current NCCN guidelines recommend CXR "as clinically indicated" for seminoma patients, and at 4 and 12 months, then annually for 5 years, for patients with NSGCT. EAU guidelines do not recommend CXR in seminoma patients, but recommend CXR twice during year 1 and 2 for patients with NSGCT, then once in year 3 and at 60 months in high-risk patients with NSGCT.

Currently, our practice for surveillance is to perform an initial chest CT for patients with NSGCT, and then perform CXR at the time of retroperitoneal imaging. In the event of symptoms or evidence of relapse, we perform a chest CT. For seminoma, we do not perform chest imaging unless there are pulmonary symptoms or evidence of relapse.

Pelvic imaging

Due to the primarily retroperitoneal initial spread of testis cancer, the need for pelvic imaging in surveillance has been questioned. However, a retrospective review by Sadow and colleagues[55] demonstrated that in a variety of settings, there was a small but appreciable risk of isolated pelvic metastases. The study found isolated pelvic relapses in both NSGCT and seminoma patients, in stage I patients on surveillance, and in patients without STM elevations (0.5%–3% isolated pelvic metastases). NCCN and EAU guidelines both recommended pelvic imaging during staging, surveillance, and follow-up.

Summary

Surveillance for stage I GCT is being increasingly used. However, 20% to 50% of patients may experience a relapse requiring therapy. Seminoma patients have a lower risk but longer average time to relapse, rarely have elevated STM at relapse, and do not have isolated intrathoracic metastases. Surveillance with CT-AP is critical for diagnosing seminoma relapse and longer surveillance regimens are required. Patients with NSGCT have a higher risk but shorter average time to relapse,

are often found by elevated STM, and may rarely have isolated intrathoracic metastases. Surveillance with STM is critical, but CT-AP also plays an important role particularly as teratoma is STM negative. Use of chest imaging in follow-up of seminoma is unnecessary, and may be unnecessary in NSGCT as well. Use of pelvic imaging is controversial although recommended by guidelines. Current studies are examining the role of less intensive and MRI-oriented regimens in surveillance for seminoma, and may allow for less burdensome surveillance regimens in the near future.

Key Points

- Controversy exists regarding the harms of medical radiation in surveillance patients.
- For NSGCT, less intensive CT regimens may be reasonable, but close follow-up with STM is necessary.
- For seminoma, imaging is more important in diagnosing relapse but relapse is less frequent. Lower intensity regimens are currently in trials.
- Chest CT imaging is not necessary in most patients, and CXR may be of limited value particularly in seminoma.
- Pelvic imaging is recommended although isolated pelvic relapse is rare.

EXPERIMENTAL IMAGING
Lymphotrophic Nanoparticle MRI

Lymphotrophic nanoparticle MRI (LNMRI) uses the increased uptake of iron oxide nanoparticles by metastatic nodal tissue as a method of MRI contrast enhancement. The technology has been used in a variety of malignancies with varying results. In testis cancer, Harisinghani and colleagues[56] performed staging LNMRI in a mixed cohort of stage I seminoma and nonseminomatous patients and compared imaging results with pathologic outcomes. Sensitivity and specificity was higher than that of CT (88% and 92% for LNMRI, 70.5% and 68% for CT). These encouraging results have not yet been validated, but seem encouraging for further stratifying true stage I patients from those with occult metastatic disease.

Intraoperative Fluorescent Techniques

Various agents have been reported on as improving the ability to discern nodal tissue from non-nodal tissue during RPLND. Most of the outcomes described are descriptive rather than oncologic, and the techniques require special equipment to visualize the fluorescent dyes. However, especially with interest in minimally invasive RPLND on the rise, further investigation/utilization of such techniques may be on the horizon.[57]

SUMMARY

Imaging plays a critical role in the diagnosis, staging, surveillance, and follow-up of patients with GCT. High-level evidence regarding intensity and duration of imaging regimens is rare, and such regimens are predominantly based on data from studies of relapse patterns. Ultrasound is the primary modality for testicular assessment, whereas MRI can be used in equivocal cases. CT-AP is used routinely in staging/surveillance/follow-up of retroperitoneal disease, although MRI can also be used particularly if contrast allergies are present. Chest imaging is controversial in the setting of normal abdominal imaging, as CXR has low sensitivity for disease, whereas chest CT has high false-positive rates. FDG-PET is useful in stratifying risk of disease in post-chemotherapy seminoma masses >3 cm in size, but has little proven use otherwise. Ongoing trials may help clarify the value of imaging in different settings (predominantly surveillance for stage I disease), whereas targeted techniques may allow for better risk stratification of patients in the future and a reduction in unnecessary treatment.

REFERENCES

1. Lenz S. Cancer of the testicle diagnosed by ultrasound and the ultrasonic appearance of the contralateral testicle. Scand J Urol Nephrol Suppl 1991;137:135–8. Available at: http://www.ncbi.nlm.nih.gov/pubmed/1947833. Accessed November 18, 2018.
2. Algaba F, Bokemeyer C, Cohn-Cedermark G, et al. Testicular cancer EAU guidelines on. 2017. Available at: https://uroweb.org/wp-content/uploads/11-Testicular-Cancer_2017_web.pdf. Accessed November 18, 2018.
3. NCCN clinical practice guidelines in oncology (NCCN guidelines ®) testicular cancer. 2019. Available at: https://www.nccn.org/professionals/physician_gls/pdf/testicular.pdf. Accessed November 18, 2018.
4. Hoei-Hansen CE, Holm M, Rajpert-De Meyts E, et al. Histological evidence of testicular dysgenesis in contralateral biopsies from 218 patients with testicular germ cell cancer. J Pathol 2003;200(3):370–4.
5. Risk MC, Masterson TA. Intratubular germ cell neoplasms of the testis and bilateral testicular tumors: clinical significance and management options. Indian J Urol 2010;26(1):64–71.
6. Lenz S, Giwercman A. Carcinoma-in-situ of the testis—is ultrasound of the testes useful as a screening method? J Med Ultrasound 2008;16(4):256–67.
7. Kim W, Rosen MA, Langer JE, et al. US–MR imaging correlation in pathologic conditions of the scrotum. Radiographics 2007;27(5):1239–53.
8. Cassidy FH, Ishioka KM, McMahon CJ, et al. MR imaging of scrotal tumors and pseudotumors. Radiographics 2010;30(3):665–83.
9. Richenberg J, Belfield J, Ramchandani P, et al. Testicular microlithiasis imaging and follow-up: guidelines of the ESUR scrotal imaging subcommittee. Eur Radiol 2015. https://doi.org/10.1007/s00330-014-3437-x.
10. Tsili AC, Tsampoulas C, Giannakopoulos X, et al. MRI in the histologic characterization of testicular neoplasms. Am J Roentgenol 2007;189(6):W331–7.
11. Cramer B, Schlegel E, Thueroff J. MR imaging in the differential diagnosis of scrotal and testicular disease. Available at: https://pubs.rsna.org/doi/pdf/10.1148/radiographics.11.1.1996400. Accessed November 18, 2018.
12. Serra AD, Hricak H, Coakley FV, et al. Inconclusive clinical and ultrasound evaluation of the scrotum: impact of magnetic resonance imaging on patient management and cost. Urology 1998;51(6):1018–21.
13. Muglia V, Tucci S, Elias J, et al. Magnetic Resonance Imaging of Scrotal Disease: When it Makes the Difference. Urology 2002;59(3):419–23.
14. Steyerberg E, Keizer H, Fossa S, et al. Prediction of residual retroperitoneal mass histology after chemotherapy for metastatic nonseminomatous germ cell tumor: multivariate analysis of individual patient data from six study groups. J Clin Oncol 2018;13(5):1177–87.
15. Ghazarian AA, Trabert B, Devesa SS, et al. Recent trends in the incidence of testicular germ cell tumors in the United States. Andrology 2015;3(1):13–8.
16. Hogeboom WR, Hoekstra HJ, Mooyaart EL, et al. The role of magnetic resonance imaging and computed tomography in the treatment evaluation of retroperitoneal lymph-node metastases of non-seminomatous testicular tumors. Eur J Radiol 1991;13(1):31–6.
17. Sohaib SA, Koh DM, Barbachano Y, et al. Prospective assessment of MRI for imaging retroperitoneal metastases from testicular germ cell tumours. Clin Radiol 2009;64(4):362–7.
18. Mosavi F, Laurell A, Ahlström H. Whole body MRI, including diffusion-weighted imaging in follow-up of patients with testicular cancer. Acta Oncol (Madr) 2015;54(10):1763–9.
19. Tandstad T, Ståhl O, Dahl O, et al. Treatment of stage I seminoma, with one course of adjuvant carboplatin or surveillance, risk-adapted recommendations implementing patient autonomy: a report from the Swedish and Norwegian Testicular Cancer Group (SWENOTECA). Ann Oncol 2016;27(7):1299–304.

20. Magnusson A. Size of normal retroperitoneal lymph nodes. Acta Radiol Diagn (Stockh) 1983;24(4): 315–8. Available at: http://www.ncbi.nlm.nih.gov/pubmed/6637570. Accessed November 19, 2018.

21. Grubnic S, Vinnicombe SJ, Norman AR, et al. MR evaluation of normal retroperitoneal and pelvic lymph nodes. Clin Radiol 2002;57(3):193–200.

22. Hilton S, Herr HW, Teitcher JB, et al. CT detection of retroperitoneal lymph node metastases in patients with clinical stage I testicular nonseminomatous germ cell cancer: assessment of size and distribution criteria. Am J Roentgenol 1997; 169(2):521–5.

23. Leibovitch I, Foster RS, Kopecky KK, et al. Improved accuracy of computerized tomography based clinical staging in low stage nonseminomatous germ cell cancer using size criteria of retroperitoneal lymph nodes. J Urol 1995;154(5): 1759–63.

24. Huddart RA, O'Doherty MJ, Padhani A, et al. [18]Fluorodeoxyglucose positron emission tomography in the prediction of relapse in patients with high-risk, clinical stage I nonseminomatous germ cell tumors: preliminary report of MRC trial TE22—the NCRI Testis Tumour Clinical Study Group. J Clin Oncol 2007;25(21):3090–5.

25. Ambrosini V, Zucchini G, Nicolini S, et al. 18F-FDG PET/CT impact on testicular tumours clinical management. Eur J Nucl Med Mol Imaging 2014;41(4): 668–73.

26. Horan G, Rafique A, Robson J, et al. CT of the chest can hinder the management of seminoma of the testis; it detects irrelevant abnormalities. Br J Cancer 2007;96(6):882–5.

27. See WA, Hoxie L. Chest staging in testis cancer patients: imaging modality selection based upon risk assessment as determined by abdominal computerized tomography scan results. J Urol 1993;150(3): 874–8.

28. White PM, Adamson DJA, Howard GCW, et al. Imaging of the thorax in the management of germ cell testicular tumours. Clin Radiol 1999;54:207–11. Available at: https://www.clinicalradiologyonline.net/article/S0009-9260(99)91152-2/pdf. Accessed November 18, 2018.

29. Feldman DR, Lorch A, Kramar A, et al. Brain metastases in patients with germ cell tumors: prognostic factors and treatment options–an analysis from the global germ cell cancer group. J Clin Oncol 2016; 34(4):345–51.

30. Mead GM, Fosså SD, Oliver RT, et al. Relapse patterns in 2,466 stage 1 seminoma patients (pts) entered into Medical Research Council randomised trials. J Clin Oncol 2008;26(15_suppl):5020.

31. Hu B, Daneshmand S. Retroperitoneal lymph node dissection as primary treatment for metastatic seminoma. Adv Urol 2018;2018:1–5.

32. Herr HW, Sheinfeld J, Puc HS, et al. Surgery for a post-chemotherapy residual mass in seminoma. J Urol 1997;157(3):860–2.

33. De Santis M, Bokemeyer C, Becherer A, et al. Predictive impact of 2 - 18 Fluoro - 2 - Deoxy - D - Glucose positron emission tomography for residual postchemotherapy masses in patients with bulky seminoma 2018;19(17):3740–4.

34. Becherer A, De Santis M, Karanikas G, et al. FDG PET is superior to CT in the prediction of viable tumour in post-chemotherapy seminoma residuals. Eur J Radiol 2005;54(2):284–8.

35. Siekiera J, Małkowski B, Jóźwicki W, et al. Can we rely on PET in the follow-up of advanced seminoma patients? Urol Int 2012;88(4):405–9.

36. Hinz S, Schrader M, Kempkensteffen C, et al. The role of positron emission tomography in the evaluation of residual masses after chemotherapy for advanced stage seminoma. J Urol 2008;179(3): 936–40.

37. Bilen MA, Hariri H, Leon C, et al. Positive FDG-PET/CT scans of a residual seminoma after chemotherapy and radiotherapy: case report and review of the literature. Clin Genitourin Cancer 2014;12(4):1–10.

38. Bachner M, Loriot Y, Gross-Goupil M, et al. 2-18fluoro-deoxy-D-glucose positron emission tomography (FDG-PET) for postchemotherapy seminoma residual lesions: a retrospective validation of the SEMPET trial. Ann Oncol 2012;23(1):59–64.

39. Rayson D, Burch PA, Richardson RL. Sarcoidosis and testicular carcinoma. Cancer 1998;83(2): 337–43.

40. Albers P, Siener R, Krege S, et al. Randomized phase III trial comparing retroperitoneal lymph node dissection with one course of bleomycin and etoposide plus cisplatin chemotherapy in the adjuvant treatment of clinical stage I nonseminomatous testicular germ cell tumors: AUO trial AH 01/94 by the German Testicular Cancer Study Group. J Clin Oncol 2008;26(18): 2966–72.

41. Al-Ahmadie HA, Carver BS, Cronin AM, et al. Primary retroperitoneal lymph node dissection in low-stage testicular germ cell tumors: a detailed pathologic study with clinical outcome analysis with special emphasis on patients who did not receive adjuvant therapy. Urology 2013;82(6): 1341–7.

42. Williams SD, Stablein DM, Einhorn LH, et al. Immediate adjuvant chemotherapy versus observation with treatment at relapse in pathological stage II testicular cancer. N Engl J Med 1987;317(23): 1433–8.

43. Kundu SD, Feldman DR, Carver BS, et al. Rates of teratoma and viable cancer at post-chemotherapy retroperitoneal lymph node dissection after

induction chemotherapy for good risk nonseminomatous germ cell tumors. J Urol 2015;193(2):513–8.

44. Beck SDW, Foster RS, Donohue JP, et al. Is full bilateral retroperitoneal lymph node dissection always necessary for postchemotherapy residual tumor? Cancer 2007;110(6):1235–40.

45. Steyerberg EW, Marshall PB, Keizer HJ, et al. Resection of small, residual retroperitoneal masses after chemotherapy for nonseminomatous testicular cancer: a decision analysis. Cancer 1999;85(6): 1331–41.

46. Kollmannsberger C, Daneshmand S, So A, et al. Management of disseminated nonseminomatous germ cell tumors with risk-based chemotherapy followed by response-guided postchemotherapy surgery. J Clin Oncol 2018;28(4). https://doi.org/10. 1200/JCO.2009.23.0755.

47. Oechsle K, Hartmann M, Brenner W, et al. [^{18} F]Fluorodeoxyglucose positron emission tomography in nonseminomatous germ cell tumors after chemotherapy: the german multicenter positron emission tomography study group. J Clin Oncol 2008; 26(36):5930–5.

48. Gietema JA, Meinardi MT, Sleijfer DT, et al. Routine chest X-rays have no additional value in the detection of relapse during routine follow-up of patients treated with chemotherapy for disseminated nonseminomatous testicular cancer. Ann Oncol 2002; 13(10):1616–20. Available at: http://www.ncbi.nlm. nih.gov/pubmed/12377651. Accessed November 19, 2018.

49. Kollmannsberger C, Tandstad T, Bedard PL, et al. Patterns of relapse in patients with clinical stage I testicular cancer managed with active surveillance. J Clin Oncol 2015;33(1):51–7.

50. van Walraven C, Fergusson D, Earle C, et al. Association of diagnostic radiation exposure and second abdominal-pelvic malignancies after testicular cancer. J Clin Oncol 2018;29(21). https://doi.org/ 10.1200/JCO.2011.34.6379.

51. Rustin GJ, Mead GM, Stenning SP, et al. Randomized trial of two or five computed tomography scans in the surveillance of patients with stage I nonseminomatous germ cell tumors of the testis: medical research council trial TE08 , ISRCTN56475197 — The National Cancer Research Institute Testis Cancer Clinical Studies Group. J Clin Oncol 2018;25(11). https://doi.org/ 10.1200/JCO.2006.08.4889.

52. Chung P, O'Malley ME, Jewett MAS, et al. Detection of relapse by low-dose computed tomography during surveillance in stage I testicular germ cell tumours. Eur Urol Oncol 2018. https://doi.org/10. 1016/j.euo.2018.08.031.

53. TRISST (MRC TE24). Available at: http://www.ctu. mrc.ac.uk/our_research/research_areas/cancer/studies/trisst_mrc_te24/. Accessed November 19, 2018.

54. La Pena HD, Sharma A, Glicksman C, et al. ScienceDirect no longer any role for routine follow-up chest x-rays in men with stage I germ cell cancer. Eur J Cancer 2017;84:354–9.

55. Sadow CA, Maurer AN, Prevedello LM, et al. CT restaging of testicular germ cell tumors: the incidence of isolated pelvic metastases. Eur J Radiol 2016; 85(8):1439–44.

56. Harisinghani MG, Saksena M, Ross RW, et al. A pilot study of lymphotrophic nanoparticle-enhanced magnetic resonance imaging technique in early stage testicular cancer: a new method for noninvasive lymph node evaluation. Urology 2005;66(5): 1066–71.

57. Joice GA, Rowe SP, Gorin MA, et al. Molecular imaging for evaluation of viable testicular cancer nodal metastases. Curr Urol Rep 2018;19(12):110.

Management of Primary Testicular Tumor

Alireza Ghoreifi, MD, Hooman Djaladat, MD, MS*

KEYWORDS

• Testicular tumor • Treatment • Orchiectomy • Organ-sparing surgery • Prosthesis

KEY POINTS

- In any man with a solid testicular mass, cancer should be considered until proven otherwise.
- Radical inguinal orchiectomy is the treatment of choice in patients with testis mass.
- Placement of a testicular prosthesis is safe with a very low complication rate and should be offered to all patients undergoing radical orchiectomy.
- In patients with widespread or life-threatening advanced disease, delayed orchiectomy following chemotherapy is recommended.
- Testis-sparing surgery can be performed in highly selected patients with solitary testicle mass, bilateral testicular tumors, or strong suspicion of a benign lesion.

INTRODUCTION

Testicular cancer is a relatively uncommon malignancy, and accounts for 1% of all cancers and 5% of urologic tumors; however, it is the most common solid malignancy in males between the ages of 15 and 35 years.[1] Its incidence has been rising during the last decades especially in developed countries.[1,2] In 2018, approximately 9310 new cases and 400 deaths from testicular cancer are expected in the US.[3] Germ cell tumors (GCTs) represent most palpable testicular tumors with the greatest incidence as clinically localized stage I disease.[4] Radical orchiectomy is the standard procedure for diagnosis and treatment of these tumors. Before the advent of new treatment strategies including platinum-based combination chemotherapy in 1970s, the 5-year survival rate of patients with testicular cancer was 64%.[5] Currently, 5-year survival rate of testicular cancers is exceeding 95% and it has become a model of curable solid neoplasms.[5,6] Most patients with clinically stage I testicular tumors are cured with orchiectomy alone, and the long-term survival rate approaches 100% regardless of the adjuvant therapy.[4] The aim of this study is to review the management of primary testicular tumors.

PREORCHIECTOMY EVALUATION

The most common presentation of testicular cancer is painless mass.[7] In any man with a solid testicular mass, cancer must be considered until proven otherwise. Expedient diagnosis of testicular cancer provides the best opportunity for cure. Nevertheless, both patient and health care providers often contribute to a delay in diagnosis. Up to 10% of patients with testicular cancer are initially diagnosed as posttraumatic pain or swelling,[8] some as infection and/or hydrocele. A mean delay up to 26 weeks from initial symptoms to surgical diagnosis has been reported in different studies.[8] Bosl and colleagues[9] reported that the median delay for patients with clinical stage I, II, and III disease was 75, 101, and 134 days, respectively. Up to 10% of patients with GCTs may present with symptoms of metastatic disease, mainly to retroperitoneum and/or lungs.[10] Also

Disclosure Statement: The authors have nothing to disclose.
Institute of Urology, Norris Comprehensive Cancer Center, University of Southern California, Los Angeles, CA, USA
* Corresponding author. 1441 Eastlake Avenue NOR 7416, Los Angeles, CA 90089.
E-mail address: djaladat@usc.edu

Urol Clin N Am 46 (2019) 333–339
https://doi.org/10.1016/j.ucl.2019.04.006

2% to 5% of GCTs arise from extragonadal origin with anterior mediastinum as the most common location.[11]

Diagnostic examinations recommended in patients with testicular tumors include physical examination, serum tumor markers AFP, β-HCG, and lactic dehydrogenase (LDH), as well as scrotal ultrasonography.[12] Recently, miRNA 371a-3p has been introduced as a novel serum tumor marker for GCTs. It is expressed by 88.7% of patients and far more sensitive and specific than classic tumor markers.[13,14] Furthermore, it correlates with tumor burden and is a helpful tool in monitoring patients undergoing surveillance, as is evaluation of residual disease following chemotherapy. Testicular ultrasonography is inexpensive and recommended in all suspicious cases, even if there is clinically evident tumor.[15] It can provide important information regarding the tumor as well as the contralateral testicle. Synchronous testicular masses have been reported in approximately 0.5% to 1% of patients.[16] Radical orchiectomy is the treatment of choice in patients with testicular mass. Placement of a testicular prosthesis (TP) should be discussed and offered to all patients undergoing radical orchiectomy.[17]

RADICAL ORCHIECTOMY

Radical inguinal orchiectomy with removal of the tumor-bearing testis and spermatic cord to the level of the internal inguinal ring is the gold standard for diagnosis and treatment of patients in whom a testicular malignancy is suspected. If feasible, it is recommended to be performed within a week of initial diagnostic evaluations.[12]

Technique

The procedure can be performed under general, spinal, or local anesthesia in supine position. Some surgeons like to have the ipsilateral thigh lightly extrarotated.[18] The standard incision is made approximately 2 cm cephalad to the pubic tubercle and extends about 5 cm laterally with an oblique orientation overlying the inguinal canal following the lines of Langer. In patients with large tumors, the hockey-stick incision can be done with extension down along the anterior scrotum.[19] Our preferred technique is fascia-preserving radical orchiectomy (FPRO), which is performed through a subinguinal incision (**Fig. 1**A). After incision of Camper and Scarpa's fascia, the external oblique fascia is exposed and the external ring is identified. In this step, many surgeons open the inguinal canal along its course between the internal and external inguinal rings.[20] FPRO technique is performed without opening the external inguinal ring; however, the spermatic cord is pulled out from the inguinal canal until the peritoneal reflection is visualized. This step includes delicate handling of cord as well as safely displacing the ilioinguinal nerve, which is lying on top of the spermatic cord. The cord then should be double clamped proximally to provide early vascular control, which can prevent any "shedding" of tumor cells during manipulation and testicular delivery (**Fig. 1**B).[21] During traction and testis delivery, great care should be taken not to rupture the mass and tumor spillage. In rare instances, in which biopsy is indicated, it can be performed at this stage after delivery of testicle. After peritoneal reflection is visualized, the vas deferens and gonadal vessels are divided (between the clamps) and ligated with nonabsorbable suture, leaving a long suture tail on the stump of the gonadal vessels to facilitate identification at the time of retroperitoneal lymph node dissection (RPLND) in future. It is usually preferred to tie the spermatic vessels and the vas deferens separately. This may decrease the chance of bleeding and facilitate retrieval of spermatic cord stump during subsequent RPLND.[20,21] Meticulous hemostasis is critical, as bleeding vessels may retract into the retroperitoneum and cause significant hematoma, which may be confused as metastatic disease on subsequent imaging.[21] A TP can be placed after

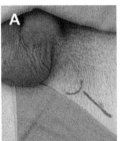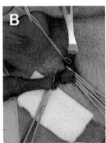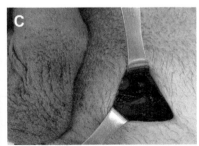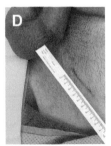

Fig. 1. Fascia-preserving radical orchiectomy for left testicular mass. (*A*) Subinguinal incision, (*B*) double clamping of the cord, (*C*) intact external oblique aponeurosis after radical orchiectomy with ilioinguinal nerve preservation, and (*D*) final view of the incision with prosthesis in place.

completion of orchiectomy. Finally, the ilioinguinal nerve is positioned safely in the floor of the inguinal canal, and closure of different layers are performed using absorbable sutures. In our fascia-preserving technique there is no need for closure of the external oblique aponeurosis (**Fig. 1**C, D).

A drain is not necessary or advisable. If desired, long-acting local anesthetics can be injected peri-incision to help with postoperative pain. Scrotal support and fluffed gauze dressings are helpful to avoid scrotal swelling and/or hematoma postoperatively.[19]

Complications

Complications after radical orchiectomy are infrequent including bleeding, wound infection, or ilioinguinal nerve injury. The most common complication is bleeding, which may occasionally cause scrotal or retroperitoneal hematoma. Unless infected, most scrotal hematomas can be treated with expectant management.[19] Significant retroperitoneal hematoma can delay further therapy or be misinterpreted as metastatic disease.[22]

CONTRALATERAL TESTIS BIOPSY

Contralateral germ cell neoplasia in situ, formerly known as intratubular germ cell neoplasia (ITGCN) or carcinoma in situ, is seen in about 3% to 5% of patients with testis cancer, which can progress to invasive malignancy in 50% and 70% of cases at 5- and 7-year follow-up, respectively.[23–26] In a European study, the risk of contralateral metachronous testicular tumors was reported at approximately 2.5%, most of which were low stage at presentation.[25] Moreover, Fossa and colleagues[26] reported that the 15-year cumulative risk of metachronous testicular cancer is 1.9% in the US population. With such a low incidence and favorable prognosis of patients diagnosed with metachronous contralateral testicular cancer, as well as the morbidity of treatment, contralateral testicular biopsy is not routinely recommended in patients with testicular cancer; however, the European Association of Urology (EAU) guidelines recommend that contralateral biopsy should be offered to patients at high risk for contralateral ITGCN, that is, testicular volume less than 12 mL, a history of cryptorchidism or poor spermatogenesis.[15]

SCROTAL VIOLATION

Despite efforts to improve quality measures in the care of testicular cancer, suboptimal approaches, such as scrotal orchiectomy, transscrotal biopsy, and fine-needle aspiration, are reported in 4% to

17% of cases.[27,28] It has been shown that prior inguinal or scrotal surgery could alter the normal lymphatic drainage of the testis.[20] Scrotal orchiectomy increases the local recurrence compared with inguinal orchiectomy (2.9% vs 0.4%), but does not affect the systemic recurrence or survival rate.[28,29] The following adjuvant treatments are recommended for patients with scrotal violation:

- In patients with low-stage seminoma, radiation should be extended to include the ipsilateral groin and scrotum.
- In patients with low-stage nonseminoma GCT, scrotal scar should be widely excised with spermatic cord remnant at the time of RPLND.
- Patients who received platinum-based chemotherapy should have the cord stump removed at the time of RPLND.[19]

PROSTHESIS PLACEMENT

Patients with testicular cancer are often young with long life expectancy. Radical orchiectomy can result in a negative change in the patients' body image, as well as their feelings. TP implantation can improve self-esteem in these patients.[30] It has been demonstrated in different studies that placement of a TP is safe with a very low complication rate. It can be inserted at the time of orchiectomy or later. Synchronous placement of a TP seems to be associated with overall satisfaction and should be offered to these patients.[17,31] In a large cohort study, Robinson and colleagues[17] showed that concurrent insertion of a TP does not increase the complication rate of radical orchiectomy (ie, length of stay, readmission, or the need for further surgery). In their study, older patients had increased risk of 30-day hospital readmission, but only 0.4% of them required prosthesis removal. The overall satisfaction rate after TP placement is remarkable and is reported as high as 83%.[31–33] A recent study showed that 89.8% of TP recipients were satisfied with the look of their prosthetic and 59.3% of respondents were satisfied with prosthetic feel.[32] Appropriate size, position, and TP comfort were significantly associated with good or excellent overall satisfaction.[31–34] Prosthesis firmness and position were the most cited reasons for dissatisfaction.[31]

DELAYED ORCHIECTOMY

The diagnosis and therapeutic approach of a testicular cancer is usually determined by histologic findings after radical orchiectomy. However, in a small subset of patients with widespread or life-threatening advanced disease, the diagnosis is made based on biopsy of a metastatic lesion or empirically based on clinical and serologic features. In these patients, initiation of systemic chemotherapy supersedes diagnostic orchiectomy.[35] This therapeutic approach is helpful for the immediate management of acute life-threatening metastatic disease. Following completion of systemic therapy, these patients may undergo delayed orchiectomy with or without dissection of retroperitoneal lymph nodes.[36]

Delayed orchiectomy is recommended for all patients with nonseminomatous germ cell tumor (NSGCT) after induction chemotherapy, even in the setting of a complete response in the retroperitoneum.[35-38] The rationale for this approach is the presence of residual testicular disease in a significant percentage of patients who cannot be distinguished by testicular ultrasonography from scar tissue. Residual viable tumor in testicular specimens is found in 39% to 66.7%.[35] In a series of 160 patients in whom chemotherapy was given before surgery, residual carcinoma and pure teratoma were identified in 25% and 31% of cases, respectively.[37] A recent review of 325 patients who underwent delayed orchiectomy also showed viable tumor in 21%, teratoma in 30.3%, and scarring/necrosis in 48.5% of patients. Complete disappearance of tumor was seen in 81.3% of seminoma and 43.4% of NSGCT cases.[39]

In patients with primary retroperitoneal or extragonadal GCT the role of (delayed) orchiectomy is controversial. Biopsy of the testis shows ITGCN in 42% of these patients,[40] in whom approximately 5% will develop a metachronous testicular cancer following chemotherapy.[41] In a small cohort series of patients with apparent extragonadal GCT who had undergone simultaneous orchiectomy with postchemotherapy-RPLND, 71% had histologic evidence of testicular teratoma or focal necrosis/fibrosis.[42] Delayed radical orchiectomy may be considered when retroperitoneal pattern of metastatic tumor spread is consistent with a primary testicular tumor.

TESTIS-SPARING SURGERY

The increasing incidence of early-stage testicular GCTs and high survival rate of these patients are encouraging the interest toward conservative treatment options.[43,44] The aim of testis-sparing surgery (TSS) is to maintain endocrine function with physiologic levels of testosterone, to preserve fertility and maintain quality of life.[45]

Indications

There is no randomized controlled trial available in the literature to compare TSS and radical orchiectomy. Several case series and retrospective studies have reported the outcome of TSS in the literature.[46-51] Heidenreich and colleagues[47,51] from the German Testicular Cancer Study Group reported the largest sample size of 73 patients in 2001, which was updated with 101 cases in 2006. According to these studies, TSS can be performed in highly selected patients who have a solitary testicle, synchronous bilateral testicular tumors, metachronous testicular GCTs, or strong suspicion of a benign lesion. Testicular mass size seems to be one of the most paramount factors for the indication of TSS. The German Cancer Study Group considered TSS as a standard approach in testis lesions less than 20 mm in diameter (or ≤50% of testicular volume) with normal preorchiectomy serum testosterone and luteinizing hormone levels.[45,47] However, the EAU guidelines consider tumor size less than 30% of testicular volume to be eligible for TSS.[15] The smaller the testis mass, the higher chance that it is benign. It has been shown that tumors less than 5 mm are benign in up to 80% of cases.[43] The location of the tumor is also important, and the polar lesions are more favorable for TSS.[52] The surgery should be done in a tertiary referral center and both patient and physician should be highly compliant. Intraoperative ultrasonography can be very helpful. Furthermore, intraoperative biopsies of the tumor bed should be negative for malignancy.[45] It is noteworthy that ITGCN may not be ruled out in frozen samples despite review by an expert pathologist. Because of the technical limitations of frozen-section examination (FSE), including suboptimal tissue preparation, as well as the possibility of skip lesions, it is recommended that ITGCN be always ruled out in permanent specimens.[43,44]

Technique

The standard approach of TSS is as the same as radical inguinal orchiectomy with early vascular control.[43] However, some experts suggest "non-clamping" technique without ischemia.[53,54] The use of hypothermia is controversial.[44] If cold ischemia is selected, it is recommended that the testis be immerged in an ice slush after cord clamping for 5 to 10 min, and then kept at 15°C to 19°C.[43,44] Use of 7.5 MHz intraoperative ultrasonography can be helpful to facilitate localization of the mass and completeness of resection.[44,45]

The tumor is enucleated and sent for FSE to identify the histology and assess the surgical margins. It is preferred to resect a small rim of surrounding parenchyma, especially when it sticks to the tumor.[46] The sensitivity and specificity of

FSE to identify malignant lesions is reported between 89.3% and 100% in different studies.[55–60] However, the experience of the pathologist is of utmost importance.[44] False-negative FSEs are caused by the nonrandom distribution of lesions as well as technical problems, that is, FSE artifacts and/or the very focal presence of malignancy.[58,61]

If FSE reveals malignancy, completion of radical orchiectomy should be considered. If radical orchiectomy is not performed, deeper resection and additional biopsies may be an option, until margins are negative.[45]

Oncological Outcome

The optimal management of patients after TSS is controversial. Some studies recommended adjuvant low-dose (18–20 Gy) radiation for all patients.[44,47] However, this treatment can cause spermatogenesis arrest and infertility, and has not become the standard of care. European Germ Cell Cancer Consensus group recommends radiation only when ITGCN is present.[12] ITGCN increases the chance of cancer recurrence and the cumulative probability for the development of a testicular tumor is 70% after 7 years.[62] Given that 30% of these patients never develop malignancy, surveillance is an alternative option in patients who accept the possible risk of recurrence. Platinum-based chemotherapy is another option that is shown to be accompanied with high recurrence rate and is no longer recommended for ITGCN. The cumulative risk of ITGCN recurrence after chemotherapy is over 40% after 10 years.[63]

SUMMARY

Testicular cancer is a relatively uncommon malignancy; it should be considered in any man with a solid testicular mass. Diagnostic evaluations include physical examination, serum tumor markers (AFP, β-HCG, and LDH, and, recently, miRNA-371a-3p), as well as scrotal ultrasonography. Radical inguinal orchiectomy with removal of the spermatic cord to the level of the internal inguinal ring is the treatment of choice. FPRO is our preferred technique; this is done through a subinguinal incision without opening the external inguinal ring. Placement of a TP is safe with a low complication rate and should be offered to all patients candidate for radical orchiectomy. In a small subset of patients with widespread or life-threatening advanced disease, delayed orchiectomy following chemotherapy is recommended. TSS can be performed in highly selected patients with solitary testicle mass, synchronous/metachronous bilateral testicular tumors or strong suspicion of a benign lesion.

REFERENCES

1. Rosen A, Jayram G, Drazer M, et al. Global trends in testicular cancer incidence and mortality. Eur Urol 2011;60(2):374–9.
2. Nigam M, Aschebrook-Kilfoy B, Shikanov S, et al. Increasing incidence of testicular cancer in the United States and Europe between 1992 and 2009. World J Urol 2015;33(5):623–31.
3. Siegel RL, Miller KD, Jemal A. Cancer statistics, 2018. CA Cancer J Clin 2018;68:7.
4. Pierorazio PM, Albers P, Black PC, et al. Non–risk-adapted surveillance for stage I testicular cancer: critical review and summary. Eur Urol 2018;73(6): 899–907.
5. Einhorn LH. Treatment of testicular cancer: a new and improved model. J Clin Oncol 1990;8(11): 1777–81.
6. Capocaccia R, Gatta G, Dal Maso L. Life expectancy of colon, breast, and testicular cancer patients: an analysis of US-SEER population-based data. Ann Oncol 2015;26(6):1263–8.
7. Germa-Lluch JR, del Muro XG, Maroto P, et al. Clinical pattern and therapeutic results achieved in 1490 patients with germ-cell tumours of the testis: the experience of the Spanish Germ-Cell Cancer Group (GG). Eur Urol 2002;42(6):553–63.
8. Moul JW. Timely diagnosis of testicular cancer. Urol Clin North Am 2007;34(2):109–17.
9. Bosl GJ, Goldman A, Lange PH, et al. Impact of delay in diagnosis on clinical stage of testicular cancer. Lancet 1981;2:970.
10. Horwich A, Nicol D, Huddart R. Testicular germ cell tumours. BMJ 2013;347:f5526.
11. Albany C, Einhorn LH. Extragonadal germ cell tumors: clinical presentation and management. Curr Opin Oncol 2013;25(3):261–5.
12. Krege S, Beyer J, Souchon R, et al. European consensus conference on diagnosis and treatment of germ cell cancer: a report of the second meeting of the European Germ Cell Cancer Consensus group (EGCCCG): part I. Eur Urol 2008;53(3):478–96.
13. Syring I, Bartels J, Holdenrieder S, et al. Circulating serum miRNA (miR-367-3p, miR-371a-3p, miR-372-3p and miR-373-3p) as biomarkers in patients with testicular germ cell cancer. J Urol 2015;193(1): 331–7.
14. Dieckmann KP, Radtke A, Spiekermann M, et al. Serum levels of microRNA miR-371a-3p: a sensitive and specific new biomarker for germ cell tumours. Eur Urol 2017;71(2):213–20.
15. Albers P, Albrecht W, Algaba F, et al. EAU guidelines on testicular cancer: 2011 update. Eur Urol 2011; 60(2):304–19.
16. Campobasso D, Ferretti S, Frattini A. Synchronous bilateral testis cancer: clinical and oncological management. Contemp Oncol (Pozn) 2017;21(1):70.

17. Robinson R, Tait CD, Clarke NW, et al. Is it safe to insert a testicular prosthesis at the time of radical orchidectomy for testis cancer: an audit of 904 men undergoing radical orchidectomy. BJU Int 2016; 117(2):249–52.

18. Pizzocaro G, Guarneri A. Inguinal orchidectomy for testicular cancer. BJU Int 2009;103(5):704–16.

19. Keane TE, Graham SD. Glenn's urologic surgery. 8th edition. Philadelphia: Lippincott Williams & Wilkins; 2015.

20. Wein AJ, Kavoussi LR, Partin AW, et al. Campbell-Walsh urology. 11th edition. Philadelphia: Elsevier; 2016.

21. Smith JA, Howards SS, Preminger GM. Hinman's atlas of urologic surgery. 3rd edition. Philadelphia: Elsevier Saunders; 2012.

22. Bochner BH, Lerner SP, Kawachi M, et al. Post-radical orchiectomy hemorrhage: should an alteration in staging strategy for testicular cancer be considered? Urology 1995;46:408–11.

23. Bazzi WM, Raheem OA, Stroup SP, et al. Partial orchiectomy and testis intratubular germ cell neoplasia: world literature review. Urol Ann 2011;3: 115–8.

24. von der Maase H, Rorth M, Walbom-Jorgensen S, et al. Carcinoma in situ of contralateral testis in patients with testicular germ cell cancer: study of 27 cases in 500 patients. Br Med J 1986;293:1398–401.

25. Andreassen KE, Grotmol T, Cvancarova MS, et al. Risk of metachronous contralateral testicular germ cell tumors: a population-based study of 7,102 Norwegian patients (1953-2007). Int J Cancer 2011;129: 2867.

26. Fosså SD, Chen J, Schonfeld SJ, et al. Risk of contralateral testicular cancer: a population-based study of 29 515 US men. J Natl Cancer Inst 2005; 97(14):1056–66.

27. Leibovitch I, Baniel J, Foster RS, et al. The clinical implications of procedural deviations during orchiectomy for nonseminomatous testis cancer. J Urol 1995;154(3):935–9.

28. Capelouto CC, Clark PE, Ransil BJ, et al. Testis cancer: a review of scrotal violation in testicular cancer: is adjuvant local therapy necessary? J Urol 1995; 153(3):981–5.

29. Aki FT, Bilen CY, Tekin MI. Is scrotal violation per se a risk factor for local relapse and metastases in stage I nonseminomatous testicular cancer? Urology 2000; 56(3):459–62.

30. Skoogh J, Steineck G, Cavallin-Stahl E, et al. Feelings of loss and uneasiness or shame after removal of a testicle by orchidectomy: a population-based long-term follow-up of testicular cancer survivors. Int J Androl 2011;34:183.

31. Clifford TG, Burg ML, Hu B, et al. Satisfaction with testicular prosthesis after radical orchiectomy. Urology 2018;114:128–32.

32. Nichols PE, Harris KT, Brant A, et al. Patient decision-making and predictors of genital satisfaction associated with testicular prostheses after radical orchiectomy: a questionnaire-based study of men with germ cell tumors of the testicle. Urology 2018;124:276–81.

33. Yossepowitch O, Aviv D, Wainchwaig L, et al. Testicular prostheses for testis cancer survivors: patient perspectives and predictors of long-term satisfaction. J Urol 2011;186(6):2249–52.

34. Dieckmann KP, Anheuser P, Schmidt S, et al. Testicular prostheses in patients with testicular cancer-acceptance rate and patient satisfaction. BMC Urol 2015;15(1):16.

35. Ondruš D, Horňák M, Breza J, et al. Delayed orchiectomy after chemotherapy in patients with advanced testicular cancer. Int Urol Nephrol 2001; 32(4):665–7.

36. Snow BW, Rowland RG, Donohue JP, et al. Review of delayed orchiectomy in patients with disseminated testis tumors. J Urol 1983;129:522.

37. Leibovitch I, Little JS, Foster RS, et al. Delayed orchiectomy after chemotherapy for metastatic nonseminomatous germ cell tumors. J Urol 1996;155:952.

38. Simmonds PD, Mead GM, Lee AHS, et al. Orchiectomy after chemotherapy in patients with metastatic testicular cancer. Is it indicated? Cancer 1995;75: 1018.

39. Reddy BV, Sivakanth A, Babu GN, et al. Role of chemotherapy prior to orchiectomy in metastatic testicular cancer—is testis really a sanctuary site? Ecancermedicalscience 2014;8:407.

40. Daugaard G, Rørth M, Von der Maase H, et al. Management of extragonadal germ-cell tumors and the significance of bilateral testicular biopsies. Ann Oncol 1992;3(4):283–9.

41. Hartmann JT, Fossa SD, Nichols CR, et al. Incidence of metachronous testicular cancer in patients with extragonadal germ cell tumors. J Natl Cancer Inst 2001;93(22):1733–8.

42. Brown JA, Bihrle R, Foster RS. Delayed orchiectomy at postchemotherapy retroperitoneal lymph node dissection due to laterality of retroperitoneal metastatic pattern consistent with testicular primary: assessment of pathologic findings. Urology 2008; 71(5):911–4.

43. Djaladat H. Organ-sparing surgery for testicular tumours. Curr Opin Urol 2015;25(2):116–20.

44. Giannarini G, Dieckmann KP, Albers P, et al. Organ-sparing surgery for adult testicular tumours: a systematic review of the literature. Eur Urol 2010; 57(5):780–90.

45. Heidenreich A, Angerer-Shpilenya M. Organ-preserving surgery for testicular tumours. BJU Int 2012; 109(3):474–90.

46. Steiner H, Höltl L, Maneschg C, et al. Frozen section analysis-guided organ-sparing approach in testicular

tumors: technique, feasibility, and long-term results. Urology 2003;62:508–13.

47. Heidenreich A, Weissbach L, Höltl W, et al. Organ sparing surgery for malignant germ cell tumor of the testis. J Urol 2001;166:2161–5.

48. Lawrentschuk N, Zuniga A, Grabowksi AC, et al. Partial orchiectomy for presumed malignancy in patients with a solitary testis due to a prior germ cell tumor: a large North American experience. J Urol 2011;185(2):508–13.

49. Gentile G, Brunocilla E, Franceschelli A, et al. Can testis-sparing surgery for small testicular masses be considered a valid alternative to radical orchiectomy? A prospective single-center study. Clin Genitourin Cancer 2013;11(4):522–6.

50. Bojanic N, Bumbasirevic U, Vukovic I, et al. Testis sparing surgery in the treatment of bilateral testicular germ cell tumors and solitary testicle tumors: a single institution experience. J Surg Oncol 2015; 111(2):226–30.

51. Heidenreich A, Albers P, Krege S. Management of bilateral testicular germ cell tumours–experience of the German testicular cancer study group (GTCSG). Eur Urol Suppl 2006;5(2):97.

52. Zuniga A, Lawrentschuk N, Jewett MA. Organ-sparing approaches for testicular masses. Nat Rev Urol 2010;7(8):454.

53. Albers P. Organ-sparing surgery for testicular lesions. Eur Urol Suppl 2006;5(6):522–4.

54. Leonhartsberger N, Pichler R, Stoehr B, et al. Organ preservation technique without ischemia in patients with testicular tumor. Urology 2014;83(5):1107–11.

55. Bozzini G, Rubino B, Maruccia S, et al. Role of frozen section examination in the management of testicular nodules: a useful procedure to identify benign lesions. Urol J 2014;11(3):1687–91.

56. Leroy XL, Rigot JM, Aubert S, et al. Value of frozen section examination for the management of non-palpable incidental testicular tumors. Eur Urol 2003;44:458–60.

57. Elert A, Olbert P, Hegele A, et al. Accuracy of frozen section examination of testicular tumors of uncertain origin. Eur Urol 2002;41:290–3.

58. Tokuc R, Sakr W, Pontes JE, et al. Accuracy of frozen section examination of testicular tumors. Urology 1992;40:512–6.

59. Connolly SS, D'Arcy FT, Bredin HC, et al. Value of frozen section analysis with suspected testicular malignancy. Urology 2006;67(1):162–5.

60. Silverio PC, Schoofs F, Iselin CE, et al. Fourteen-year experience with the intraoperative frozen section examination of testicular lesion in a tertiary university center. Ann Diagn Pathol 2015;19(3):99–102.

61. Dieckmann KP, Loy V. False-negative biopsies for the diagnosis of testicular intraepithelial neoplasia (TIN)—an update. Eur Urol 2003;43(5):516–21.

62. Hoei-Hansen CE, Rajpert-De Meyts E, Daugaard G, et al. Carcinoma in situ testis, the progenitor of testicular germ cell tumors: a clinical review. Ann Oncol 2005;16:863–8.

63. Hoei-Hansen CE, Holm M, Rajpert-De Meyts E, et al. Histological evidence of testicular dysgenesis in contralateral biopsies from 218 patients with testicular germ cell cancer. J Pathol 2003;200:370–4.

Preservation of Fertility in Testis Cancer Management

Robert Craig Sineath, MPH, Akanksha Mehta, MD, MS*

KEYWORDS

- Testicular neoplasms • Testis cancer • Leydig cell • Sertoli cell • Synchronous neoplasms
- Metachronous neoplasms • Fertility preservation

KEY POINTS

- Testicular cancer affects men during their prime reproductive years, and physicians treating these patients should be familiar with available options for fertility preservation.
- Testicular cancer can significantly and permanently affect fertility potential, so fertility preservation should be offered to all men with testicular cancer before initiating treatment.
- Cryopreservation of ejaculated or surgically retrieved sperm is currently the only established method of fertility preservation for postpubertal men.
- Methods for fertility preservation in prepubertal boys are still experimental, with current research suggesting a promising future for use of spermatogonial stem cells.
- Many barriers exist to accessing specialized fertility care, including race and ethnic disparities, cost, and geographic availability of providers.

INTRODUCTION

Neoplasms of the testes are unique in that they affect men at a young age, and have high survival rates. Testicular cancer is the most common cancer in men aged 14 to 44 years.[1] Although testis cancer is more common among white men compared with African American men (6.9 vs 1.2 per 100,000 men, respectively),[2,3] African American men are more likely to present at a later stage of disease compared with white men.[4] The incidence for testicular cancer has been increasing over the last several decades in the United States and Europe.[5] Because of a combination of increased awareness, earlier detection, and advancements in the treatment of testicular cancer, overall survival rate is more than 95%.[6]

Given that testicular cancer generally affects men during their prime reproductive years, it is important to understand how this disease and its treatments affect the patients' ability to father offspring. Loss of reproductive potential caused by a diagnosis of cancer has been shown to be associated with impaired quality of life and psychological distress.[7–9] Most men with a cancer diagnosis are interested in fertility preservation.[10] One survey of cancer survivors showed that 51% of participants overall wanted children in the future, including 77% of men who were childless at cancer diagnosis.[11] Physicians treating patients with testicular cancer need to be familiar with available options for fertility preservation. This article discusses the effects of testicular cancer diagnosis and treatment on male fertility potential, and options for maintaining fertility after disease treatment.

TESTICULAR CANCER DIAGNOSIS AND TREATMENT

Most testicular cancers are detected as palpable masses during self-examination of the testes or

Disclosure: Neither of the authors have any relationships with a commercial company that has a direct financial interest in subject matter or materials discussed in this article or with a company making a competing product.
Department of Urology, Emory University School of Medicine, 1365 Clifton Road, Building B, Suite 1400, Atlanta, GA 30322, USA
* Corresponding author.
E-mail address: akanksha.mehta@emory.edu

Urol Clin N Am 46 (2019) 341–351
https://doi.org/10.1016/j.ucl.2019.04.010

physical examinations performed by a health care provider. Rarely, patients present with symptoms of more advanced disease that include hemoptysis, cachexia, and breathlessness.[1]

The work-up for suspected testicular cancer includes scrotal ultrasonography and laboratory evaluation of tumor markers: alpha fetoprotein (AFP), beta human chorionic gonadotropin (beta-hCG), and lactose dehydrogenase.[12] If a tumor is suspected during this work-up, a radical orchiectomy is indicated for histologic confirmation of the diagnosis and treatment planning. Cross-sectional imaging to evaluate for metastatic disease is also indicated. Synchronous bilateral testicular cancer is rare, accounting for only 0.5% to 1% of all testicular cancers, and occurs when the neoplasm is found in both testicles at the same time.[13] Between 5% and 6% of men who have unilateral testis cancer develop testis cancer in the contralateral testis at a later time point, termed metachronous bilateral testicular cancer.[14] Men with bilateral testicular cancer have special considerations for treatment and

fertility preservation, as discussed later in this article.

The World Health Organization (WHO) classifies testicular cancer into 2 major groups, depending on whether or not they are germ cell derived. Germ cell neoplasia in situ is primarily, but not always, found in postpubertal testes, and includes both seminomas and nonseminomas. In contrast, non–germ cell neoplasia is situ, typically arises in prepubertal testes and includes both benign and malignant tumors.[15] **Fig. 1** provides an overview of the WHO classification of testicular cancer. Seminomas are the most commonly diagnosed type of testicular cancer, accounting for about half of all cases.[1] Nonseminomas can be pure, or histologically mixed, to include elements of embryonal carcinoma, teratoma, yolk sac tumor, and choriocarcinoma; seminomatous elements may be present as well.[1]

Staging, in combination with histologic typing, is used to guide treatment choice. Patients with germ cell neoplasia in situ are treated either with radical inguinal orchiectomy or radiation to the

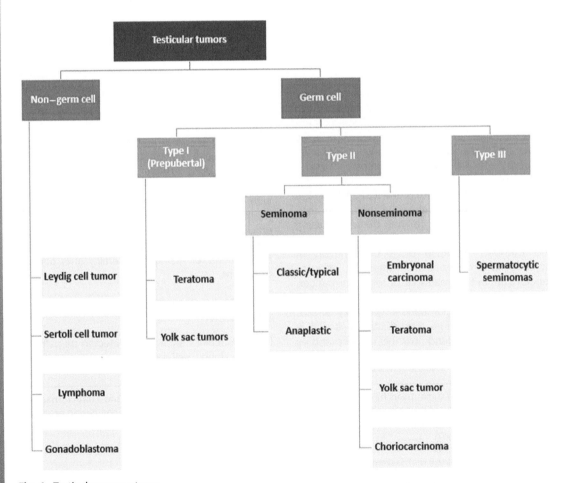

Fig. 1. Testicular cancer types.

affected testis. All patients with disease of stage I or beyond are offered a radical inguinal orchiectomy. Adjuvant postorchiectomy therapies include surgery (ie, retroperitoneal lymph node dissection [RPLND]), radiation therapy, and chemotherapy. Chemotherapeutic agents commonly used for testicular cancer are bleomycin, etoposide, and cisplatin. Staging and typical postorchiectomy treatment options are outlined in **Table 1**. Patients with residual disease after these treatments may be offered salvage chemotherapy, which consists of paclitaxel, ifosfamide, and cisplatin (TIP), or vinblastine, ifosfamide, and cisplatin (VIP).[1]

TESTICULAR CANCER EFFECTS ON FERTILITY

Male fertility requires a normal-functioning testis, an intact hypothalamic-pituitary axis, and normal ejaculation of sperm from the body (**Fig. 2**). Affecting any of these can reduce a man's chances of producing offspring.

Testicular Cancer Intrinsic Effects on Fertility

The presence of cancer in the testes has been shown to intrinsically reduce fertility, even before any medical or surgical treatments are introduced.[16] Spermatogenesis can even be impaired in the contralateral testis in the setting of unilateral testis cancer.[17] A recent study showed that men with testicular cancer have lower sperm concentrations and lower sperm motility compared with men with other types of cancer before treatments are started.[18] Furthermore, men with testicular cancer are less likely to have a total motile count (TMC) of sperm greater than 5 million compared with men with other types of cancer.[19] Predictors of a higher postthaw TMC include nonseminomatous germ cell tumor histology, use of density gradient purification, and higher prefreeze TMC.[20]

The reduction in sperm count and motility in the setting of testis cancer has been attributed to 1 or more of several possible reasons. Histologic studies of orchiectomy specimens from patients with testicular cancer have shown that spermatogenesis occurs throughout the testicle, including the diseased portion, in two-thirds of patients and in areas located away from the tumor in 94% of patients.[21] However, other studies of patients with disease affecting a larger proportion of the testicle have shown that those with a tumor involving greater than 50% of the testis have less than a 50% chance of that testis having functional spermatogenesis.[21] Both of these studies show a reduction in normal spermatogenesis in tissue samples from patients with testicular cancer; direct invasion of a tumor into the testis reduces the amount of normal testicular tissue that is available to produce sperm.

The presence of malignancy also activates a systemic cytokine-mediated inflammatory response, resulting in fever, malnutrition, and stress on the body.[22] Fluctuation in core body and testicular temperature further affects spermatogenesis.[23] This systemic response likely explains why bilateral testicular function is affected in the setting of unilateral testis cancer.

Table 1
Overview of testicular cancer staging and postorchiectomy treatments options

Clinical Stage	Location of Disease	Treatment	
		Seminoma	Nonseminoma
Stage I	Confined to testis	Surveillance Chemotherapy (single-agent carboplatin) Radiation therapy	Surveillance Chemotherapy (1–2 cycles of BEP) Prophylactic RPLND
Stage II	Testis and lymph node involvement	Chemotherapy (3 cycles of BEP or 4 cycles of EP) Radiation therapy	Chemotherapy (3 cycles of BEP or 2–4 cycles of EP) RPLND
Stage III	Testis and distant metastasis (ie, nonregional lymph nodes, pulmonary or visceral organs)	Chemotherapy • Good prognosis: 3 cycles of BEP or 4 cycles of EP • Intermediate or poor prognosis: 4 cycles of BEP or VIP or clinical trial RPLND Radiation therapy	Chemotherapy • Good prognosis: 3 cycles of BEP or 4 cycles of EP • Intermediate or poor prognosis: 4 cycles of BEP or clinical trial RPLND

Abbreviations: BEP, bleomycin, etoposide, cisplatin; EP, etoposide, cisplatin; VIP, vincristine, ifosfamide, cisplatin.
Adapted from the MD Anderson Cancer Center Testicular[67] Cancer Algorithm and American Cancer Society.[68]

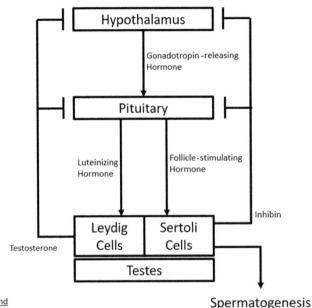

Fig. 2. The hypothalamic-pituitary-gonadal axis.

Tumor histology, tumor stage, presence of microcalcification, and increased levels of tumor markers are not significant predictors of spermatogenesis in patients with testicular cancer.[21] Cryptorchidism, a risk factor for testicular cancer, has been shown to be associated with lower sperm count in patients with testicular cancer.[24]

Endocrine Effects

A diagnosis of testicular cancer is associated with aberration of the hypothalamic-pituitary-gonadal (HPG) axis.[25] Compared with matched controls, patients with testicular cancer are more likely to have increased follicle-stimulating hormone and luteinizing hormone levels, and low testosterone level, an endocrine pattern that is commonly seen in subfertile men.[26] Increase of follicle-stimulating hormone level has also been associated with lack of return of normal spermatogenesis after testis cancer treatment.[27,28]

Testicular tumors are known to cause increases in the levels of certain tumor markers, including beta-hCG and AFP.[29] Increased beta-hCG level is associated with reduced spermatogenesis and increased levels of estradiol, testosterone, and prolactin.[30,31] In addition, increased serum alpha-fetoprotein level is correlated with decreased sperm count.[24] The exact causal pathway of this disruption of spermatogenesis has yet to be fully understood; however, it is thought to be caused by either a direct effect on the testis or an indirect effect through disruption of the HPG axis.[30]

Cancer Diagnosis Effects on Sexual Function

Men with testicular cancer are more likely to have changes in their sexual life, decreased sexual enjoyment, and decreased sexual desire.[32] In addition, men are known to have increased risk of erectile dysfunction after testicular cancer treatment, independent of the presence of hypogonadism.[33] These conditions can, in turn, substantially affect a man's ability to father offspring.

TREATMENT OF TESTIS CANCER AND THEIR EFFECTS ON FERTILITY
Medical Cancer Treatments

As mentioned previously, medical treatment of testicular cancer includes gonadotoxic systemic chemotherapeutic agents and radiation therapy.[34] Chemotherapy drugs act by destroying rapidly dividing cells, such as cancer cells. However, these drugs do not discriminate between cancer and noncancer cells, and also adversely affect rapidly dividing spermatocytes.

There does seem to be a difference in how these drugs affect different types of spermatogonia. Type A spermatogonia serve as a population of self-renewing cells that divide mitotically. These cells also give rise to type B spermatogonia, which are capable of differentiating into mature sperm.

Type A spermatogonia have been shown to sometimes survive after chemotherapy (CT) and radiotherapy (RT), thereby allowing for eventual restoration of some level of spermatogenesis.[35] However, men who recover spermatogenesis remain more likely to produce sperm with DNA damage, compared with men not exposed to CT and RT.[36,37]

It is important to recognize that there are no fertility-friendly chemotherapeutic agents, although some agents can have a more profound effect on testicular function than others. For example, platinum-based drugs usually cause a temporary azoospermia. Spermatogenesis can recover in up to 50% of these patients after 2 years, and 80% after 5 years.[38] However azoospermia can be permanent with higher doses (400–600 mg/m^2).[35] Alkylating agents are more toxic to the germinal epithelium than platinum-based drugs, and fertility can be irreversible even with lower doses.[35]

Damage caused by radiation seems to be dose dependent. Studies have shown that men receiving less than 0.2 Gy had no effect on sperm counts, 0.2 to 0.7 Gy had transient decrease in sperm counts with a return to normal values by 12 to 24 months posttreatment, and more than 1.2 Gy were unlikely to recover spermatogenesis.[38]

Surgery

Surgical treatment of testicular cancer affects fertility in more obvious ways. First, orchiectomy removes diseased and healthy testicular tissue. In adults, there has been a compensatory mechanism seen in the sperm production in the remaining testicular tissue; however, this has not been studied in prepubertal boys.[39] In rare cases of bilateral disease in which both testicles must be removed, the patient is rendered sterile with no chances of producing sperm in the future for conception. Therefore, sperm cryopreservation is ideally performed before orchiectomy. Partial orchiectomy, combined with intraoperative testicular sperm extraction or testicular tissue banking, may be possible in certain cases of synchronous or metachronous bilateral testis cancers, depending on extent of disease and possibility of close patient follow-up.

Patients with more advanced disease that requires RPLND may have damage to the postganglionic sympathetic nerves affecting ejaculatory function during this surgery, leading to anejaculation or retrograde ejaculation.[40] Modified surgical templates provide some degree of nerve sparing to reduce the risk of ejaculatory dysfunction,

preserving anterograde ejaculation in 79% of patients without compromising survival.[41,42] Nerve-sparing approaches to RPLND have further reduced the risk of retrograde ejaculation to less than 10%.[43–45] Nevertheless, sperm cryopreservation should be encouraged before RPLND, if not already completed.

Sperm recovery is possible in men who maintain or recover some degree of spermatogenesis after cancer treatment, even in the setting of retrograde ejaculation. Medical treatment options for these men include the use of alpha agonists, with the goal of temporarily restoring antegrade ejaculation.[40] Postejaculatory sperm extraction from the bladder is also possible, for men who fail medical therapy or are unable to tolerate it. Sperm recovered in this manner can be washed and prepared for use with intrauterine insemination.

FERTILITY PRESERVATION TECHNIQUES

Recovery of spermatogenesis is theoretically possible in men who have completed systemic therapy for testicular cancer. Thus, the first step in fertility preservation in patients with testicular cancer is to prevent the harmful effects of cancer therapies and maximize the amount of viable tissue available for spermatogenesis.

There are currently no interventions to protect testicular tissue from the harmful effects of systemic chemotherapeutic agents. In patients undergoing radiation, gonadal shielding can reduce the amounts of radiation delivered to the unaffected testicle.[10] In addition, there have been case reports of pediatric patients in whom the remaining unaffected testicular tissue was wrapped in a radioprotective sheath and repositioned to the anterior abdominal wall for protection during radiation treatment.[46]

For surgical interventions, there are a few considerations that may help preserve long-term fertility. First, if oncologically safe, surgeons may consider a partial orchiectomy to preserve as much testicular tissue as possible. A partial orchiectomy is a technically challenging procedure that requires the tumor to be less than 2 cm in size, maintenance of cold ischemia during the procedure, meticulous dissection of testicular blood supply, and biopsies of adjacent testicular tissue to ensure negative margins.[47,48] The procedure is conducted via an inguinal approach. Intraoperative ultrasonography may be used to help define the margins of the tumor for excision planning; after the tumor is removed, the tunica albuginea is carefully reconstructed with an absorbable suture to ensure hemostasis and is placed back into the scrotum.[49] Patients must then also undergo radiotherapy to the affected testicle, which affects fertility but maintains Leydig cell function, reducing the need for lifelong assisted reproductive technology (ART).[49]

Although partial orchiectomy is not universally accepted as standard of care, nor is it endorsed by practice guidelines, this procedure should only be considered if radical orchiectomy would negatively and irreversibly affect a patient's quality of life. This choice should be an informed, shared decision made between the physician and patient, with the patient being educated and counseled on potential recurrence outcomes and the need for close long-term follow-up. Long-term outcome data for recurrences in patients undergoing this procedure are lacking. In one small study of 73 partial orchiectomy patients with a mean follow-up time of 91 months, 4 patients who did not receive postsurgical radiation had a local recurrence of disease between 3 and 165 months after resection and were subsequently treated with a radical orchiectomy eliminating the disease.[50] One patient from this series had systemic recurrence and died of the disease.[50] A contraindication to providing this procedure to patients includes the inability to reliably have long-term follow-up for laboratory tests and imaging as surveillance for recurrence.

At present, the only established fertility preservation method available for men is sperm cryopreservation,[34] which has been shown to be effective and should be discussed with all postpubertal men diagnosed with testicular cancer.[34,37] Sperm can be collected for cryopreservation through several methods.

Ejaculated sperm can be used for intrauterine insemination if concentration and quality is appropriate. The easiest and most commonly used method of stimulating an ejaculation is through masturbation. Patients who are unwilling or unable to provide a specimen this way may be offered other means of inducing an ejaculated sample, such as penile vibratory stimulation (PVS) or electroejaculation (EEJ).[51] These approaches are commonly used in men with spinal cord injuries, but can be applied in other clinical settings as well.

PVS involves using a vibratory device placed at the head of the penis to induce an ejaculation. This method requires an intact ejaculatory reflex arc. The success of PVS can vary with different amplitudes of vibration; the use of high-amplitude vibrators has been associated with higher success rates.[52] PVS may be done either in a clinical setting or at home.

EEJ involves using electrodes that are placed rectally onto the seminal vesicles and trigger an ejaculation via electrical stimulation of sympathetic nerves. This method involves some pain and is usually done in a clinical setting under sedation[53] and has a potential risk of rectal mucosal injury.

Patients with spinal cord injuries above T6 are at risk for having episodes of autonomic dysreflexia (AD) after the triggering of an ejaculation; this presents as acute increase in blood pressure, bradycardia, severe headache, profuse sweating, flushing, and piloerection in the dermatomes above the area of injury.[54] AD is treated first conservatively with removal of the stimulus and repositioning the patient in the upright position; if the blood pressure remains increased or the patient is symptomatic, sublingual nifedipine, a calcium channel blocker, can be used as pharmacologic treatment.[55]

In addition, men with azoospermia or who are not willing or able to use these previously discussed methods can be offered surgical approaches to sperm extraction. These methods include epididymal aspiration and testicular sperm extraction. Surgically extracted sperm are not mature or capable of fertilizing an egg without assistance. With these methods, patients must use in vitro fertilization or intracytoplasmic sperm injection for egg fertilization. **Table 2** provides an overview of fertility preservation options for men.

Fertility Considerations in Prepubertal Boys

In the case of prepubertal boys, options for fertility preservation are more limited. Certain institutions offer testicular tissue cryopreservation; however, this method is experimental and should only be offered under an approved research protocol with patient assent and parental/guardian consent.[37] Scientists have been able to induce in vitro spermatogenesis with the successful production of offspring in mice using neonatal testicular tissue.[56] In addition, investigators have been able to restore fertility in adult and prepubertal rhesus macaques with the autotransplant of preserved spermatogonial stem cells.[57] However, neither of these techniques have been reproduced in humans. The goal of collecting testicular tissue in prepubertal boys desiring fertility preservation is the hope of future use of the stem cells present in the sample for one of these techniques or future fertility preservation techniques that are discovered. In patients who opt for testicular tissue preservation, surgical extraction of testicular tissue should be considered to be completed at the time of other medically indicated procedures (ie, orchiectomy) to reduce costs, anesthetic risks, and inconvenience.[58]

Table 2
Summary of fertility preservation options in men

Intervention	Definition	Comment	Considerations
Sperm cryopreservation (S) after masturbation	Freezing sperm obtained through masturbation	The most established technique for fertility preservation in men; large studies in men with cancer	Outpatient procedure Approximately $1500 for 3 samples stored for years, storage fees for additional years[a]
Sperm cryopreservation (S) after alternative methods of sperm collection	Freezing sperm obtained through testicular aspiration or extraction, electroejaculation under sedation, or from postmasturbation urine sample	Small case series and case reports	Testicular sperm extraction: outpatient surgical procedure
Gonadal shielding during radiation therapy (S)	Use of shielding to reduce the dose of radiation delivered to the testicles	Case series	Only possibly with selected radiation fields and anatomy Expertise is required to ensure shielding does not increase dose delivered to the reproductive organs
Testicular tissue cryopreservation, testis xenografting, spermatogonial isolation (I)	Freezing testicular tissue or germ cells and reimplantation after cancer treatment or maturation in animals	Has not been tested in humans; successful application in animal models	Outpatient surgical procedure
Testicular suppression with gonadotropin-releasing hormone analogs or antagonists (I)	Use of hormonal therapies to protect testicular tissue during chemotherapy or radiation therapy	Studies do not support the effectiveness of this approach	—

Abbreviations: I, investigational; S, standard.
[a] Cost is an estimate.
Reproduced with permission from the American Society of Clinical Oncology Recommendations on Fertility Preservation in Cancer Patients.

TIMING OF FERTILITY PRESERVATION AND THE APPROACH TO THE CONVERSATION

Men with testicular cancer are more likely to be referred to a fertility specialist compared with men with other types of cancer, possibly because they are already under the care of a urologist.[19] Guidelines published by the American Society of Clinical Oncology (ASCO),[37] the American Society for Reproductive Medicine (ASRM),[59] and the American Academy of Pediatrics (AAP)[60] all recommend that the discussion about fertility preservation with patients, or their parents/guardians in the case of children with cancer, should be initiated as soon as possible after the initial diagnosis of cancer.[37] Furthermore, providers should refer patients who have an interest in preserving fertility or are unsure about fertility preservation to reproductive specialists.[37] Cryopreservation of sperm after the initiation of systemic gonadotoxic therapies is not recommended, because sperm exposed to these treatments have a higher risk of harboring genetic damage.[37] **Fig. 3** provides a decision flowchart for providers to use in aiding the conversation on fertility preservation with men who have testicular cancer.

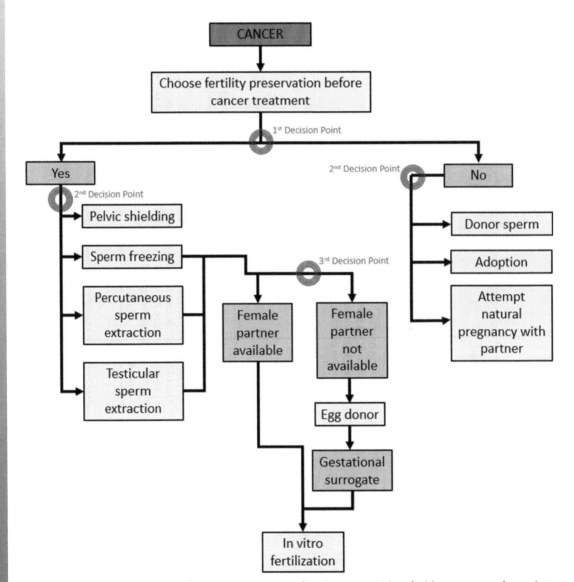

Fig. 3. Male fertility preservation decision tree. *From* Gardino S, Jeruss J. Using decision trees to enhance interdisciplinary team work: the case of oncofertility. Journal of Assisted Reproduction and Genetics 2010;27:230; with permission.

BARRIERS TO FERTILITY PRESERVATION

Ideally, all patients undergoing care for testicular cancer should be offered fertility preservation. However, there are several barriers that can make this process difficult for patients to access.

Sperm cryopreservation before cancer treatment has been shown to be more cost-effective than deferring fertility treatment until after cancer treatment, which includes surgical sperm extraction and ART.[61] However, it is estimated that 3 samples stored for 3 years costs about $1500, with additional storage fees for additional years.[10] This upfront cost is prohibitive for many patients.[62]

Furthermore, racial and ethnic minorities in the United States have higher rates of being uninsured and have more difficulty accessing care, including fertility care.[63] Specialized fertility care also tends to be offered in urban centers. In patients without access to specialized reproductive care for geographic reasons, the use of telemedicine could be considered to facilitate care.[34]

Factors shown to influence whether someone banks sperm before cancer treatment include discussion of fertility preservation options by a health care provider, the desire to father biological children, involvement of a parent or partner in the decision, attitudes toward survival at the time of diagnosis, and cost of sperm banking.[64] In a recent survey of oncologists, although most participants (91%) acknowledged that sperm banking should be offered to all men who are at risk of infertility because of upcoming cancer treatment, half admitted to never bringing up the topic during consultation.[65] Barriers for oncologists in referring a patient to fertility specialists included lack of time for discussion, perceived high cost of fertility preservation, and lack of convenient facilities for patient referral.[66] Oncologists were less likely to offer sperm banking to men who were homosexual, human immunodeficiency virus positive, had a poor prognosis, or had aggressive tumors.[65]

There are instances when cytotoxic therapies must be initiated as soon as possible, making it challenging for patients to bank multiple semen specimens for cryopreservation. However, timing should not be a deterrent from offering patient cryopreservation; even a single vial of cryopreserved sperm can be sufficient for use with ART for family building at a later date.[37]

One study showed that only 60% of men remembered being informed that infertility was a side effect of cancer treatment, and only half were offered sperm banking.[11] These men confirmed that lack of information about sperm banking is the most common reason for not pursuing fertility preservation.[11]

SUMMARY

Testicular cancer affects men during their prime reproductive years. The presence of cancer in the testes intrinsically reduces fertility. The medical and surgical treatments available for testis cancer lead to high survival rates but can have an additional adverse impact on fertility potential. Although strategies such as the use of gonadal shielding during radiation therapy can limit cytotoxic exposures and the impact on fertility potential, the only established method of fertility preservation currently available to men is cryopreservation of sperm. Sperm for cryopreservation can be acquired through masturbation, PVS, or EEJ, or surgically extracted from the testis or epididymis. Depending on sperm source, quality, and quantity, cryopreserved sperm can be used with or without assisted reproductive technologies to allow paternity among cancer survivors. Methods for fertility preservation in prepubertal boys are still experimental, but research on future technology development is promising. Many barriers exist to accessing specialized fertility care, including health care system issues, race and ethnic disparities, cost, and geographic availability or providers. Physicians treating patients with testicular cancer should have an understanding of how this disease affects fertility, how fertility can be preserved, and who to refer patients to for these services.

REFERENCES

1. Cheng L, Albers P, Berney DM, et al. Testicular cancer. Nat Rev Dis Primers 2018;4(1):29.
2. Rosen A, Jayram G, Drazer M, et al. Global trends in testicular cancer incidence and mortality. Eur Urol 2011;60(2):374–9.
3. Ghazarian AA, Trabert B, Devesa SS, et al. Recent trends in the incidence of testicular germ cell tumors in the United States. Andrology 2015;3(1):13–8.
4. Gajendran VK, Nguyen M, Ellison LM. Testicular cancer patterns in African-American men. Urology 2005;66(3):602–5.
5. Nigam M, Aschebrook-Kilfoy B, Shikanov S, et al. Increasing incidence of testicular cancer in the United States and Europe between 1992 and 2009. World J Urol 2015;33(5):623–31.
6. Trama A, Foschi R, Larrañaga N, et al. Survival of male genital cancers (prostate, testis and penis) in Europe 1999–2007: results from the EUROCARE-5 study. Eur J Cancer 2015;51(15):2206–16.
7. Tonsing KN, Ow R. Quality of life, self-esteem, and future expectations of adolescent and young adult cancer survivors. Health Soc Work 2018;43(1): 15–21.

8. Benedict C, Thom B, Kelvin JF. Fertility preservation and cancer: challenges for adolescent and young adult patients. Curr Opin Support Palliat Care 2016;10(1):87–94.

9. Dohle GR. Male infertility in cancer patients: review of the literature. Int J Urol 2010;17(4):327–31.

10. Lee SJ, Schover LR, Partridge AH, et al. American Society of Clinical Oncology recommendations on fertility preservation in cancer patients. J Clin Oncol 2006;24(18):2917–31.

11. Schover LR, Brey K, Lichtin A, et al. Knowledge and experience regarding cancer, infertility, and sperm banking in younger male survivors. J Clin Oncol 2002;20(7):1880–9.

12. Murray MJ, Huddart RA, Coleman N. The present and future of serum diagnostic tests for testicular germ cell tumours. Nat Rev Urol 2016;13(12): 715–25.

13. Campobasso D, Ferretti S, Frattini A. Synchronous bilateral testis cancer: clinical and oncological management. Contemp Oncol (Pozn) 2017;21(1): 70–6.

14. Kier MG, Hansen MK, Lauritsen J, et al. Second malignant neoplasms and cause of death in patients with germ cell cancer: a Danish Nationwide Cohort Study. JAMA Oncol 2016;2(12):1624–7.

15. Williamson SR, Delahunt B, Magi-Galluzzi C, et al. The World Health Organization 2016 classification of testicular germ cell tumours: a review and update from the International Society of Urological Pathology Testis Consultation Panel. Histopathology 2017;70(3):335–46.

16. Petersen PM, Skakkebaek NE, Rorth M, et al. Semen quality and reproductive hormones before and after orchiectomy in men with testicular cancer. J Urol 1999;161(3):822–6.

17. Berthelsen JG, Skakkebaek NE. Gonadal function in men with testis cancer. Fertil Steril 1983;39(1): 68–75.

18. Williams DHt, Karpman E, Sander JC, et al. Pretreatment semen parameters in men with cancer. J Urol 2009;181(2):736–40.

19. Hotaling JM, Lopushnyan NA, Davenport M, et al. Raw and test-thaw semen parameters after cryopreservation among men with newly diagnosed cancer. Fertil Steril 2013;99(2):464–9.

20. Hotaling JM, Patel DP, Vendryes C, et al. Predictors of sperm recovery after cryopreservation in testicular cancer. Asian J Androl 2016;18(1):35–8.

21. Moody JA, Ahmed K, Horsfield C, et al. Fertility preservation in testicular cancer - predictors of spermatogenesis. BJU Int 2018;122(2):236–42.

22. Ostrowski KA, Walsh TJ. Infertility with testicular cancer. Urol Clin North Am 2015;42(3):409–20.

23. Marmor D, Elefant E, Dauchez C, et al. Semen analysis in Hodgkin's disease before the onset of treatment. Cancer 1986;57(10):1986–7.

24. Hansen PV, Trykker H, Andersen J, et al. Germ cell function and hormonal status in patients with testicular cancer. Cancer 1989;64(4):956–61.

25. Carroll PR, Whitmore WF Jr, Herr HW, et al. Endocrine and exocrine profiles of men with testicular tumors before orchiectomy. J Urol 1987;137(3):420–3.

26. Sprauten M, Brydoy M, Haugnes HS, et al. Longitudinal serum testosterone, luteinizing hormone, and follicle-stimulating hormone levels in a population-based sample of long-term testicular cancer survivors. J Clin Oncol 2014;32(6):571–8.

27. Fossa SD, Theodorsen L, Norman N, et al. Recovery of impaired pretreatment spermatogenesis in testicular cancer. Fertil Steril 1990;54(3):493–6.

28. Brennemann W, Stoffel-Wagner B, Wichers M, et al. Pretreatment follicle-stimulating hormone: a prognostic serum marker of spermatogenesis status in patients treated for germ cell cancer. J Urol 1998; 159(6):1942–6.

29. Dieckmann KP, Linke J, Pichlmeier U, et al. Spermatogenesis in the contralateral testis of patients with testicular germ cell cancer: histological evaluation of testicular biopsies and a comparison with healthy males. BJU Int 2007;99(5):1079–85.

30. de Bruin D, de Jong IJ, Arts EG, et al. Semen quality in men with disseminated testicular cancer: relation with human chorionic gonadotropin beta-subunit and pituitary gonadal hormones. Fertil Steril 2009; 91(6):2481–6.

31. Cochran JS, Walsh PC, Porter JC, et al. The endocrinology of human chorionic gonadotropin-secreting testicular tumors: new methods in diagnosis. J Urol 1975;114(4):549–55.

32. Joly F, Heron JF, Kalusinski L, et al. Quality of life in long-term survivors of testicular cancer: a population-based case-control study. J Clin Oncol 2002;20(1):73–80.

33. Eberhard J, Stahl O, Cohn-Cedermark G, et al. Sexual function in men treated for testicular cancer. J Sex Med 2009;6(7):1979–89.

34. Loren AW, Mangu PB, Beck LN, et al. Fertility preservation for patients with cancer: American Society of Clinical Oncology clinical practice guideline update. J Clin Oncol 2013;31(19):2500–10.

35. Colpi GM, Contalbi GF, Nerva F, et al. Testicular function following chemo-radiotherapy. Eur J Obstet Gynecol Reprod Biol 2004;113(Suppl 1):S2–6.

36. Kim C, McGlynn KA, McCorkle R, et al. Fertility among testicular cancer survivors: a case-control study in the U.S. J Cancer Surviv 2010;4(3):266–73.

37. Oktay K, Harvey BE, Partridge AH, et al. Fertility preservation in patients with cancer: ASCO clinical practice guideline update. J Clin Oncol 2018; 36(19):1994–2001.

38. Howell SJ, Shalet SM. Spermatogenesis after cancer treatment: damage and recovery. J Natl Cancer Inst Monogr 2005;(34):12–7.

39. Rombaut C, Faes K, Goossens E. The effect of a unilateral orchiectomy before gonadotoxic treatment on the contralateral testis in adult and prepubertal rats. PLoS One 2016;11(10):e0164922.

40. Mehta A, Sigman M. Management of the dry ejaculate: a systematic review of aspermia and retrograde ejaculation. Fertil Steril 2015;104(5):1074–81.

41. Pearce S, Steinberg Z, Eggener S. Critical evaluation of modified templates and current trends in retroperitoneal lymph node dissection. Curr Urol Rep 2013;14(5):511–7.

42. Winter C, Raman JD, Sheinfeld J, et al. Retroperitoneal lymph node dissection after chemotherapy. BJU Int 2009;104(9 Pt B):1404–12.

43. Beck SDW, Bey AL, Bihrle R, et al. Ejaculatory status and fertility rates after primary retroperitoneal lymph node dissection. J Urol 2010;184(5):2078–80.

44. Syan-Bhanvadia S, Bazargani ST, Clifford TG, et al. Midline extraperitoneal approach to retroperitoneal lymph node dissection in testicular cancer: minimizing surgical morbidity. Eur Urol 2017;72(5):814–20.

45. Donohue JP, Foster RS, Rowland RG, et al. Nerve-sparing retroperitoneal lymphadenectomy with preservation of ejaculation. J Urol 1990;144(2 Pt 1):287–91 [discussion: 291–2].

46. Acosta JM, Tiao G, Stein JE, et al. Temporary relocation of testes to the anterior abdominal wall before radiation therapy of the pelvis or perineum. J Pediatr Surg 2002;37(8):1232–3.

47. Weissbach L. Organ preserving surgery of malignant germ cell tumors. J Urol 1995;153(1):90–3.

48. Heidenreich A, Bonfig R, Derschum W, et al. A conservative approach to bilateral testicular germ cell tumors. J Urol 1995;153(1):10–3.

49. Bazzi WM, Raheem OA, Stroup SP, et al. Partial orchiectomy and testis intratubular germ cell neoplasia: World literature review. Urol Ann 2011;3(3):115–8.

50. Heidenreich A, Weissbach L, Holtl W, et al. Organ sparing surgery for malignant germ cell tumor of the testis. J Urol 2001;166(6):2161–5.

51. Abram McBride J, Lipshultz LI. Male fertility preservation. Curr Urol Rep 2018;19(7):49.

52. Sonksen J, Biering-Sorensen F, Kristensen JK. Ejaculation induced by penile vibratory stimulation in men with spinal cord injuries. The importance of the vibratory amplitude. Paraplegia 1994;32(10):651–60.

53. Lucas MG, Hargreave TB, Edmond P, et al. Sperm retrieval by electro-ejaculation. Preliminary experience in patients with secondary anejaculation. Br J Urol 1991;67(2):191–4.

54. Elliott S, Krassioukov A. Malignant autonomic dysreflexia in spinal cord injured men. Spinal Cord 2006;44(6):386–92.

55. Courtois F, Rodrigue X, Côté I, et al. Sexual function and autonomic dysreflexia in men with spinal cord injuries: how should we treat? Spinal Cord 2012;50:869.

56. Yokonishi T, Sato T, Komeya M, et al. Offspring production with sperm grown in vitro from cryopreserved testis tissues. Nat Commun 2014;5:4320.

57. Hermann BP, Sukhwani M, Winkler F, et al. Spermatogonial stem cell transplantation into rhesus testes regenerates spermatogenesis producing functional sperm. Cell Stem Cell 2012;11(5):715–26.

58. Babayev SN, Arslan E, Kogan S, et al. Evaluation of ovarian and testicular tissue cryopreservation in children undergoing gonadotoxic therapies. J Assist Reprod Genet 2013;30(1):3–9.

59. Ethics Committee of the American Society for Reproductive Medicine. Fertility preservation and reproduction in cancer patients. Fertil Steril 2005;83(6):1622–8.

60. Fallat ME, Hutter J, American Academy of Pediatrics Committee on Bioethics; American Academy of Pediatrics Section on Hematology/Oncology; American Academy of Pediatrics Section on Surgery. Preservation of fertility in pediatric and adolescent patients with cancer. Pediatrics 2008;121(5):e1461–9.

61. Gilbert K, Nangia AK, Dupree JM, et al. Fertility preservation for men with testicular cancer: is sperm cryopreservation cost effective in the era of assisted reproductive technology? Urol Oncol 2018;36(3):92.e91-9.

62. Meropol NJ, Schrag D, Smith TJ, et al. American Society of Clinical Oncology guidance statement: the cost of cancer care. J Clin Oncol 2009;27(23):3868–74.

63. Mead H, Cartwright-Smith L, Jones K, et al. Racial and ethnic disparities in U.S. Health care: a chartbook. The Commonwealth Fund 2008. Available at: https://www.commonwealthfund.org/publications/publication/2008/mar/racial-and-ethnic-disparities-us-health-care-chartbook.

64. Achille MA, Rosberger Z, Robitaille R, et al. Facilitators and obstacles to sperm banking in young men receiving gonadotoxic chemotherapy for cancer: the perspective of survivors and health care professionals. Hum Reprod 2006;21(12):3206–16.

65. Schover LR, Brey K, Lichtin A, et al. Oncologists' attitudes and practices regarding banking sperm before cancer treatment. J Clin Oncol 2002;20(7):1890–7.

66. Micaux Obol C, Armuand GM, Rodriguez-Wallberg KA, et al. Oncologists and hematologists' perceptions of fertility-related communication - a nationwide survey. Acta Oncol 2017;56(8):1103–10.

67. Center TUoTMAC. MD Anderson Cancer Center testicular cancer algorithm. 2017 2018. Available at: https://www.mdanderson.org/documents/for-physicians/algorithms/cancer-treatment/ca-treatment-testicular-web-algorithm.pdf. Accessed November 28, 2018.

68. Society AC. Treatment options for testicular cancer, by type and stage 2018. Available at: https://www.cancer.org/cancer/testicular-cancer/treating/by-stage.html. Accessed November 28, 2018.

Management of Clinical Stage I Germ Cell Tumors

Bruce J. Roth, MD

KEYWORDS

- Germ cell tumors • Stage I • Cancer • Testicular cancer

KEY POINTS

- Several decades of experience have demonstrated that there are multiple paths to cure for patients with clinical stage I testicular cancer.
- Since all available options provides disease-specific survival near 100%, factors other than overall survival become dominant in evaluation of therapeutic options.
- This allows practitioners to factor in quality of life, toxicity, cost, impact on compliance, and so on, when deciding what will best serve their patients.
- The appropriate treatment of a rare, highly curable malignancy should involve all appropriate resources, including potential referral to a regional center of excellence.
- Appropriate treatment might also involve nothing more than pathologic review or possibly a second opinion regarding management.

INTRODUCTION

Germ cell neoplasms of the testicle overall remain relatively uncommon, with 9300 cases estimated by the American Cancer Society in 2018. However, it remains the most common malignancy in males aged 15 to 35, and the incidence is increasing in Northern Europe and North America, as it has since the 1940s. Clinical stage I disease is characterized by disease confined to the testicle, with postorchiectomy normalization of tumor markers; negative imaging of the chest, abdomen, and pelvis; and a normal physical examination and is the most common clinical presentation, accounting for more than 70% of cases.[1] As such, decisions regarding the management of these patients have an outsized impact on the testis cancer population as a whole. A number of postorchiectomy adjuvant approaches have developed over the years for both seminoma and nonseminoma and will be discussed elsewhere in this article in detail. However, the overwhelming curability of recurrent disease with systemic chemotherapy allows us the luxury of interpreting the results of these approaches in terms of factors other than survival, including quality of life. Key to choosing an appropriate therapy for a patient is establishing an accurate pathologic diagnosis from the testicle (including risk assignment based on pathologic variables), and accurate staging. This process can be challenging for a relatively rare tumor type, and even a highly trained treating physician may be limited by ancillary service providers who do not have as much experience with this disease, leading some to argue that patients with this disease should be treated primarily at high-volume centers of excellence.[2] A number of factors have contributed over the past 20 years to a shift away from active intervention with surgery, radiation therapy, or chemotherapy to a now dominant strategy of surveillance. The evolutionary path to this noninterventional approach is outlined herein.

Disclosure Statement: The author has nothing to disclose.
Division of Oncology/BMT, Department of Medicine, Washington University in St. Louis, 660 South Euclid Avenue, CB 8056, St Louis, MO 63110, USA
E-mail address: broth@dom.wustl.edu

Urol Clin N Am 46 (2019) 353–362
https://doi.org/10.1016/j.ucl.2019.04.001

urologic.theclinics.com

SEMINOMA

Clinical stage I seminoma represents the most common clinical presentation in germ cell tumor patients overall. Early reports of orchiectomy alone in unselected patients with clinical stage I disease suggested a 15% to 20% recurrence rate, reflecting the frequency of occult metastatic disease at the time of presentation, with the bulk of recurrences in the retroperitoneum. Approaches to this situation have ranged from radiotherapy to the retroperitoneum with or without ipsilateral pelvis, single-agent chemotherapy, and surveillance with combination chemotherapy at relapse.

Prognostic Factors

Obviously, any clinical situation in which 85% of unselected patients will be cured without additional therapy would benefit from identification of prognostic factors predictive of recurrent disease. In 2002, Warde and colleagues[3] looked at data from 4 separate surveillance studies in clinical stage I seminoma, and a pooled analysis revealed that a tumor diameter of more than 4 cm and the presence of rete testis invasion were independently predictive of a higher relapse rate. In this study, patients with neither risk factor, 1 risk factor, or both risk factors had 5-year relapse rates of 12%, 16%, and 32%, respectively, allowing for the assignment of patients in subsequent studies into low-, intermediate-, or high-risk categories. Subsequent prognostic models developed using various cutpoints for tumor size, from 3 cm[4] up to 6 cm,[5] and some multivariable models have confirmed tumor size as a prognostic factor, but have not been able to confirm independent significance for rete testis invasion.[4] A systematic review by a European guidelines panel concluded that the prognostic value of these 2 factors had "significant limitations," and that the "prognostic power of these two factors in the published literature is too low to advocate for their routine use in clinical practice and to drive the choice on adjuvant treatment in clinical stage I seminoma testis patients."[6]

These pathologic factors clearly have their limitations and there is much room for improvement to accurately identify those patients at the highest risk of relapse after orchiectomy. Perhaps as we continue in the molecular age, novel factors (eg, a specific microRNA signature[7]) may be identified and provide additional accuracy to our existing models.

Radiotherapy

For decades, radiotherapy had been recommended as adjuvant therapy for clinical stage I seminoma, owing to seminoma's exquisite radiosensitivity compared with nonseminoma, and the predictable pattern of relapse, allowing for localized treatment to paraaortic and ipsilateral iliac lymph nodes (standard dogleg field). Results with adjuvant radiotherapy have resulted in a lowering of the relapse rate to 3% to 4%, with the vast majority occurring outside the irradiated field,[8] most commonly in the mediastinum, lungs, and left supraclavicular fossa, and yields a disease-specific survival of close to 100%. This approach effectively removes the retroperitoneum as a potential site of relapse, obviating the need for routine computed tomography (CT) imaging of the abdomen during follow-up, decreasing the cumulative radiation exposure and cost during subsequent follow-up. Although radiation therapy in this setting is clearly safe and effective, it is not devoid of toxicity. Nausea and lethargy are common acute side effects, but there are also long-term concerns regarding infertility related to scatter radiation to the remaining testicle, cardiovascular disease, and second primary malignancies. In 1 retrospective analysis, subdiaphragmatic radiotherapy increased the risk of either cardiovascular disease or a second malignancy 1.8-fold, and a 2.6-fold increase in the risk of second primary cancer alone.[9] A separate review of the Surveillance, Epidemiology and End Results database found a 19% increase in second malignancies in seminoma patients receiving radiotherapy compared with the general population.[10] There were increased risks of developing thyroid and pancreatic cancers, urothelial malignancies, hematologic malignancies, and non-Hodgkin's lymphoma, with persistently elevated risk out to 15 years after radiotherapy.

Attempts to minimize toxicity have focused on modification of the radiotherapy field or decreasing the overall dose and number of fractions, with outcomes defined by 2 large randomized, noninferiority trials conducted by the Medical Research Council and European Organization for Research and Treatment of Cancer. In trial TE10, 468 patients were randomly assigned to receive 30 Gy in 15 fractions to the standard paraaortic and ipsilateral iliac lymph node fields (dogleg), or the same total dose and schedule to the paraaortic lymph nodes alone.[6] Updated data with a median follow-up of 10.7 years in the dogleg arm and 12.0 years in the paraaortic arm showed 5-year relapse-free survival rates to be equivalent (96.2% for dogleg, 96.1% for paraaortic).[11] Not surprisingly, all 4 pelvic relapses occurred in the paraaortic only arm.

In a subsequent TE18 trial, 1094 patients (625 from TE18 and the remainder from the radiotherapy arm of a subsequent trial TE19) were given predominant paraaortic radiotherapy and randomized to 20 Gy in 10 fractions or 30 Gy in 15 fractions.[12,13] With a median follow-up of 7 years, the 5-year relapse-free rate was 95.1% in the 30 Gy arm (with 2 deaths) and 96.8% in the 20 Gy arm (with 1 death). There were fewer adverse events in the lower dose arm. Clearly, the majority of patients can be cured with lower doses, smaller fields, and less toxicity, although paraaortic radiotherapy alone increases the pelvic recurrence rate, necessitating routine CT imaging of the pelvis in follow-up.

Chemotherapy

Carboplatin has been studied as a single agent in the adjuvant setting for clinical stage I seminoma, primarily because of a more favorable toxicity profile than cisplatin, with more convenience for patients. However, it should be noted that in 2 large randomized studies in advanced germ cell cancer, carboplatin-based regimens were found to be significantly inferior to cisplatin-based regimens in terms of disease outcome. In the TE19 trial, 1477 unselected patients were randomly assigned to adjuvant radiotherapy (n = 904) or a single dose of carboplatin at an area under the curve of 7 (n = 573). At the time of the initial report in 2005,[14] with a median follow-up of 4 years, the 3-year relapse-free survival rates were similar (95.9% for radiotherapy, 94.8% for carboplatin). From a toxicity standpoint, the authors reported less lethargy and less time taken off work for those receiving carboplatin. They also claimed a decrease in the number of second primary testicular neoplasms in the remaining testicle in those receiving carboplatin, although it is interesting to note that all 10 second testicular primary tumors in the radiotherapy arm occurred in patients who had received paraaortic radiotherapy without ipsilateral pelvic radiotherapy. The relapse rate in the radiotherapy arm was 3.5% (32/904 patients) and for carboplatin 4.7%. A predefined noninferiority margin of 3% was selected, leading the authors to conclude that carboplatin was not inferior to radiotherapy.

Updated results with a median follow-up of 5 years was reported in 2011,[15] and the 5-year relapse-free survival rates were 96.0% for radiotherapy and 94.7% for carboplatin. The conclusion of noninferiority for carboplatin in this analysis could only be reached after adjustment of the noninferiority margin to 5% absolute difference. Despite the longer follow-up in this analysis, it remains insufficient to figure in the effects of late relapses, or late toxicities, including cardiovascular

disease, or the incidence of second primary (treatment-related) tumors, as has been noted by others.[16] Additionally, 74% of relapses occurred in the retroperitoneum, indicating a need for routine abdominal and pelvic imaging after carboplatin therapy. Finally, patients relapsing after single-agent carboplatin, although usually having good risk disease at the time of recurrence, may not experience same low relapse rate/high cure rate compared with historical controls treated with cisplatin-based combination chemotherapy without prior exposure to carboplatin.[17] Thus, there remains serious doubt regarding the noninferiority (much less equivalence) of single-dose carboplatin compared with radiotherapy given as an adjuvant for unselected patients with clinical stage I seminoma. This finding has led a number of testicular cancer experts recently to call for elimination of this as a treatment option.[18]

Although these trials used unselected (non–risk-stratified) patients, a number of others have attempted a risk-adapted approach, using the prognostic factors of tumor size and rete testis invasion to select the highest risk patients. Tandstad and colleagues[19] reported the results from the Swedish and Norwegian Testicular Cancer Group (SWENOTECA), in which 897 patients received either a single dose of carboplatin at an area under the curve of 7 (n = 469) or surveillance (n = 422). Using rete testis invasion (hazard ratio [HR], 1.9) and tumor diameter 4 cm (HR, 2.7), patients had either 0, 1, or 2 of these risk factors. This was not a randomized trial, because patients with 0 or 1 risk factor were recommended to undergo surveillance whereas those with both risk factors were recommended to receive carboplatin, the ultimate choice was left up to the patient. The median follow-up was 5.6 years and again rete testis invasion (HR, 1.9) and tumor diameter of greater than 4 cm (HR, 2.7) were predictive of relapse. In patients with neither risk factor, the relapse rate with surveillance was 4.0% and with carboplatin 2.2%. In patients having either of the risk factors present, 15.5% of those on surveillance relapsed compared with 9.3% of those receiving carboplatin. Finally, in patients with both risk factors, 31.5% of surveillance patients relapsed, compared with 10.4% in patients receiving carboplatin.

There are 3 important take-home messages from this trial. First, overall, a single dose of carboplatin only reduced the relapse rate by 50%. Second, consistent with the previously mentioned trials, the bulk of relapses (90% in this case) occurred in the retroperitoneum, once again highlighting the need for prolonged abdominal imaging with CT scans during follow-up. Third, even in the highest risk patients, almost 70% of patients are cured with their orchiectomy and would not benefit from additional therapy.

In toto, the trials with single-agent carboplatin have not demonstrated noninferiority when compared with radiotherapy, and when compared with surveillance, only reduce the relapse rate by one-half, with no decrease in the need for subsequent abdominal imaging. The role of carboplatin in this clinical situation is dubious, and has led to a number of testicular cancer experts to call for its elimination as a treatment option,[18] despite its wide adoption as an equivalent treatment option by many guideline panels.

Surveillance

Certainly in any disease such as clinical stage I seminoma, where the recurrence rate is only 5% to 30% (15% in unselected patients) after orchiectomy, surveillance as a strategy needs to be evaluated to minimize the risk of overtreatment. Unlike many other solid tumors, the high curability of recurrent disease with combination chemotherapy allows for the ethical consideration of this strategy. Early reports of surveillance after orchiectomy date to the late 1980s and early 1990s from the United Kingdom,[20,21] the Princess Margaret Hospital,[22,23] and multiple institutions in Denmark.[24] In 2007, a systematic review of the publications on the subject at that time identified 23 publications, including 14 descriptive, and 9 comparative studies, including 7 cohort studies.[25] These pooled data represented 2060 patients with a relapse rate of 17% (n = 356) and only 6 deaths, and showed remarkable consistency among patient cohorts. A subsequent metaanalysis in 2015 analyzed 13 trials with more than 12,000 patients and could not find an overall survival benefit of active therapy compared with surveillance.[26] Individual reports with this approach are summarized in **Table 1**.

The most extensive international experience has come from Denmark, where a protocol of surveillance for clinical stage I seminoma has been in place since 1984, and a number of nationwide databases have provided meticulous follow-up (including cause of death) in all patients since that time. Mortensen and colleagues[27] reported on 1954 patients followed for at least 5 years, with a median follow-up of 15.1 years. The relapse rate was 18.8%, with a median time to relapse of 13.7 months but, most important, disease-specific survival after 15 years was 99.3%. Similarly, Tandstad and colleagues[28] reported the results for SWENOTECA after establishment of a protocol for surveillance in clinical stage I disease in Norway and Sweden. Over a 6-year period ending in 2006, 1384 patients with seminoma (including 1181 with clinical stage I disease) were followed with surveillance (n = 512), adjuvant carboplatin (n = 188), or adjuvant radiotherapy (481), with relapse rates of 14.3%, 3.9%, and 0.8%, respectively. Again, most notably, the 5-year cause-specific survival was 99.6%.

This approach has gained in popularity over the past decade, with some evidence that the increased use of surveillance has been accompanied by a decrease in the number of patients receiving adjuvant radiotherapy.[29] Increased use of surveillance as a strategy worldwide has allowed the pooling of patients from large databases. In 1 such report,[30] 1344 patients with clinical stage I seminoma managed with surveillance were analyzed for patterns of relapse and ultimate outcome. The median time to relapse was 14 months, and 92% of relapses occurred within 3 years. A frequent argument against surveillance is the possibility that patients will recur with larger volume disease and a correspondingly lower cure rate with salvage chemotherapy. However, in this analysis, 99% of recurrences exhibited International Germ Cell Collaborative Group[31] good-risk features. None of the patients died of seminoma, and 1 patient died of

Table 1 Reports of surveillance in clinical stage I seminoma				
Author (Ref)	Organization	Patient Number (n)	Relapse Rate (%)	Deaths (n)
Ramakrishnan et al[20] 1992	Weston Park Hospital	72	18	0
Duchesne et al[21] 1990	Royal Marsden	113	15.8	0
Warde et al[23] 1995	Princess Margaret	172	18.1	1
Mortensen et al[27] 2014	Multi-Center Denmark	1954	18.9	9
Kollmannsberger[30] 2015	Pooled Multinational	1344	13	1

Data from Petrelli F, Coinu A, Cabiddu M, et.al. Surveillance or adjuvant treatment with chemotherapy or radiotherapy in stage I seminoma: a systematic review and meta-analysis of 13 studies. Clin Genitourin Cancer 2015; 13(5):428-434.

treatment-related complications, for an overall 5-year disease-specific survival of 99.7%.

The virtual 100% cure rate with surveillance argues strongly against recommending routine active intervention in patients with stage I disease, prompting many testicular cancer experts to argue that surveillance represents not just one viable option, but is actually the preferred approach in both unselected and risk-adapted patients.[32]

Surveillance has clearly become the most attractive option in dealing with patients with clinical stage I seminoma disease, avoiding unnecessary therapy in the 85% of patients already cured with their orchiectomy, with no compromise of the overall cure rate. Although current recommendations for follow-up[30] are less intense than what was recommended even a decade ago, the approach still requires a long-term commitment from the patient and ongoing compliance with recommended visits and imaging. Although there will always be a small number of patients judged by their physicians to be potentially noncompliant, the vast majority of patients will be served well by a surveillance approach. In those few noncompliant patients, radiotherapy represents a reasonable and effective alternative. If given, however, it must include ipsilateral pelvic radiation (dogleg field) because paraaortic strip only treatment is associated with a higher pelvic recurrence rate, indicating a need for long-term pelvic imaging (and compliance with that recommendation).

NONSEMINOMA

There are several notable differences in patients with clinical stage I nonseminoma compared with similar stage patients with seminoma. These include that (1) the relative radioresistance of nonseminoma has resulted in primary retroperitoneal lymph node dissection (RPLND) being offered for the past 50 years as focal adjuvant therapy instead of radiation; (2) the percentage of patients with occult retroperitoneal metastases at presentation (or the relapse rate after orchiectomy alone) is roughly 30%, compared with 15% for seminoma; and (3) systemic adjuvant therapy has been much more aggressive, generally involving 1 or 2 courses of cisplatin-based combination chemotherapy compared with a single dose of carboplatin in seminoma.

Prognostic Factors

In unselected patients with clinical stage I nonseminoma, only 30% will have recurrent disease after orchiectomy and, by definition, 70% of patients who receive any adjuvant therapy will get that therapy unnecessarily. Attempts to identify histopathologic features predictive of relapse to identify risk groups more or less likely to benefit from additional therapy have spanned 4 decades. Factors that in univariate analysis that have been identified as significant include:

- Vascular invasion,
- Lymphatic invasion,
- Percentage of the specimen containing embryonal carcinoma,
- Pathologic T stage, and
- Tumor size, among others.[33–41]

The most reproducible reported results seem to be with vascular invasion, a factor that, in the hands of a reference pathologist, can identify a relatively high-risk population with a relapse rate of 50% (vascular invasion positive) and a low-risk group with a relapse rate of 15% (vascular invasion negative). Thus, high-volume centers of excellence may use this discriminating factor to some benefit and it frequently appears in published guidelines. Unfortunately, even VI has serious prognostic limitations; 1 study reported a positive predictive value of only 52.7%; more than one-third of the patients predicted to have pathologic stage II disease (or relapse) did not end up having metastatic disease.[42] Another study found a poor correlation between local pathologists and central pathology review for several histopathologic features, including VI.[43] Such observations raise serious questions regarding the ability to broadly apply such histopathologic prognostic factors or use them in a risk-adapted approach anywhere except a high-volume center of excellence.

Primary Retroperitoneal Lymph Node Dissection

In the late 1950s and 1960s, the development of an approach that involved the aggressive dissection of retroperitoneal lymph nodes in clinical stage I nonseminomatous disease provided important diagnostic and staging information. In the prechemotherapy era (up to the mid-1970s), it also offered some therapeutic benefit, because some patients found to have positive lymph nodes did not subsequently develop distant metastatic disease at a time when no other therapeutic options were available. In patients who had uninvolved lymph nodes at the time of RPLND (pathologic stage I) had distant recurrence rates of less than 10%, and in those with involved lymph nodes (pathologic stage II) recurrence rates ranged from 15% to 30%.[44,45]

Even in high-risk patients who have nearly a 50% chance of having positive lymph nodes, RPLND maintains some therapeutic benefit with two-thirds of such patients cured with surgery alone. Early on in the application of this maneuver, full bilateral node dissections resulted in the loss of emission and ejaculation in 65% to 70% of patients with resultant infertility owing to the resection of postganglionic sympathetic fibers. Exquisite mapping studies[46] were performed and defined primary landing zones associated with the laterality of the primary tumor, and led to the development of modified templates for resection. Additionally, the development of true nerve-sparing techniques with prospective preservation of the aforementioned sympathetic fibers allowed virtually 100% of patients postoperatively to maintain antegrade ejaculation, and to some degree preservation of fertility.[47] Although the bulk of the literature deals with open procedures, more recently there is accumulating evidence using a laparoscopic approach, with similar staging results for high-volume surgeons.[48]

In the hands of experienced urologists, RPLND should have a mortality rate of less than 0.5%,[49] with a very low incidence of major morbidities, such as hemorrhage, renal injury, or small bowel obstruction.[50] This technique effectively removes the retroperitoneum as a subsequent site of relapse,[51] with the majority of subsequent relapse occurring in the lung. This relapse pattern removes the necessity of routine abdominal imaging during follow-up.

Although an RPLND in experienced hands offers several advantages, its heyday in clinical stage I disease has probably come and gone. As the overall number of these procedures declines, even at high-volume centers, the number of trainees being exposed to sufficient volumes of cases to garner expertise decrease as well. As the number of urologists capable of doing the procedure declines, fewer procedures will be done, and so on. Although there will always be a demand for this surgical procedure in patients after chemotherapy who have residual abdominal masses, its demise in patients with clinical stage I disease becomes a self-fulfilling prophecy and is inevitable.

Chemotherapy

The majority of trials using chemotherapy as an adjuvant treatment in clinical stage I nonseminoma have used 1 to 2 cycles of cisplatin-based chemotherapy, most frequently cisplatin + etoposide + bleomycin (BEP).[52–64] Data from the studies has been pooled by Vaughn,[65] with some interesting observations. The relapse rate in pooled data was 2.7% in patients who had received adjuvant combination chemotherapy, a decrease of more than 90%, particularly

impressive given that these patients were labeled as high risk by available prognostic factors, although as has been discussed elsewhere in this article, there are significant limitations to these factors. Such observations prompted the inclusion of this as a treatment strategy in treatment guidelines and certainly increased the use of chemotherapy in this situation over the years. One randomized trial conducted by the German Testicular Cancer Study Group compared an RPLND with 1 course of adjuvant BEP in patients with clinical stage I disease and claimed superiority for chemotherapy in terms of relapse in unselected patients.[45] However, this trial has been criticized because of the elevated relapse rate in the RPLND arm, including retroperitoneal relapse, likely owing to the fact that the trial was conducted at 61 centers, including community hospitals, reinforcing the observation above that such surgery, if performed, must be done at a high-volume center of excellence.

The downsides of chemotherapy in this situation needs to be fully considered and raise many questions.

1. Chemotherapy represents overtreatment for 70% of patients and the acute and long-term toxicities of 1 or 2 courses of cisplatin-based combination chemotherapy are certainly likely to be more significant than a single dose of carboplatin in patients with seminoma. Long-term toxicities might include permanent infertility, the appearance of treatment-related second neoplasms, or cardiovascular toxicity, although 1 small series documented rates of oligospermia that are less than that normally reported after 3 or 4 cycles of similar chemotherapy in disseminated disease.[66]

2. Two cycles of BEP in this setting will reduce relapse rates to 1% to 2%, although the results with 1 cycle are less reproducible. Because good-risk recurrent disease is treated routinely with 3 cycles of BEP, is giving 2 cycles of therapy to 70% of patients unnecessarily justified to save the other 30% of patients a third cycle of therapy?

3. Are 2 courses of therapy sufficient for the 30% who are destined to recur after orchiectomy? From sequential randomized trials in small volume good-risk disseminated disease (perhaps serologic-only persistence/recurrence), we have already defined the minimum amount of therapy that can be given without compromising outcome. In 1 trial, 3 cycles of EP was inferior to 3 cycles of BEP,[67] defining 3 cycles of 3 drugs as the minimum therapy required to cure virtually all of the patients. Is it not

Table 2
Reports of surveillance in clinical stage I nonseminoma

Author (Ref)	Organization	Patient Number (n)	Relapse Rate (%)	Deaths (n)
Daugaard et al[70] 2014	Multi-Institutional Denmark	1226	30.6	6
Johnson et al[71] 1984	M.D. Anderson	31	16	0
Sogani et al[72] 1984	Memorial Sloan Kettering	45	20	NR
Peckham and Brada[73] 1987	ICRF/Royal Marsden	132	27	0
Read et al[74] 1992	Medical Research Council	373	27	5
Nicolai and Pizzocaro[75] 1995	Instituto Nazionale Tumori	85	29.4	3
Kollmannsberger et al[30] 2015	Pooled Multinational	1139	19	3

Abbreviation: NR, not reported.

reasonable to ask whether 2 cycles of this therapy for microscopic disease after orchiectomy might not be enough? As a corollary, what do we tell a patient who relapses within a year after 2 such cycles of therapy regarding his curative potential with subsequent therapy? The answer is that we simply do not know.

Surveillance

Because the treatment options for adjuvant therapy in nonseminoma are more toxic than those in seminoma, it certainly seems at least as reasonable to consider surveillance as an option in these patients as well. Single-institution and cooperative group reports over 2 decades have demonstrated the efficacy of this approach with excellent long-term outcomes.[68] Individual reports are summarized in **Table 2**. In 1 report pooling data from testicular cancer centers of excellence worldwide,[30] 1139 patients with clinical stage I nonseminoma disease underwent active surveillance. Relapse occurred in 19% of patients at a median of 4 months (range, 2–61 months) and 8 months (range, 2–61 months) for lymphovascular invasion positive and lymphovascular invasion negative patients, respectively, with 90% of relapses occurring by 24 months, and 90% of recurrences exhibiting International Germ Cell Collaborative Group good-risk features. Only 3 patients (0.3%) died of testicular cancer, and 2 patients died of treatment-related toxicity. Five-year disease-specific survival was 99.7%, the most important outcome measure of a specific approach in clinical stage I disease.

An important aspect of this report was defining the pattern of relapse in clinical stage I disease in terms of timing of relapse (which, in turns out, is different in seminoma and nonseminoma), and the testing procedure that first detected the relapse (ie, serum tumor markers vs imaging studies). Such information is critical to developing an optimal design for a follow-up schedule with the appropriate frequency of visits and testing procedures to maximize early detection, maintain compliance, and minimize toxicity (eg, radiation exposure from frequent CT scans). Such evidence-based guidelines for follow-up should be considered the standard of care.

SUMMARY

Several decades of experience have demonstrated that there are multiple paths to cure for patients with clinical stage I testicular cancer. Because all of the options available should provide a long-term cure rate near 100%, overall survival is no longer a relevant factor in making a decision among these options. This allows practitioners to consider quality of life, toxicity, cost, impact on compliance, and other factors when deciding what will best serve their patients. Many of us have come to the conclusion that surveillance for all patients with clinical stage I seminoma and clinical stage I nonseminoma represents not merely 1 potential option among several, but the preferred option.[32] The contrarian view, held by some, is that a risk-adapted approach should persist, with surveillance for low-risk individuals and active therapy for those at high risk.[69] The results obtained in unselected patients (99.7% 5-year disease-free survival) provides a strong argument against the need for such an approach.

Finally, it is clear that case volume of individual treating physicians, as well as institutions, matters and that high-volume institutions achieve superior results,[2] and expectations to obtain results similar to those in the published literature are achievable only with a similar level of expertise, not merely on the part of the urologist but pathologists and diagnostic radiologists as well. The appropriate treatment of a rare, highly curable malignancy should involve all appropriate resources, including potential referral to a regional center of excellence.

REFERENCES

1. Powles TB, Bhardwa J, Shamash J, et al. The changing presentation of germ cell tumours of the testis between 1983 and 2002. BJU Int 2005;95:1197–200.
2. Tandstad T, Kollmannsberger CK, Roth BJ, et al. Practice makes perfect: the rest of the story in testicular cancer as a model curable neoplasm. J Clin Oncol 2017;35(31):3525–8.
3. Warde P, Specht L, Horwich A, et al. Prognostic factors for relapse in stage I seminoma managed by surveillance: a pooled analysis. J Clin Oncol 2002; 20:4448–52.
4. Chung P, Daugaard G, Tyldesley S, et al. Evaluation of a prognostic model for risk of relapse in stage I seminoma surveillance. Cancer Med 2015;4(1): 155–60.
5. Mortensen MS, Bandak M, Kier MG, et al. Surveillance versus adjuvant radiotherapy for patients with high-risk stage I seminoma. Cancer 2017;123: 1212–8.
6. Boormans JL, Mayor de Castro J, Marconi L, et al. Testicular tumor size and rete testis invasion as prognostic factors for the risk of relapse of clinical stage I seminoma testis patients under surveillance: a systematic review by the Testicular Cancer Guidelines panel. Eur Urol 2018;73:394–405.
7. Van Agthoven T, Eijkenboom WMH, et al. microRNA-371a-3p as informative biomarker for the follow-up of testicular germ cell cancer patients. Cell Oncol 2017;40:379–88.
8. Schmoll HJ, Souchon R, Krege S, et al. European consensus on diagnosis and treatment of germ cell cancer: a report of the European Germ Cell Cancer Consensus Group (EGCCCG). Ann Oncol 2004; 15:1377–99.
9. Van den Belt-Dusebout AW, de Wit R, Gietema JA, et al. Treatment-specific risks of second malignancies and cardiovascular disease in 5-year survivors of testicular cancer. J Clin Oncol 2007;25(28): 4370–8.
10. Lewinshtein D, Gulati R, Nelson PS, et al. Incidence of second malignancies after external beam radiotherapy for clinical stage I seminoma. BJU Int 2011;109:706–12.
11. Fossa SD, Horwich A, Russell JM, et al. Optimal planning target volume for stage I testicular seminoma: a Medical Research Council Randomized Trial. J Clin Oncol 1999;17(4):1146–54.
12. Jones WG, Fossa SD, Mead GM, et al. Randomized trial of 30 versus 20 Gy in the adjuvant treatment of stage I testicular seminoma: a report on Medical Research Council trial TE18, European Organization for the Research and Treatment of Cancer trial 30942. J Clin Oncol 2005;23:1200–8.
13. Mead GM, Fossa SD, Oliver TD, et al. Randomized trials in 2466 patients with stage I seminoma: patterns of relapse and follow-up. J Natl Cancer Inst 2011;103:241–9.
14. Oliver RTD, Mason MD, Mead GM, et al. Radiotherapy versus single-dose carboplatin in adjuvant treatment of stage I seminoma: a randomized trial. Lancet 2005;366:293–300.
15. Oliver TD, Mead GM, Rustin GJS, et al. Randomized trial of carboplatin versus radiotherapy for stage I seminoma: mature results on relapse and contralateral testis cancer rates in MRC TE19/EORTC 30982 study. J Clin Oncol 2011;29(8):957–62.
16. Fischer S, Tandstad T, Wheater M, et al. Outcome of men with relapse after adjuvant carboplatin for clinical stage I seminoma. J Clin Oncol 2016;35: 194–200.
17. Powles T, Robison D, Shamash J, et al. The long-term risks of adjuvant carboplatin treatment of stage I seminoma of the testis. Ann Oncol 2008; 19:443–7.
18. Van der Wetering RAW, Sleijfer S, Feldman DR, et al. Controversies in the management of clinical stage I seminoma: carboplatin a decade in – time to start backing out. J Clin Oncol 2018;36(9):837–40.
19. Tandstad T, Stahl O, Dahl O, et al. Treatment of stage I seminoma, with one course of adjuvant carboplatin or surveillance, risk-adapted recommendations implementing patient autonomy: a report from the Swedish and Norwegian Testicular Cancer Group (SWENOTECA). Ann Oncol 2016;27:1299–304.
20. Ramakrishnan S, Champion AE, Dorreen MS, et al. Stage I seminoma of the testis: is post-orchiectomy surveillance a safe alternative to routine postoperative radiotherapy? Clin Oncol 1992;4:284–6.
21. Duchesne GM, Horwich A, Dearnaley DP, et al. Orchidectomy alone for stage I seminoma of the testis. Cancer 1990;65(5):1115–8.
22. Thomas GM, Sturgeon JF, Alison R, et al. A study of post-orchiectomy surveillance in stage I testicular seminoma. J Urol 1989;142(2 Pt 1):313–6.
23. Warde P, Gospodarowicz MK, Panzarella T, et al. Stage I testicular seminoma: results of adjuvant irradiation and surveillance. J Clin Oncol 1995;13(9): 2255–62.
24. Von der Maase H, Specht L, Jacobsen GK, et al. Surveillance following orchidectomy for stage I seminoma of the testis. Eur J Cancer 1993; 29A(14):1931–4.
25. Groll RJ, Warde P, Jewett MAS. A comprehensive systematic review of testicular germ cell tumor surveillance. Crit Rev Oncol Hematol 2007;64:182–97.
26. Petrelli F, Coinu A, Cabiddu M, et al. Surveillance or adjuvant treatment with chemotherapy or radiotherapy in stage I seminoma: a systematic review

and meta-analysis of 13 studies. Clin Genitourin Cancer 2015;13(5):428–34.

27. Mortensen MS, Lauritsen J, Gundgaard MG, et al. A nationwide cohort study of stage I seminoma patients followed on a surveillance program. Eur Urol 2014;66:1172–8.

28. Tandstad T, Smaaland R, Solberg A, et al. Management of seminomatous testicular cancer: a binational prospective population-based study from the Swedish Norwegian Testicular Cancer Group. J Clin Oncol 2011;29(6):719–25.

29. Kollmannsberger C, Tyldesley S, Moore C, et al. Evolution in management of testicular seminoma: population-based outcomes with selective utilization of active therapies. Ann Oncol 2018;22:808–14.

30. Kollmannsberger C, Tandstad T, Bedard PL, et al. Patterns of relapse in patients with clinical stage I testicular cancer managed with active surveillance. J Clin Oncol 2015;33(1):51–7.

31. International Germ Cell Cancer Collaborative Group. International germ cell consensus classification: a prognostic factor-based staging system for metastatic germ cell cancers. J Clin Oncol 1997;15(2):594–603.

32. Nichols CR, Roth B, Albers P, et al. Active surveillance is the preferred approach to clinical stage I testicular cancer. J Clin Oncol 2013;31(28):3490–3.

33. Moriyama N, Daly JJ, Keating MA, et al. Vascular invasion as a prognosticator of metastatic disease in nonseminomatous germ cell tumors of the testis: importance in "surveillance only" protocols. Cancer 1985;56:2492–8.

34. NHoskin P, Dilly S, Easton D, et al. Prognostic factors in stage I non-seminomatous germ-cell testicular tumors managed by orchiectomy and surveillance: implications for adjuvant chemotherapy. J Clin Oncol 1986;4:1031–6.

35. Rodriguez PN, Hafez GR, Messing EM. Nonseminomatous germ cell tumor of the testicle: does extensive staging of the primary tumor predict the likelihood of metastatic disease? J Urol 1986;136:604–8.

36. Fung CY, Kalish LA, Brodsky GL, et al. Stage I nonseminomatous germ cell testicular tumor: prediction of metastatic potential by primary histology. J Clin Oncol 1988;6:1467–73.

37. Dunphy CH, Ayala AG, Swanson DA, et al. Clinical stage I nonseminomatous and mixed germ cell tumors of the testis: a clinicopathologic study of 93 patients on a surveillance protocol after orchiectomy alone. Cancer 1988;62:1202–6.

38. Pont J, Holtl W, Kosak D, et al. Risk-adapted treatment choice in stage I nonseminomatous testicular germ cell cancer by regarding vascular invasion in the primary tumor: a prospective trial. J Clin Oncol 1990;8(1):16–20.

39. Klepp O, Olsson AM, Henrikson H, et al. Prognostic factors in clinical stage I nonseminomatous germ cell tumors of the testis: multivariate analysis of a prospective multicenter study. J Clin Oncol 1990;8(3):509–18.

40. Moul JW, McCarthy WF, Fernandez EB, et al. Percentage of embryonal carcinoma and of vascular invasion predicts pathological stage in clinical stage I nonseminomatous testicular cancer. Cancer Res 1994;54:362–4.

41. Vergouwe Y, Steyerberg EW, Eijkemans JC, et al. Predictors of occult metastasis in clinical stage I nonseminoma: a systematic review. J Clin Oncol 2003;21:4092–9.

42. Albers P, Siemer R, Kliesch S, et al. Risk factors for relapse in clinical stage I nonseminomatous testicular germ cell tumors: results of the German Cancer Study Group trial. J Clin Oncol 2003;21(8):1503–12.

43. Sesterhenn IA, Weiss RB, Mosofi FK, et al. Prognosis and other clinical correlates of pathologic review in stage I and II testicular carcinoma: a report from the Testicular Cancer Intergroup Study. J Clin Oncol 1992;10(1):69–78.

44. Donohue JP, Thornhill JA, Foster RS, et al. Primary retroperitoneal lymph node dissection in clinical stage A nonseminomatous germ cell testis cancer: a review of the Indiana University experience 1965-1989. Br J Urol 1993;71(3):326–35.

45. Albers P, Siener R, Krege S, et al. Randomized phase III trial comparing retroperitoneal lymph node dissection with one course of bleomycin and etoposide plus cisplatin chemotherapy in the adjuvant treatment of clinical stage I nonseminomatous testicular germ cell tumors: AUO trial AH 01/94 by the German Testicular Cancer Study Group. J Clin Oncol 2008;26:2966–72.

46. Donohue JP, Sachary FM, Maynard BR. Distribution of nodal metastases in nonseminomatous testis cancer. J Urol 1982;128:315–20.

47. Foster RS, McNulty A, Rubin LR. The fertility of patients with clinical stage I testis cancer managed by nerve-sparing retroperitoneal lymph node dissection. J Urol 1994;152:1139–44.

48. Janetschek G, Hobisch A, Holtl L, et al. Retroperitoneal lymphadenectomy for clinical stage I nonseminomatous testicular tumor: laparoscopy versus open surgery and impact of learning curve. J Urol 1996;156:89–94.

49. Fraley EE, Narayan P, Vogelzang NJ, et al. Surgical treatment of patients with stages I and II nonseminomatous testicular cancer. J Urol 1985;134:70–3.

50. Staubitz WJ, Early KS, Magoss IV, et al. Surgical treatment of non-seminomatous germinal testes tumors. Cancer 1973;32:1206–11.

51. Johnson DE, Bracken RB, Blight EM. Prognosis for pathologic stage I nonseminomatous germ cell

tumors of the testis managed by retroperitoneal lymphadenectomy. J Urol 1976;116:63–5.

52. Made G, Pawinski A. Risk-related adjuvant chemotherapy for stage I non-seminoma of the testis. Clin Oncol 1991;3:270–2.

53. Studer UE, Fey MF, Calderoni A, et al. Adjuvant chemotherapy after orchiectomy in high-risk patients with clinical stage I non-seminomatous testicular cancer. Eur Urol 1993;23:444–9.

54. Cullen MH, Stenning SP, Parkinson MC, et al. Short-course adjuvant chemotherapy in high-risk stage I nonseminomatous germ cell tumors of the testis: a Medical Research council report. J Clin Oncol 1996;14(4):1106–13.

55. Pont J, Albrecht W, Postner G, et al. Adjuvant chemotherapy for high-risk clinical stage I nonseminomatous testicular germ cell cancer: long-term results of a prospective trial. J Clin Oncol 1996;14:441–8.

56. Klepp O, Dahl O, Flodgren P, et al. Risk-adapted treatment of clinical stage I non-seminoma testis cancer. Eur J Cancer 1997;33(7):1038–44.

57. Bohlen D, Borner M, Sonntag RW, et al. Long-term results following adjuvant chemotherapy in patients with clinical stage I testicular nonseminomatous germ cell tumors with high risk factors. J Urol 1999;161:1148–52.

58. Amato RJ, Ro JY, Ayala AG, et al. Risk-adapted treatment for patients with clinical stage I nonseminomatous germ cell tumor of the testis. Urology 2004;63:144–9.

59. Chevreau C, Mazerolles C, Soulie M, et al. Long-term efficacy of two cycles of BEP regimen in high-risk stage I nonseminomatous testicular germ cell tumors with embryonal carcinoma and/or vascular invasion. Eur Urol 2004;46(2):209–14.

60. Oliver RTD, Ong J, Shamash J, et al. Long-term follow-up of Anglian Germ Cell Cancer Group surveillance versus patients with stage I nonseminoma treated with adjuvant chemotherapy. Urology 2004;63:556–61.

61. Dearnaley DP, Fossa SD, Kaye SB, et al. Adjuvant bleomycin, vincristine and cisplatin (BOP) for high-risk stage I non-seminomaous germ cell tumours: a prospective trial (MRC TE17). Br J Cancer 2005;92(12):2107–13.

62. Maroto P, Garcia del Muro X, Aparicio J, et al. Multicentre risk-adapted management for stage I non-seminomaous germ cell tumours. Ann Oncol 2005;16:1915–20.

63. Westerman DH, Schefer H, Thalmann GN, et al. Long-term follow-up results of 1 cycle of adjuvant bleomycin, etoposide, and cisplatin chemotherapy for high-risk clinical stag I nonseminomatous germ cell tumors of the testis. J Urol 2008;179:163–6.

64. Guney S, Guney N, Sonmez NC, et al. Risk-adapted management for patients with clinical stage I nonseminomatous germ cell tumour of the testis. Med Oncol 2009;6(2):136–42.

65. Vaughn DJ. Chemotherapy for clinical stage I nonseminomatous germ cell tumours. BJU Int 2009;104:1381–6.

66. Bohlen D, Burkhard FC, Mills R, et al. Fertility and sexual function following orchiectomy and 2 cycles of chemotherapy for stage I high risk nonseminomatous germ cell cancer. J Urol 2001;165:441–4.

67. Loehrer PJ, Johnson D, Elson P, et al. Importance of bleomycin in favorable-prognosis disseminated germ cell tumors: an Eastern Cooperative Oncology Group trial. J Clin Oncol 1995;13(2):470–6.

68. Kollmannsberger C, Moore C, Chi KN, et al. Non-risk-adapted surveillance for patients with stage I nonseminomatous testicular germ-cell tumors: diminishing treatment related morbidity while maintaining efficacy. Ann Oncol 2010;21:1296–301.

69. De Wit R, Bosl GJ. Optimal management of clinical stage I testis cancer: one size does not fit all. J Clin Oncol 2013;31(28):3477–9.

70. Daugaard G, Gundgaard MG, Mortensen MS, et al. Surveillance for stage I nonseminoma testicular cancer: outcomes and long-term follow-up in a population-based cohort. J Clin Oncol 2014;32(34):3817–23.

71. Johnson DE, Lo RK, von Eschenbach AC, et al. Surveillance alone for patients with clinical stage I nonseminomatous germ cell tumors of the testis: preliminary results. J Urol 1984;131:491–3.

72. Sogani PC, Whitmore WF, Herr HW, et al. Orchiectomy alone in the treatment of clinical stage I nonseminomatous germ cell tumor of the testis. J Clin Oncol 1984;2(4):267–70.

73. Peckham MJ, Brada M. Surveillance following orchidectomy for stage I testicular cancer. Int J Androl 1987;10:247–54.

74. Read G, Stenning SP, Cullen MH, et al. Medical research council prospective study of surveillance for stage I testicular teratoma. J Clin Oncol 1992;10(11):1762–8.

75. Nicolai N, Pizzocaro G. A surveillance study of clinical stage I nonseminomatous germ cell tumors of the testis: 10-year followup. J Urol 1995;154:1045–9.

Management of Stage II Germ Cell Tumors

Rashed A. Ghandour, MD[1], Nirmish Singla, MD[1], Aditya Bagrodia, MD*

KEYWORDS

- Germ cell tumor • Seminoma • Nonseminoma • Retroperitoneal lymph node dissection
- Chemotherapy

KEY POINTS

- Stage II germ cell tumor (GCT) represents a highly curable disease state that necessitates careful consideration of treatment-related morbidity while maintaining excellent oncologic control.
- Standard options for managing stage II seminoma include induction chemotherapy or radiation therapy; active surveillance is an option in select cases and investigation into the role of primary retroperitoneal lymph node dissection (RPLND) is underway.
- Options for managing stage II nonseminoma GCT include primary RPLND with or without adjuvant chemotherapy or induction chemotherapy with or without postchemotherapy RPLND; active surveillance is an option in select cases.
- Expert multidisciplinary care is mandatory for optimal management of this nuanced disease state.

INTRODUCTION
Staging and Relevance to Proper Management

In most cases, testicular germ cell tumors (GCTs) predictably metastasize to retroperitoneal lymph nodes before spreading elsewhere in the body. According to the American Joint Committee on Cancer (AJCC) TNM Staging Classification for Testis Cancer, stage II GCT is defined as any local T stage with nodal metastasis to the retroperitoneum in the absence of distant metastasis and without significant increase in serum tumor marker (STM) levels.[1] Stage II disease is further subdivided into stages IIA (cTanyN1M0S0-1), IIB (cTanyN2M0S0-1), and IIC (cTanyN3M0S0-1) according to nodal status. Clinical (c) and pathologic (p) nodal staging is fairly nuanced and varies by the size (c and p), number (p), and/or extent (p) of involved lymph nodes. Briefly, cN1 involves lymph node enlargement up to 2 cm in greatest dimension, cN2 involves at least 1 lymph node between

2 and 5 cm but none greater than 5 cm, and cN3 involves any lymph node greater than 5 cm. Pathologic staging is based on the histopathologic assessment of the retroperitoneal lymph node dissection (RPLND) specimen and includes pN1 (no more than 5 involved lymph nodes, with greatest diameter 2 cm), pN2 (>5 involved lymph nodes of any size up to 5 cm, or at least 1 node between 2 and 5 cm, or evidence of extranodal extension), and pN3 (any node >5 cm).

Because multimodal treatment strategies for GCT vary by stage, a thorough understanding of the complexities and nuances of the staging classification is critical for urologists, medical oncologists, and radiation oncologists in appropriately managing this disease. Furthermore, approaches to management differ based on the histology, classified broadly as pure seminoma and nonseminomatous GCT (NSGCT) disease, given differences in biological behaviors and therapeutic responses.

Disclosures: None.
Department of Urology, University of Texas Southwestern Medical Center, 2001 Inwood Road, 4th Floor, Dallas, TX 75390-9110, USA
[1] These authors contributed equally to this article.
* Corresponding author.
E-mail address: Aditya.bagrodia@utsouthwestern.edu

Urol Clin N Am 46 (2019) 363–376
https://doi.org/10.1016/j.ucl.2019.04.002

This article discusses contemporary management strategies for stage II GCT, which may encompass RPLND, chemotherapy, radiotherapy, or (less often) surveillance. It begins by reviewing patterns of lymphatic drainage in GCT; it then discusses specific considerations in the management of stage II seminoma and stage II NSGCT separately. In addition, it concludes with a discussion of surgical considerations during RPLND, including modified templates, nerve-sparing approaches, and minimally invasive techniques.

Patterns of Lymphatic Drainage in Germ Cell Tumors

Lymphatic drainage of GCTs follows the path of venous flow from the testicles, which originates embryologically in the retroperitoneum. Although GCT can also spread hematogenously, the predictable lymphatic drainage system may be leveraged to allow for locoregional treatment in the context of suspected or known nodal metastatic disease. Knowledge of the primary landing zone in testicular GCT is paramount to determine the proper staging, with its implications for therapeutic decision making. Attempts to identify the proper landing zone started in the early 1900s, when Cuneo[2] reported the first successful example of a curative RPLND and long-term survival despite nodal involvement with teratoma. This report was followed by one by Hinman[3] from Johns Hopkins on 4 long-term survivors of nodally metastatic GCT that had surgically resected disease. The achievement of cure with surgery hence depended on accurate identification of the landing zones to achieve proper resection of potentially involved lymph nodes.

The first in vitro lymphatic drainage study was described in 1910 by Jamieson and Dobson.[4] Prussian blue was used to show the efferent plexus of vessels in the respiratory and genitourinary tracts. In 1963, Busch and Sayegh[5] reported on the use of Evans blue injected in the testicle to identify testicular lymphatics. Following this report, several mapping studies were performed to establish primary landing zones for right and left testicular tumors.[6–8] These early studies provided evidence that although right-sided testicular tumors have the ability to involve both sides of the retroperitoneum, left-sided tumors typically spread to the ipsilateral retroperitoneal lymph nodes.[9] Based on this information, the modern concept of primary landing zones for right-sided (ie, interaortocaval, precaval, and paracaval nodes) and left-sided (para-aortic and preaortic nodes) tumors emerged and forms the basis for templated approaches to treatment.

MANAGEMENT OF STAGE II SEMINOMA
General Overview of Treatment Options

Recommendations for the management of stage II pure seminoma are largely influenced by the extent and bulkiness of retroperitoneal lymphadenopathy. Preferred primary options generally include either chemotherapy or radiation therapy. Unlike NSGCT, seminoma uniquely shows radiosensitivity, which introduces radiation therapy into the armamentarium of effective treatment options for patients with stage II pure seminoma.[10] In contrast, primary RPLND for seminoma has not been a standard approach, unlike the case for NSGCT. In an effort to mitigate toxicities related to chemotherapy and radiation, including secondary malignancies and cardiovascular effects,[11] there are 2 ongoing prospective trials evaluating the role of primary RPLND to treat seminoma: the SEMS (NCT02537548) and PRIMETEST (NCT02797626) trials.[12] Interim results from the latter have been presented recently, but, for now, primary RPLND in patients with stage II seminoma should be considered investigational.

Unlike in stage I GCT, active surveillance is less favored in stage II seminomas, given the tumor's remarkable chemosensitivity/radiosensitivity. However, in select cases of stage IIA disease with isolated, borderline lymph node enlargement, some clinicians advocate waiting 6 weeks and reimaging to confirm clinical stage classification before pursuing treatment. This article primarily focuses on radiation therapy and chemotherapy, given their more widespread acceptance in the treatment paradigm for stage II seminomas, and discusses the management of residual masses following chemotherapy.

Radiation Therapy or Chemotherapy?

Although chemotherapy is more widely used than radiation therapy in stage II seminoma, patient selection dictates both candidacy for and anticipated benefit from radiation therapy. In general, chemotherapy is considered the standard of care for stage IIC disease, which by definition is considered good-risk disease per the International Germ-Cell Cancer Collaborative Group (IGCCCG) classification.[13] Chemotherapy also tends to be preferred for stage IIA/B disease, particularly in the setting of multiple enlarged lymph nodes or bulky nodes larger than 3 cm.[14–17] Three cycles of bleomycin, etoposide, and cisplatin (BEP) or 4 cycles of etoposide and cisplatin (EP) in bleomycin-ineligible patients are considered standard.[18–23] Contraindications to receipt of radiation therapy, including horseshoe kidney, inflammatory bowel disease, prior radiation treatment, and renal hilar lymphadenopathy, naturally favor chemotherapy, as would a salvage setting involving persistently increased STM levels following radiation.[24–27]

Radiation dosing and portals have been well described.[14,28,29] Previously, extensive treatment portals covered the entire ipsilateral iliac and inguinal chains and contralateral pelvis.[27,30–32] However, in a prospective multicenter clinical trial of patients with stage IIA/B seminoma treated with radiotherapy, Classen and colleagues[14] found that reduced portals involving the para-aortic/paracaval nodes from T10-11 to L4-S1 with coverage of the cisterna chyli and ipsilateral high iliac nodes in a hockey-stick or dogleg configuration yielded excellent tumor control with low toxicity. Furthermore, they used a cumulative total dose of 30 Gy and 36 Gy for stage IIA and IIB disease, respectively, which were comparable with prior studies[27,31,32] and remain the preferred dosing strategy of the National Comprehensive Cancer Network (NCCN).[33] Notably, prophylactic mediastinal or supraclavicular radiotherapy is ill-advised.[34]

Outcomes for radiotherapy in stage II seminoma depend primarily on tumor bulk,[15–17] with approximately 90% 5-year recurrence-free survival reported for stage IIA/B compared with only 44% in IIC disease[27]; in contrast, none of the patients receiving chemotherapy for stage IIC disease in this study relapsed at 5 years. Two recent independent retrospective studies using the National Cancer Database (NCDB) compared radiotherapy and chemotherapy for patients with stage IIA/B seminoma and notably found that 5-year overall survival was significantly higher with radiotherapy than with chemotherapy in stage IIA patients, whereas survival outcomes were comparable between the two treatment modalities in stage IIB patients.[35,36] Although these studies may lend additional support to radiotherapy in managing stage IIA patients, these studies are inherently limited by their retrospective, nonrandomized nature of analysis and inhomogeneous treatment allocation per the discretion of individual physicians. The decision to pursue chemotherapy versus radiotherapy for stage IIA/B seminoma ultimately should involve a shared decision between provider and patient, taking into account tumor bulk, toxicity profiles of both treatment modalities, and potential contraindications to radiotherapy candidacy.

Late treatment-related toxicities also must be considered in long-term GCT survivors, and they are particularly compounded for those who receive salvage chemotherapy following radiation. The risk of both solid and hematologic secondary malignancies is significantly increased from exposure to either chemotherapy or radiation alone, as is the risk of cardiovascular disease and metabolic syndrome.[37] Cardiovascular morbidity may arise from acute cardiovascular toxicity induced by platinum-based chemotherapy or a late chronic vascular toxicity and is further increased by receipt of mediastinal radiation therapy[38]; however, subdiaphragmatic radiation is associated with an increased cardiovascular risk too.[39,40] Use of less toxic chemotherapy regimens, reduction of radiation dose, and modification of radiation portals have been used in an effort to mitigate these life-threatening toxic effects[38] (**Fig. 1**).

Management of residual masses following chemotherapy

Following the receipt of chemotherapy, patients should undergo contrast-enhanced restaging with computed tomography (CT) chest/abdomen/pelvis and STMs to evaluate response. Subsequent management recommendations vary based on the presence and size of residual masses and status of STMs, with the following discussion unique to pure seminomas.

In the SEMPET trial, 2-[18]fluorodeoxy-D-glucose (FDG) PET was found to be a reliable predictor for viable tumor in residual masses following chemotherapy for seminoma.[41] A 3-cm cutoff was established as an appropriate size threshold for the utility of PET imaging based on a sensitivity, specific, negative predictive value, and positive predictive value of 82%, 90%, 95%, and 69%, respectively.[42] Based on these findings, international guidelines recommend observation for residual tumors less than or equal to 3 cm with normal STM levels and further work-up of residual masses larger than 3 cm with an FDG-PET scan. The recommended timing of a PET scan is at least 6 to 8 weeks following completion of the chemotherapy regimen to reduce false-positives,[43] and it should ideally provide coverage from at least the skull base to the midthigh.[41,44–48]

In the setting of a positive FDG-PET scan, surgical excision is considered the mainstay and the preferred approach at our institution. However, some groups advocate short-term observation for initially positive scans and recommend considering repeat PET scans 6 to 8 weeks later because of the often-extensive fibrosis and desmoplastic reaction, which may increase technical difficulty, surgical morbidity, and the chance of incomplete resection after chemotherapy for seminomatous disease.[49] Furthermore, although less common, granulomatous conditions, such as sarcoidosis, may cause false-positive FDG-PET scans. If surgical resection seems too challenging,

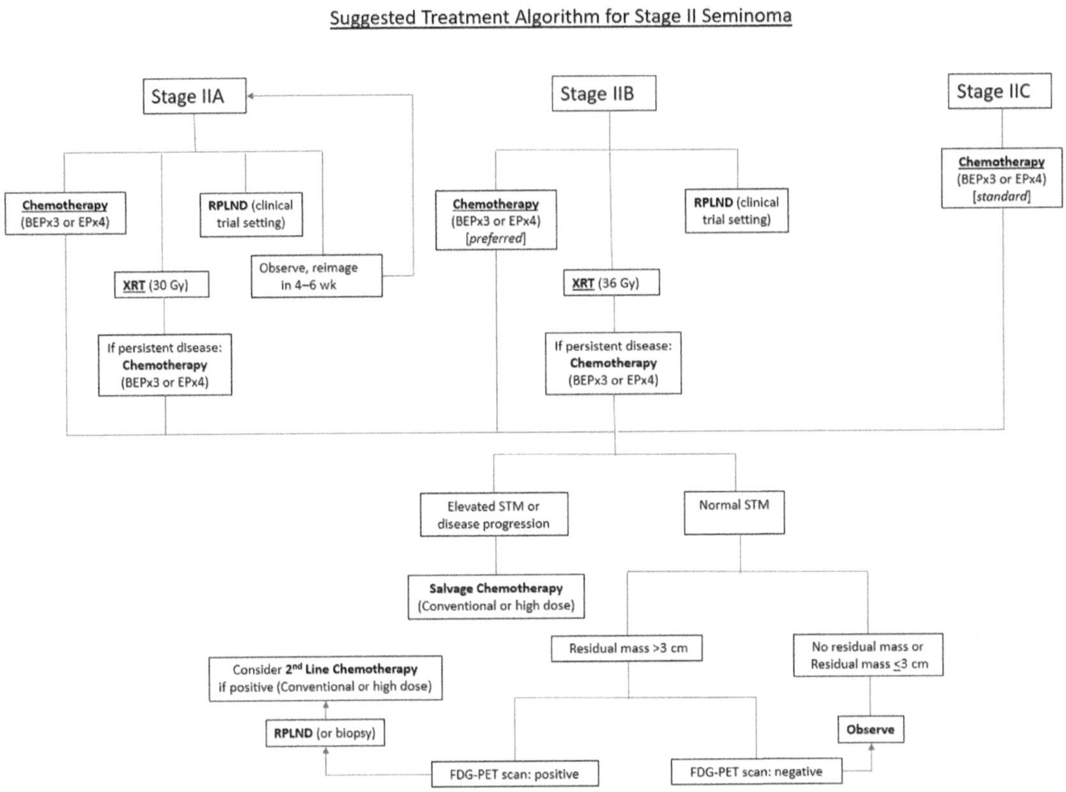

Suggested Treatment Algorithm for Stage II Seminoma

Fig. 1. Treatment options for retroperitoneal involvement in seminoma (stage II). FDG, 2-^{18}fluorodeoxy-D-glucose; XRT, radiation therapy.

percutaneous biopsy of the residual mass is reasonable. Second-line chemotherapy with either conventional (paclitaxel, ifosfamide, and cisplatin[50] or vinblastine, ifosfamide, and cisplatin[51,52]) or high-dose chemotherapy with stem cell rescue is appropriate if either the surgical specimen or biopsy results show viable seminoma.

As a cautionary note, even despite a negative postchemotherapy FDG-PET scan, viable tumors have been occasionally found in tumors greater than 3 cm (false-negative),[53,54] and thus the NCCN recommends continued radiographic surveillance in these patients with CT abdomen/pelvis every 6 months for the first year and then annually for at least 5 years.[33]

INITIAL MANAGEMENT OF STAGE II NONSEMINOMATOUS GERM CELL TUMOR
General Overview of Treatment Options

Matched for stage, NSGCT is biologically more aggressive than pure seminomas, often requiring multimodal approaches to treatment in advanced stages.[10] The choice of primary therapy is largely based on postorchiectomy STMs, the extent and

bulkiness of retroperitoneal lymphadenopathy, and the presence of attributable symptoms (eg, back pain). Although active surveillance is an acceptable option for stage I NSGCT, it is a less favorable approach in stage II disease. According to the NCCN guidelines, only in select cases of stage IIA disease with isolated, borderline lymph node enlargement is it acceptable to wait 6 weeks and repeat imaging to confirm clinical stage classification before initiating treatment.[33] Furthermore, unlike seminomas, NSGCT shows radioresistance, thereby rendering radiotherapy ineffective. Thus, in the present discussion, primary RPLND with or without adjuvant chemotherapy, upfront chemotherapy with or without postchemotherapy RPLND, and combinations of both constitute the central treatment paradigm of stage II NSGCT and are divided by clinical substage.

Stage IIA/IIB Nonseminomatous Germ Cell Tumor

Primary retroperitoneal lymph node dissection
The NCCN guidelines recommend primary RPLND as a treatment option for stage IIA and IIB NSGCT in the setting of normal STM levels after

orchiectomy, absence of multifocal spread, symptomatic metastasis, and disease with aberrant lymphatic drainage outside the primary landing zones.[33] The decision to perform a primary RPLND is based on historically favorable cure rates and the avoidance of toxicity associated with chemotherapy. The main rationale for primary RPLND is based on historical data that support avoiding chemotherapy in pathologically negative lymph nodes, pathologic teratoma resistant to chemotherapy and curable with surgical excision, 98% to 100% long-term cancer-specific survival after primary RPLND with or without adjuvant chemotherapy, and the evolution of surgical techniques to preserve ejaculation and fertility.[55–59] In contrast, RPLND might not be curative in nearly half, 13% to 15% of whom might have persistent disease requiring induction chemotherapy, and a high-quality RPLND might be only obtained in centers of excellence well experienced with the management of advanced testicular cancer[55,58,59] (**Fig. 2**).

In prior studies, RPLND was curative in 60% to 92% of patients with pN1 disease and 50% of those with pN2 disease, whereas the cure rate increased to 98% following the administration of 2 cycles of adjuvant cisplatin-based chemotherapy.[60,61] Patient selection for primary RPLND is paramount to minimize the need for full-course chemotherapy following surgery. STM levels that remain increased after orchiectomy, multifocal nodal disease or disease outside the primary landing zone, and related back pain that could signify psoas invasion or unresectable disease are all factors that make primary RPLND a less attractive option.[60,62]

Given reported relapse rates of 5% and 35% after RPLND for stage IIA and IIB, respectively, some groups advocate primary RPLND followed by observation for stage IIA patients and primary RPLND followed by adjuvant chemotherapy for stage IIB patients.[56,63] In a multicenter prospective trial from Germany and Austria that included 109 patients who underwent primary RPLND and 78 who received primary chemotherapy, the pN0 rate in the surgical arm was 12%, whereas the relapse rate was comparable (7% vs 11%); however, because chemotherapy was more toxic in the definitive setting compared with the adjuvant setting and postchemotherapy (PC) RPLND was associated with higher complications, the investigators recommended that primary RPLND be performed in stage IIA/IIB patients.[58] In another

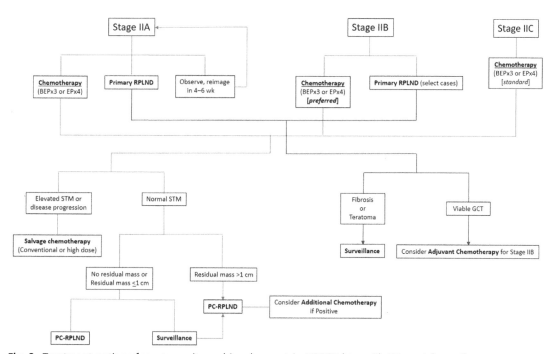

Fig. 2. Treatment options for retroperitoneal involvement in NSGCT (stage II). PC, postchemotherapy.

trial, patients with stage II testicular cancer were treated with RPLND and randomly assigned to either immediate adjuvant cisplatin-based chemotherapy or observation and salvage chemotherapy for recurrences.[64] Only 1 out of 97 patients in the adjuvant chemotherapy arm recurred, compared with 48 of 98 in the observation arm. There were no differences in disease-specific survival between the groups, and observation was accordingly deemed acceptable only with low risk of recurrence and adequate patient compliance.

Adjuvant chemotherapy following retroperitoneal lymph node dissection for stage IIA/B nonseminomatous germ cell tumor

Given the risk of relapse in stage IIA/B disease, adjuvant chemotherapy has been advocated in this setting, especially for stage IIB. Furthermore, patients with stage IIA disease who are poorly compliant are also recommended to receive adjuvant chemotherapy.[33,65]

The accepted adjuvant protocols have evolved historically. In 1987, a trial comparing adjuvant and salvage chemotherapy allowed for a regimen of cisplatin/vinblastine/bleomycin (PVB) at the University of Indiana or a cyclophosphamide/dactinomycin/cisplatin/vinblastine/bleomycin regimen at Memorial Sloan Kettering.[64] The triple therapy currently widely used, BEP, was found in the same year to be superior to the previously used PVB in disseminated disease.[66] In 1995, Motzer and colleagues[67] published the results of 50 patients with pathologic N2 and N3 disease treated with 2 cycles of EP, with all 50 alive and recurrence free at a median follow-up of 35 months. The protocol used was 2 cycles of etoposide (100 mg/m^2) plus cisplatin (20 mg/m^2) per day, administered on days 1 to 5 at a 21-day interval. Kondagunta and colleagues[61] published in 2004 the updated results of 87 patients who received the adjuvant EP regimen, with 99% recurrence-free survival at a median follow-up of 8 years. Behnia and colleagues[68] from the Indiana University published their experience with 86 patients with stage IIA or IIB NSGCT who received 2 cycles of BEP adjuvant chemotherapy. The regimen consisted of bleomycin, 30 units weekly for 8 weeks, etoposide (100 mg/m^2), and cisplatin (20 mg/m^2) each for 5 days every 28 days for 2 cycles. All patients were alive at last follow-up and only 1 patient had a cervical node relapse, which was later treated with surgery. Given this evidence, the current NCCN guidelines recommend 2 cycles of BEP or EP as the preferred adjuvant chemotherapy regimen for stage IIA or IIB disease.[33]

Definitive chemotherapy for stage IIA/B nonseminomatous germ cell tumor

Definitive chemotherapy is an alternative option to surgery for the primary treatment of stage IIA and IIB GCT.[33] Induction chemotherapy has been widely used because of the advantages related to the high rate of complete response, the ease of delivering treatment in community-based facilities, and a cancer-specific survival approaching 100% for patients receiving the induction chemotherapy.[55,58,69] In contrast, this approach subjects all patients to the long-term toxicity of a full course of chemotherapy, and, whenever not properly evaluated for PC-RPLND, patients might be at risk of relapse with chemorefractory GCT or teratoma.[55]

Several trials were conducted to determine the optimal regimen combination, dosage, and duration of treatment of good-risk metastatic GCTs.[19,21,22,70,71] Initially, 3 cycles of BEP were established as equivalent to 4 cycles with less toxicity.[22,70] Three other trials compared BEP with EP. The first, by Loehrer and colleagues,[21] compared 3 cycles of EP with 3 cycles of BEP and showed inferior failure-free (69 vs 86%; $P = .01$) and overall survival (86% vs 95%, $P = .01$) in the EP arm. The second trial, by de Wit and colleagues,[19] compared 3 cycles of BEP with 3 cycles of BEP plus a fourth cycle of EP and showed equivalent efficacy and toxicity. In 2007, a third trial, by Culine and colleagues,[71] compared 3 cycles of BEP with 4 cycles of EP in 257 patients. Although the primary end point of favorable response (91% vs 86%) and the 4-year overall survival (96% vs 90%) were equivalent, the study was underpowered for the latter, and BEP became the regimen of choice for metastatic NSGCT. The NCCN guidelines consider both 3 cycles of BEP and 4 cycles of EP to be acceptable options with excellent survival following either regimen.[33] The choice between the two regimens depends largely on the toxicity profile, with bleomycin known to harbor toxic pulmonary effects and Raynaud phenomenon,[72] whereas the dose of cisplatin varies between the two.

As primary therapy in stage IIA/B GCT, platinum-based chemotherapy was found to be an effective alternative to RPLND. Horwich and colleagues[73] published in 1994 their experience with 122 patients (58 stage IIA, 64 stage IIB) who achieved an overall 97% disease-free survival at a median follow-up of 5.5 years after receipt of chemotherapy alone. PC-RPLND for residual disease was performed in 17% of stage IIA patients and in 39% of stage IIB, with most yielding pathology findings of mature teratoma. Since then, chemotherapy for stage IIA/B has been increasingly used, and, in a nonrandomized comparison at Memorial Sloan Kettering Cancer Center (MSKCC), a strategy of primary chemotherapy followed by PC-RPLND when indicated improved the relapse-free survival over time from 84% to 98%, and from 79% to 98% compared with primary RPLND.[59] Similarly, this strategy allowed a better selection of patients for primary RPLND, with relapse-free survival rates improving from 78% to 100% for selected patients undergoing primary RPLND. Based on the current evidence, the NCCN and European guidelines tend to favor primary RPLND for stage IIA GCT in centers with significant expertise and primary chemotherapy with PC-RPLND as indicated for stage IIB GCT.[33,65]

Stage IIC Nonseminomatous Germ Cell Tumor

International germ-cell cancer collaborative group risk of stage IIC
According to the IGCCCG risk stratification, stage IIC GCT is classified as favorable-risk disease.[13] Primary RPLND is ill-advised in this group, and instead definitive chemotherapy is the recommended treatment strategy for clinical stage IIC GCT.[13,33] The rationale for this recommendation is to minimize the morbidity of a noncurative surgery in metastatic or locally unresectable disease that would result in a high relapse rate requiring salvage chemotherapy.[60]

Adjuvant chemotherapy following retroperitoneal lymph node dissection for pathologic stage IIC nonseminomatous germ cell tumor
Although 2 cycles of cisplatin-based adjuvant chemotherapy is an option for stage IIA disease and a recommendation for stage IIB disease, adjuvant chemotherapy cannot compensate for incomplete resection and high risk of relapse in stage IIC disease.[74] Following an RPLND that yields pN3 disease, a full course of chemotherapy with 3 cycles of BEP or 4 cycles of EP is recommended post-RPLND in this setting.[33,60,65]

Management of Stage II Nonseminomatous Germ Cell Tumor Following Definitive Chemotherapy

Follow-up schedules
After completion of definitive chemotherapy, patients are followed with physical examinations, STMs, and cross-sectional imaging of the chest, abdomen, and pelvis. The NCCN recommends STMs every 2 months for the first year, every 3 months for the second year, and every 6 months thereafter. Contrast-enhanced CT scans of the chest, abdomen, and pelvis are recommended every 6 months in the first year of follow-up, every 6 to 12 months in the second year, and annually thereafter.[33]

Management of postchemotherapy complete response
Following definitive chemotherapy, there is controversy regarding how complete response of retroperitoneal adenopathy is best managed. The rationale behind PC-RPLND is to excise any microscopic residual disease not visible by radiographic imaging, particularly given the purported chemoresistance of teratoma. However, there are no accurate and widely used predictive tools to help delineate who may be safely observed and who should receive PC-RPLND.[75–78] Carver and colleagues[79] published the MSKCC experience of PC-RPLND for 154 patients who had no residual masses greater than 1 cm following chemotherapy, and they found teratoma and viable GCT in the RPLND specimen of 22% and 5% of patients, respectively. The investigators concluded that the risks of an uncontrolled retroperitoneum are unacceptably high, including a risk of malignant transformation, late relapse, and growing teratoma syndrome. Based on the fact that 27% of patients have a combined risk of teratoma and viable GCT and may derive benefit from PC-RPLND, the group advocates aggressive use of PC-RPLND even in the context of residual masses smaller than 1 cm. Advocates of surveillance for masses smaller than 1 cm believe such microscopic foci of tumors will not affect the excellent survival in complete responders to induction chemotherapy, with a 15-year recurrence-free survival of 90% and disease-specific survival of 100%.[80] The rationale for surveillance is the generally indolent course of microscopic teratoma and the ability to avoid an unnecessary PC-RPLND in most patients with no residual microscopic disorder. The Indiana University group reported on 141 patients who achieved a complete response and who underwent surveillance following chemotherapy with a median follow-up of 15.5 years. Twelve patients (9%) had recurrence at a median of 11 months. Of these, 8 patients were ostensibly cured after further intervention at a median of 11 years of follow-up, whereas 4 patients died, all within 12 months after chemotherapy.[80]

Kollmannsberger and colleagues[81] published the joint experience of British Columbia Cancer Agency and the Oregon Testis Cancer Program over 10 years and identified 161 patients with complete response after definitive chemotherapy, including 83% with good-risk disease and 40% with teratoma in the testicular specimen, who underwent observation. Ten patients relapsed, 3 of whom had initial stage IS, 5 had stage II, and 3 had stage III disease. In addition, 5 of the relapsed patients had a teratoma component in their gonadal GCT histology. Ultimately, there are philosophically different opinions regarding the approach to the management of patients with complete radiographic response to chemotherapy. Although some clinicians favor being surgically aggressive to salvage a few, others favor observation while understanding the risks that a small fraction of patients may have missed a window of opportunity for cure.

Management of postchemotherapy residual mass

Residual disease following chemotherapy for NSGCT poses a challenge and may involve persistently increased STM levels or a growing mass despite normalized STM levels. Unlike for seminomas, PET scans hold limited utility for NSGCT given the poor discrimination between fibrosis and teratoma. Most guidelines recommend resecting any residual mass larger than 1 cm following normalization or plateauing of STM levels, preferably using a full bilateral template PC-RPLND, although modified templates have been proposed and advocated by some clinicians.[33,65,75–78,82,83] Even with residual masses larger than 1 cm, nearly half of patients receive a negative PC-RPLND, with associated risks and toxicities. Although significant efforts have been made to determine whether and when PC-RPLND may be avoided, no predictive tools have gained widespread usage.[75–78] Given the technical challenges of this surgery, ideally it should be limited to high-volume centers with clinical expertise in managing these patients.[6,33,74,84]

Occasionally, a teratoma can begin to grow rapidly in uncontrolled fashion if not resected promptly. Referred to as growing teratoma syndrome, this phenomenon may arise during or after chemotherapy and can obstruct and invade adjacent vital organs, rendering resection exceedingly difficult with considerable morbidity.[85] Malignant transformation of teratomatous elements is another possibility, giving rise to secondary malignancies that are resistant to conventional chemotherapy for GCT. Inadequate resection may amount to a poor prognosis in such settings.[86,87] Further discussion of growing teratoma syndrome and malignant transformation are outside the scope of the present article.

SURGICAL CONSIDERATIONS
Retroperitoneal Lymph Node Dissection Templates and Nerve-sparing Approaches

The limits of the standard bilateral RPLND template traditionally span to include the renal hila superiorly, ureters bilaterally, and common iliacs inferiorly, with further refinement based on mapping studies of the distribution of lymph node metastases in these patients.[6–8] Despite favorable oncologic control, complications related to bowel obstruction, renovascular or ureteral injury, or chylous ascites are risks of this approach[88] in addition to potential overtreatment by resection of fibrotic or necrotic disease.[7,89] Furthermore, anejaculation related to extensive dissection of paravertebral sympathetic trunks and postganglionic sympathetic fibers converging in the hypogastric plexus[90] represents a considerable source of morbidity for many of these patients.[91–94] To help preserve rates of antegrade ejaculation while potentially decreasing surgical morbidity and operative times,[95–97] 2 general strategies have been described: (1) developing modified dissection templates to minimize contralateral dissection, and (2) prospectively identifying and preserving sympathetic nerves using a nerve-sparing approach that can be implemented in either modified or full bilateral RPLND templates.

The concept of meticulous dissection to improve ejaculation by prospectively preserving postganglionic sympathetic fibers was initially described in the 1980s.[94,98,99] Thereafter, based on an improved understanding of side-specific landing zones, the notion of modifying the traditional bilateral full-template RPLND emerged for low-stage NSGCT in an effort to avoid dissection of the contralateral sympathetic trunk and region below the inferior mesenteric artery while removing ipsilateral lymph nodes extending from the renal hilum superiorly to the bifurcation of the common iliac artery inferiorly.[100] Initial side-specific modified templates were shown to preserve antegrade ejaculation in more than 90% of patients without compromising oncologic outcomes in patients with low-stage NSGCT.[7,100] There have since emerged several modified RPLND templates without a clear consensus on the optimal modification approach or patient candidacy.[101] Two reports from MSKCC evaluated the risk of extratemplate disease when modified templates were used for both primary RPLND and PC-RPLND. When 5 modified templates were applied to 191 patients who underwent primary RPLND for stage II NSGCT, extratemplate disease ranged from 3% to 23% for all patients, and was 1% to 11% for those with clinical stage

IIA.[102] Similarly, when those 5 templates were applied for 532 patients with metastatic GCT who underwent PC-RPLND, 7% to 32% of patients had extratemplate disease. The incidence varied from 8% extratemplate disease when residual retroperitoneal masses less than 1 cm were identified radiologically to 25% when the residual masses were larger than 5 cm.[103]

Patient selection is perhaps the most important factor in determining the appropriateness of offering modified-template RPLND. In the postchemotherapy setting, the standard of care remains the full-template bilateral RPLND, but modified templates may be considered in highly selected patients without compromising oncologic outcomes.[89] Heidenreich and colleagues[104] suggested an algorithm to select patients for unilateral RPLND after chemotherapy based on the presence of a residual mass less than or equal to 5 cm in the primary landing zone, which was externally validated in a series by Vallier and colleagues.[105] At our institution, we prefer a full-template bilateral RPLND in cases of bulky adenopathy, enlargement of multiple lymph nodes, or presence of lymphadenopathy outside the primary landing zone. In the postchemotherapy setting, we consider a modified RPLND template only if STM levels have normalized and there is either no or low-volume residual disease confined to the primary landing zone both before and after chemotherapy. In a recent study on 100 patients who underwent modified-template postchemotherapy RPLND at Indiana University using selection criteria similar to those practiced at our institution, Cho and colleagues[106] reported favorable recurrence-free survival rates (93% and 92% at 5 and 10 years, respectively) with 99% overall survival at 10 years. They noted that all recurrences in their series occurred outside the boundaries of a full bilateral RPLND template.

Although nerve-sparing approaches and modified RPLND templates may improve surgical morbidity and antegrade ejaculation compared with traditional full bilateral template RPLND, the authors again stress the importance of patient selection in order to achieve similar oncologic outcomes, especially in the postchemotherapy setting. Postchemotherapy RPLND can be technically challenging and ought to be performed primarily in high-volume centers with a general surgeon and vascular surgeon available on standby. Furthermore, pursuit of a modified template, especially for higher-stage disease, carries the risk of extratemplate disease recurrence, and surgeons should have a low threshold for conversion to bilateral dissection should nodal involvement be detected intraoperatively.[79,89,102,103]

Minimally Invasive Approaches

Traditionally, open RPLND has been accomplished through a sizable midline laparotomy incision. In an effort to reduce morbidity, minimally invasive approaches to RPLND with either conventional laparoscopy or robotic assistance have emerged. Although there are currently no randomized trials directly comparing open and minimally invasive approaches, several retrospective series have shown the safety and feasibility of the latter in low-stage disease, with reduced blood loss, faster convalescence, and shorter hospital length of stay.[107–111] Nakamura and colleagues[112] recently published their institutional series on postchemotherapy nerve-sparing, bilateral template, laparoscopic RPLND in patients with clinical stage IIA/B disease and found this approach to be safe with preservation of antegrade ejaculation and improved blood loss and postoperative recovery compared with the open approach. Longer-term outcomes are needed to evaluate oncologic efficacy of minimally invasive RPLND approaches, and such approaches should be restricted to experienced, high-volume centers on selected patients.

SUMMARY

There are several treatment strategies available for stage II GCT, either alone or in combination. Patient selection, histology, and extent of lymphadenopathy are all factors that drive management. Although chemotherapy is perhaps the most widely used treatment option for both seminoma and NSGCT, overtreatment and unfavorable toxicity profile remain legitimate concerns. Radiation therapy is an alternative option for low-volume seminoma, whereas RPLND retains an integral role in the multidisciplinary approach to treating NSGCT. PET scans have a defined role, primarily limited to residual sizable masses following chemotherapy for pure seminoma. As both treatment and detection strategies continue to emerge and be refined, the management of patients with stage II GCT continues to evolve.

REFERENCES

1. Amin MB, Edge SB, Greene FL. American Joint Committee on Cancer. Springer(UK): AJCC cancer staging manual; 2018. p. 327–32.
2. Cuneo B. Note sur les lymphatiques du testicule. Bull et Mem Soc Anat de Paris 1901;(76):105.
3. Hinman F. The operative treatment of tumors of the testicle. JAMA 1914;(58):2009–15.
4. Jamieson JK, Dobson JF. On the injection of lymphatics by Prussian blue. J Anat Physiol 1910; 45(Pt 1):7–10.

5. Busch FM, Sayegh ES. Roentgenographic visualization of human testicular lymphatics: a preliminary report. J Urol 1963;89:106–10.

6. Donohue JP, Zachary JM, Maynard BR. Distribution of nodal metastases in nonseminomatous testis cancer. J Urol 1982;128(2):315–20.

7. Weissbach L, Boedefeld EA. Localization of solitary and multiple metastases in stage II nonseminomatous testis tumor as basis for a modified staging lymph node dissection in stage I. J Urol 1987;138(1):77–82.

8. Ray B, Hajdu SI, Whitmore WF Jr. Proceedings: distribution of retroperitoneal lymph node metastases in testicular germinal tumors. Cancer 1974;33(2):340–8.

9. Sogani PC. Evolution of the management of stage I nonseminomatous germ-cell tumors of the testis. Urol Clin North Am 1991;18(3):561–73.

10. Stutzman RE, McLeod DG. Radiation therapy: a primary treatment modality for seminoma. Urol Clin North Am 1980;7(3):757–64.

11. Beyer J, Albers P, Altena R, et al. Maintaining success, reducing treatment burden, focusing on survivorship: highlights from the third European consensus conference on diagnosis and treatment of germ-cell cancer. Ann Oncol 2013;24(4):878–88.

12. Lusch A, Grobe Siemer R, Albers P. The PRIMET-EST trial - interim results for a phase II trial for primary retroperitoneal lymph node dissection (RPLND) in Stage II A/B seminoma patients without adjuvant treatment. Eur Urol Suppl 2018;17(2):e1136.

13. International germ cell consensus classification: a prognostic factor-based staging system for metastatic germ cell cancers. International Germ Cell Cancer Collaborative Group. J Clin Oncol 1997;15(2):594–603.

14. Classen J, Schmidberger H, Meisner C, et al. Radiotherapy for stages IIA/B testicular seminoma: final report of a prospective multicenter clinical trial. J Clin Oncol 2003;21(6):1101–6.

15. Garcia-del-Muro X, Maroto P, Gumà J, et al. Chemotherapy as an alternative to radiotherapy in the treatment of stage IIA and IIB testicular seminoma: a Spanish Germ Cell Cancer Group Study. J Clin Oncol 2008;26(33):5416–21.

16. Gordon W Jr, Siegmund K, Stanisic TH, et al. A study of reproductive function in patients with seminoma treated with radiotherapy and orchidectomy: (SWOG-8711). Southwest Oncology Group. Int J Radiat Oncol Biol Phys 1997;38(1):83–94.

17. Mason BR, Kearsley JH. Radiotherapy for stage 2 testicular seminoma: the prognostic influence of tumor bulk. J Clin Oncol 1988;6(12):1856–62.

18. Bajorin DF, Sarosdy MF, Pfister DG, et al. Randomized trial of etoposide and cisplatin versus etoposide and carboplatin in patients with good-risk germ cell tumors: a multiinstitutional study. J Clin Oncol 1993;11(4):598–606.

19. de Wit R, Roberts JT, Wilkinson PM, et al. Equivalence of three or four cycles of bleomycin, etoposide, and cisplatin chemotherapy and of a 3- or 5-day schedule in good-prognosis germ cell cancer: a randomized study of the European Organization for Research and Treatment of Cancer Genitourinary Tract Cancer Cooperative Group and the Medical Research Council. J Clin Oncol 2001;19(6):1629–40.

20. Kondagunta GV, Bacik J, Bajorin D, et al. Etoposide and cisplatin chemotherapy for metastatic good-risk germ cell tumors. J Clin Oncol 2005;23(36):9290–4.

21. Loehrer PJ Sr, Johnson D, et al. Importance of bleomycin in favorable-prognosis disseminated germ cell tumors: an Eastern Cooperative Oncology Group trial. J Clin Oncol 1995;13(2):470–6.

22. Saxman SB, Finch D, Gonin R, et al. Long-term follow-up of a phase III study of three versus four cycles of bleomycin, etoposide, and cisplatin in favorable-prognosis germ-cell tumors: the Indian University experience. J Clin Oncol 1998;16(2):702–6.

23. Xiao H, Mazumdar M, Bajorin DF, et al. Long-term follow-up of patients with good-risk germ cell tumors treated with etoposide and cisplatin. J Clin Oncol 1997;15(7):2553–8.

24. Culine S, Abs L, Terrier-Lacombe MJ, et al. Cisplatin-based chemotherapy in advanced seminoma: the Institut Gustave Roussy experience. Eur J Cancer 1998;34(3):353–8.

25. Gholam D, Fizazi K, Terrier-Lacombe MJ, et al. Advanced seminoma–treatment results and prognostic factors for survival after first-line, cisplatin-based chemotherapy and for patients with recurrent disease: a single-institution experience in 145 patients. Cancer 2003;98(4):745–52.

26. Mencel PJ, Motzer RJ, Mazumdar M, et al. Advanced seminoma: treatment results, survival, and prognostic factors in 142 patients. J Clin Oncol 1994;12(1):120–6.

27. Warde P, Gospodarowicz M, Panzarella T, et al. Management of stage II seminoma. J Clin Oncol 1998;16(1):290–4.

28. Choo R, Sandler H, Warde P, et al. Survey of radiation oncologists: practice patterns of the management of stage I seminoma of testis in Canada and a selected group in the United States. Can J Urol 2002;9(2):1479–85.

29. Jones WG, Fossa SD, Mead GM, et al. Randomized trial of 30 versus 20 Gy in the adjuvant treatment of stage I Testicular Seminoma: a report on Medical Research Council Trial TE18, European Organisation for the Research and Treatment of

Cancer Trial 30942 (ISRCTN18525328). J Clin Oncol 2005;23(6):1200–8.

30. Patterson H, Norman AR, Mitra SS, et al. Combination carboplatin and radiotherapy in the management of stage II testicular seminoma: comparison with radiotherapy treatment alone. Radiother Oncol 2001;59(1):5–11.

31. Vallis KA, Howard GC, Duncan W, et al. Radiotherapy for stages I and II testicular seminoma: results and morbidity in 238 patients. Br J Radiol 1995;68(808):400–5.

32. Zagars GK, Pollack A. Radiotherapy for stage II testicular seminoma. Int J Radiat Oncol Biol Phys 2001;51(3):643–9.

33. National Comprehensive Cancer Network. NCCN clinical practice guidelines in oncology, testicular cancer 2018. 2.2018. Available at: https://www.nccn.org/professionals/physician_gls/pdf/testicular.pdf.

34. Gospodarwicz MK, Sturgeon JF, Jewett MA. Early stage and advanced seminoma: role of radiation therapy, surgery, and chemotherapy. Semin Oncol 1998;25(2):160–73.

35. Glaser SM, Vargo JA, Balasubramani GK, et al. Stage II testicular seminoma: patterns of care and survival by treatment strategy. Clin Oncol (R Coll Radiol) 2016;28(8):513–21.

36. Paly JJ, Lin CC, Gray PJ, et al. Management and outcomes of clinical stage IIA/B seminoma: Results from the National Cancer Data Base 1998-2012. Pract Radiat Oncol 2016;6(6):e249–58.

37. Haugnes HS, Wethal T, Aass N, et al. Cardiovascular risk factors and morbidity in long-term survivors of testicular cancer: a 20-year follow-up study. J Clin Oncol 2010;28(30):4649–57.

38. Gugic J, Zaletel LZ, Oblak I. Treatment-related cardiovascular toxicity in long-term survivors of testicular cancer. Radiol Oncol 2017;51(2):221–7.

39. Huddart RA, Norman A, Shahidi M, et al. Cardiovascular disease as a long-term complication of treatment for testicular cancer. J Clin Oncol 2003;21(8):1513–23.

40. Maroto P, Anguera G, Martin C. Long-term toxicity of the treatment for germ cell-cancer. A review. Crit Rev Oncol Hematol 2018;121:62–7.

41. De Santis M, Becherer A, Bokemeyer C, et al. 2-18fluoro-deoxy-D-glucose positron emission tomography is a reliable predictor for viable tumor in postchemotherapy seminoma: an update of the prospective multicentric SEMPET trial. J Clin Oncol 2004;22(6):1034–9.

42. Bachner M, Loriot Y, Gross-Goupil M, et al. 2-(1)(8) fluoro-deoxy-D-glucose positron emission tomography (FDG-PET) for postchemotherapy seminoma residual lesions: a retrospective validation of the SEMPET trial. Ann Oncol 2012;23(1):59–64.

43. Hinz S, Schrader M, Kempkensteffen C, et al. The role of positron emission tomography in the evaluation of residual masses after chemotherapy for advanced stage seminoma. J Urol 2008;179(3):936–40 [discussion: 940].

44. Albers P, Bender H, Yilmaz H, et al. Positron emission tomography in the clinical staging of patients with Stage I and II testicular germ cell tumors. Urology 1999;53(4):808–11.

45. Becherer A, De Santis M, Karanikas G, et al. FDG PET is superior to CT in the prediction of viable tumour in post-chemotherapy seminoma residuals. Eur J Radiol 2005;54(2):284–8.

46. Cremerius U, Wildberger JE, Borchers H, et al. Does positron emission tomography using 18-fluoro-2-deoxyglucose improve clinical staging of testicular cancer?–Results of a study in 50 patients. Urology 1999;54(5):900–4.

47. De Santis M, Pont J. The role of positron emission tomography in germ cell cancer. World J Urol 2004;22(1):41–6.

48. Spermon JR, De Geus-Oei LF, Kiemeney LA, et al. The role of (18)fluoro-2-deoxyglucose positron emission tomography in initial staging and restaging after chemotherapy for testicular germ cell tumours. BJU Int 2002;89(6):549–56.

49. Decoene J, Winter C, Albers P. False-positive fluorodeoxyglucose positron emission tomography results after chemotherapy in patients with metastatic seminoma. Urol Oncol 2015;33(1):23 e15–21.

50. Kondagunta GV, Bacik J, Donadio A, et al. Combination of paclitaxel, ifosfamide, and cisplatin is an effective second-line therapy for patients with relapsed testicular germ cell tumors. J Clin Oncol 2005;23(27):6549–55.

51. Loehrer PJ Sr, Lauer R, et al. Salvage therapy in recurrent germ cell cancer: ifosfamide and cisplatin plus either vinblastine or etoposide. Ann Intern Med 1988;109(7):540–6.

52. Miller KD, Loehrer PJ, Gonin R, et al. Salvage chemotherapy with vinblastine, ifosfamide, and cisplatin in recurrent seminoma. J Clin Oncol 1997;15(4):1427–31.

53. Flechon A, Bompas E, Biron P, et al. Management of post-chemotherapy residual masses in advanced seminoma. J Urol 2002;168(5):1975–9.

54. Herr HW, Sheinfeld J, Puc HS, et al. Surgery for a post-chemotherapy residual mass in seminoma. J Urol 1997;157(3):860–2.

55. Rice KR, Cary CK, Masterson TA, et al. Surgery of Testicular Tumors. Campbell-Walsh Urology, Philadelphia: Elsevier Saunders; 2016.

56. Pizzocaro G. Retroperitoneal lymph node dissection in clinical stage IIA and IIB nonseminomatous germ cell tumours of the testis. Int J Androl 1987;10(1):269–75.

57. Donohue JP, Thornhill JA, Foster RS, et al. Clinical stage B non-seminomatous germ cell testis cancer: the Indiana University experience (1965-1989) using routine primary retroperitoneal lymph node dissection. Eur J Cancer 1995;31a(10):1599–604.

58. Weissbach L, Bussar-Maatz R, Flechtner H, et al. RPLND or primary chemotherapy in clinical stage IIA/B nonseminomatous germ cell tumors? Results of a prospective multicenter trial including quality of life assessment. Eur Urol 2000;37(5):582–94.

59. Stephenson AJ, Bosl GJ, Motzer RJ, et al. Nonrandomized comparison of primary chemotherapy and retroperitoneal lymph node dissection for clinical stage IIA and IIB nonseminomatous germ cell testicular cancer. J Clin Oncol 2007;25(35): 5597–602.

60. Stephenson AJ, Sheinfeld J. The role of retroperitoneal lymph node dissection in the management of testicular cancer. Urol Oncol 2004;22(3):225–33 [discussion: 234–5].

61. Kondagunta GV, Sheinfeld J, Mazumdar M, et al. Relapse-free and overall survival in patients with pathologic stage II nonseminomatous germ cell cancer treated with etoposide and cisplatin adjuvant chemotherapy. J Clin Oncol 2004;22(3):464–7.

62. Bosl GJ, Motzer RJ. Testicular germ-cell cancer. N Engl J Med 1997;337(4):242–53.

63. Stephenson AJ, Bosl GJ, Bajorin DF, et al. Retroperitoneal lymph node dissection in patients with low stage testicular cancer with embryonal carcinoma predominance and/or lymphovascular invasion. J Urol 2005;174(2):557–60 [discussion: 560].

64. Williams SD, Stablein DM, Einhorn LH, et al. Immediate adjuvant chemotherapy versus observation with treatment at relapse in pathological stage II testicular cancer. N Engl J Med 1987;317(23): 1433–8.

65. Albers P, Albrecht W, Algaba F, et al. Guidelines on testicular cancer: 2015 update. Eur Urol 2015; 68(6):1054–68.

66. Williams SD, Birch R, Einhorn LH, et al. Treatment of disseminated germ-cell tumors with cisplatin, bleomycin, and either vinblastine or etoposide. N Engl J Med 1987;316(23):1435–40.

67. Motzer RJ, Sheinfeld J, Mazumdar M, et al. Etoposide and cisplatin adjuvant therapy for patients with pathologic stage II germ cell tumors. J Clin Oncol 1995;13(11):2700–4.

68. Behnia M, Foster R, Einhorn LH, et al. Adjuvant bleomycin, etoposide and cisplatin in pathological stage II non-seminomatous testicular cancer. the Indiana University experience. Eur J Cancer 2000;36(4):472–5.

69. Culine S, Theodore C, Court BH, et al. Evaluation of primary standard cisplatin-based chemotherapy for clinical stage II non-seminomatous germ cell tumours of the testis. Br J Urol 1997;79(2):258–62.

70. Einhorn LH, Williams SD, Loehrer PJ, et al. Evaluation of optimal duration of chemotherapy in favorable-prognosis disseminated germ cell tumors: a Southeastern Cancer Study Group protocol. J Clin Oncol 1989;7(3):387–91.

71. Culine S, Kerbrat P, Kramar A, et al. Refining the optimal chemotherapy regimen for good-risk metastatic nonseminomatous germ-cell tumors: a randomized trial of the Genito-Urinary Group of the French Federation of Cancer Centers (GETUG T93BP). Ann Oncol 2007;18(5):917–24.

72. Feldman DR, Bosl GJ, Sheinfeld J, et al. Medical treatment of advanced testicular cancer. JAMA 2008;299(6):672–84.

73. Horwich A, Norman A, Fisher C, et al. Primary chemotherapy for stage II nonseminomatous germ cell tumors of the testis. J Urol 1994;151(1): 72–7 [discussion: 77–8].

74. Tarin T, Carver B, Sheinfeld J. The role of lymphadenectomy for testicular cancer: indications, controversies, and complications. Urol Clin North Am 2011;38(4):439–49, vi.

75. Albers P, Weissbach L, Krege S, et al. Prediction of necrosis after chemotherapy of advanced germ cell tumors: results of a prospective multicenter trial of the German Testicular Cancer Study Group. J Urol 2004;171(5):1835–8.

76. Spiess PE, Brown GA, Liu P, et al. Predictors of outcome in patients undergoing postchemotherapy retroperitoneal lymph node dissection for testicular cancer. Cancer 2006;107(7):1483–90.

77. Steyerberg EW, Keizer HJ, Fosså SD, et al. Prediction of residual retroperitoneal mass histology after chemotherapy for metastatic nonseminomatous germ cell tumor: multivariate analysis of individual patient data from six study groups. J Clin Oncol 1995;13(5):1177–87.

78. Leão R, Nayan M, Punjani N, et al. A new model to predict benign histology in residual retroperitoneal masses after chemotherapy in nonseminoma. Eur Urol Focus 2018;4(6):995–1001.

79. Carver BS, Bianco FJ Jr, Shayegan B, et al. Predicting teratoma in the retroperitoneum in men undergoing post-chemotherapy retroperitoneal lymph node dissection. J Urol 2006;176(1):100–3 [discussion: 103–4].

80. Ehrlich Y, Brames MJ, Beck SD, et al. Long-term follow-up of Cisplatin combination chemotherapy in patients with disseminated nonseminomatous germ cell tumors: is a postchemotherapy retroperitoneal lymph node dissection needed after complete remission? J Clin Oncol 2010;28(4):531–6.

81. Kollmannsberger C, Daneshmand S, So A, et al. Management of disseminated nonseminomatous germ cell tumors with risk-based chemotherapy followed by response-guided postchemotherapy surgery. J Clin Oncol 2010;28(4):537–42.

82. Oldenburg J, Fosså SD, Nuver J, et al, ESMO Guidelines Working Group. Testicular seminoma and non-seminoma: ESMO Clinical Practice Guidelines for diagnosis, treatment and follow-up. Ann Oncol 2013;24(Suppl 6):vi125–32.

83. Lakes J, Lusch A, Nini A, et al. Retroperitoneal lymph node dissection in the setting of elevated markers. Curr Opin Urol 2018;28(5):435–9.

84. Woldu SL, Matulay JT, Clinton TN, et al. Impact of hospital case volume on testicular cancer outcomes and practice patterns. Urol Oncol 2018; 36(1):14.e7-15.

85. Logothetis CJ, Samuels ML, Trindade A, et al. The growing teratoma syndrome. Cancer 1982;50(8): 1629–35.

86. Motzer RJ, Amsterdam A, Prieto V, et al. Teratoma with malignant transformation: diverse malignant histologies arising in men with germ cell tumors. J Urol 1998;159(1):133–8.

87. Donadio AC, Motzer RJ, Bajorin DF, et al. Chemotherapy for teratoma with malignant transformation. J Clin Oncol 2003;21(23):4285–91.

88. Mosharafa AA, Foster RS, Koch MO, et al. Complications of post-chemotherapy retroperitoneal lymph node dissection for testis cancer. J Urol 2004;171(5):1839–41.

89. Beck SD, Foster RS, Bihrle R, et al. Is full bilateral retroperitoneal lymph node dissection always necessary for postchemotherapy residual tumor? Cancer 2007;110(6):1235–40.

90. Lange PH, Narayan P, Fraley EE. Fertility issues following therapy for testicular cancer. Semin Urol 1984;2(4):264–74.

91. Baniel J, Foster RS, Rowland RG, et al. Complications of primary retroperitoneal lymph node dissection. J Urol 1994;152(2 Pt 1):424–7.

92. Donohue JP, Rowland RG. Complications of retroperitoneal lymph node dissection. J Urol 1981; 125(3):338–40.

93. Pettus JA, Carver BS, Masterson T, et al. Preservation of ejaculation in patients undergoing nerve-sparing postchemotherapy retroperitoneal lymph node dissection for metastatic testicular cancer. Urology 2009;73(2):328–31 [discussion: 331–2].

94. Narayan P, Lange PH, Fraley EE. Ejaculation and fertility after extended retroperitoneal lymph node dissection for testicular cancer. J Urol 1982; 127(4):685–8.

95. Fosså SD, Klepp O, Ous S, et al. Unilateral retroperitoneal lymph node dissection in patients with non-seminomatous testicular tumor in clinical stage I. Eur Urol 1984;10(1):17–23.

96. Foster RS, Donohue JP, Bihrle R. Stage A nonseminomatous testis carcinoma: rationale and results of nerve-sparing retroperitoneal lymphadenectomy. Urol Int 1991;46(3):294–7.

97. Pizzocaro G, Salvioni R, Zanoni F. Unilateral lymphadenectomy in intraoperative stage I nonseminomatous germinal testis cancer. J Urol 1985; 134(3):485–9.

98. Colleselli K, Poisel S, Schachtner W, et al. Nerve-preserving bilateral retroperitoneal lymphadenectomy: anatomical study and operative approach. J Urol 1990;144(2 Pt 1):293–7 [discussion: 297–8].

99. Jewett MA, Kong YS, Goldberg SD, et al. Retroperitoneal lymphadenectomy for testis tumor with nerve sparing for ejaculation. J Urol 1988;139(6): 1220–4.

100. Donohue JP, Thornhill JA, Foster RS, et al. Retroperitoneal lymphadenectomy for clinical stage A testis cancer (1965 to 1989): modifications of technique and impact on ejaculation. J Urol 1993; 149(2):237–43.

101. Pearce S, Steinberg Z, Eggener S. Critical evaluation of modified templates and current trends in retroperitoneal lymph node dissection. Curr Urol Rep 2013;14(5):511–7.

102. Eggener SE, Carver BS, Sharp DS, et al. Incidence of disease outside modified retroperitoneal lymph node dissection templates in clinical stage I or IIA nonseminomatous germ cell testicular cancer. J Urol 2007;177(3):937–42 [discussion: 942–3].

103. Carver BS, Shayegan B, Eggener S, et al. Incidence of metastatic nonseminomatous germ cell tumor outside the boundaries of a modified postchemotherapy retroperitoneal lymph node dissection. J Clin Oncol 2007;25(28):4365–9.

104. Heidenreich A, Pfister D, Witthuhn R, et al. Postchemotherapy retroperitoneal lymph node dissection in advanced testicular cancer: radical or modified template resection. Eur Urol 2009;55(1): 217–24.

105. Vallier C, Savoie PH, Delpero JR, et al. External validation of the Heidenreich criteria for patient selection for unilateral or bilateral retroperitoneal lymph node dissection for post-chemotherapy residual masses of testicular cancer. World J Urol 2014;32(6):1573–8.

106. Cho JS, Kaimakliotis HZ, Cary C, et al. Modified retroperitoneal lymph node dissection for postchemotherapy residual tumour: a long-term update. BJU Int 2017;120(1):104–8.

107. Abdul-Muhsin HM, L'esperance JO, Fischer K, et al. Robot-assisted retroperitoneal lymph node dissection in testicular cancer. J Surg Oncol 2015;112(7):736–40.

108. Hyams ES, Pierorazio P, Proteek O, et al. Laparoscopic retroperitoneal lymph node dissection for clinical stage I nonseminomatous germ cell tumor: a large single institution experience. J Urol 2012; 187(2):487–92.

109. Janetschek G, Hobisch A, Peschel R, et al. Laparo-scopic retroperitoneal lymph node dissection for clinical stage I nonseminomatous testicular carcinoma: long-term outcome. J Urol 2000;163(6):1793–6.

110. Pearce SM, Golan S, Gorin MA, et al. Safety and early oncologic effectiveness of primary robotic retroperitoneal lymph node dissection for nonseminomatous germ cell testicular cancer. Eur Urol 2017;71(3):476–82.

111. Nielsen ME, Lima G, Schaeffer EM, et al. Oncologic efficacy of laparoscopic RPLND in treatment of clinical stage I nonseminomatous germ cell testicular cancer. Urology 2007;70(6):1168–72.

112. Nakamura T, Kawauchi A, Oishi M, et al. Post-chemotherapy laparoscopic retroperitoneal lymph node dissection is feasible for stage IIA/B non-seminoma germ cell tumors. Int J Clin Oncol 2016;21(4):791–5.

Current Management of Disseminated Germ Cell Tumors

Jean-Michel Lavoie, MD, FRCPC[a],
Christian K. Kollmannsberger, MD, FRCPC[b],*

KEYWORDS

- Testis cancer • Management guidelines • Chemotherapy • Disseminated germ cell tumor

KEY POINTS

- Disseminated germ cell tumors are highly curable cancers due to their sensitivity to a cisplatin-containing regimen, and patients who relapse may still be successfully salvaged.
- The cornerstone of systemic treatment is a combination of bleomycin, etoposide, and cisplatin, individualized based on the International Germ Cell Cancer Collaborative Group prognostic group and with adjustments for patients who have contraindications to cisplatin.
- Patients are at risk of long-term complications and will need lifelong medical care.
- Treatment in high-volume expert centers and given in adherence with current guidelines leads to improved outcomes.

INTRODUCTION

Cancer of the testis is a relatively uncommon disease, accounting for only approximately 1% of all cancers in male patients. However, germ cell tumors (GCT) almost always affect young men. GCTs represent a highly curable malignancy, and overall, more than 90% of GCT patients are cured. Curative treatment requires a combination of cisplatin-containing multiagent chemotherapy and surgery for the appropriate management of residual disease.[1,2] For patients who relapse, tandem high-dose chemotherapy followed by stem cell rescue may still be curative.[3] The objective of front-line therapy in metastatic GCT is always cure and never palliation.

FIRST-LINE TREATMENT

The curative potential of cisplatin-based chemotherapy was initially demonstrated in 1977 by Einhorn and Donohue[4] with a regimen of cisplatin, vinblastine, and bleomycin (PVB). In this phase 2 study, a complete remission was achieved in 85% of patients with a combination of chemotherapy and resection of residual masses. These data led to a series of studies aimed at optimizing outcomes and minimizing toxicity from these multidrug regimens.[5] In 1987, a landmark study[6] established the combination of bleomycin, etoposide, and cisplatin (BEP; described in **Table 1**) as a new standard of care in the management of disseminated testicular cancer. To this day, BEP remains the cornerstone of the authors' management in the first-line setting, with some refinements.

Malignant GCTs are rare diseases, of which only a subset are disseminated. To achieve optimal outcomes, following the fundamental principles of testis cancer treatment is of critical importance. Several retrospective analyses have

---

Disclosure Statement: The authors have nothing to disclose.
[a] Genitourinary Service, Division of Medical Oncology, Department of Medicine, BC Cancer- Vancouver Cancer Center, University of British Columbia, 600 West 10th Avenue, Vancouver, British Columbia V5Z 4E6, Canada;
[b] Division of Medical Oncology, Department of Medicine, BC Cancer–Vancouver Cancer Center, University of British Columbia, 600 West 10th Avenue, Vancouver, British Columbia V5Z 4E6, Canada
* Corresponding author.
E-mail address: ckollmannsberger@bccancer.bc.ca

Table 1
Common chemotherapy regimens used in the management of disseminated germ cell tumors

Regimen	Schedule	Dose (per day)[a]
BEP (21-d protocol)		
Cisplatin	Days 1–5	20 mg/m^2
Etoposide	Days 1–5	100 mg/m^2
Bleomycin	Days 1, 8, and 15	30 units
VIP (21-d protocol)		
Cisplatin	Days 1–5	20 mg/m^2
Etoposide	Days 1–5	100 mg/m^2
Ifosfamide	Days 1–4	1500 mg/m^2
Mesna	Days 1–4	900 mg/m^2 (intravenous [IV])
EP (21-d protocol)		
Cisplatin	Days 1–5	20 mg/m^2
Etoposide	Days 1–5	100 mg/m^2
Attenuated EP		
Cisplatin	Days 1–3	20 mg/m^2
Etoposide	Days 1–3	100 mg/m^2
TIP (21-d protocol)		
Paclitaxel	Day 1	175 mg/m^2
Cisplatin	Days 2–6	20 mg/m^2
Ifosfamide	Days 2–6	1200 mg/m^2
Mesna	Days 2–6	900 mg/m^2 (IV)

Abbrevaitions: EP, etoposide and cisplatin; TIP, paclitaxel, ifosfamide and cisplatin.
[a] Dose adjustments may apply.

demonstrated significantly improved outcomes for patients treated correctly according to guidelines, and for those treated in high-volume centers. Paffenholz and colleagues[7] examined adherence to European Association of Urology guidelines[2] in patients referred to a tertiary center after initial treatment in the community. Patients who were undertreated (n = 10/115) had significantly worse relapse-free survival ($P = .005$). Similarly, in a review of the US National Cancer Database, Woldu and colleagues[8] showed that patients treated in high-volume centers (defined as 99th percentile; more than 26 cases per year) had significantly improved survival, despite their patients having worse disease characteristics. This difference was driven by patients with disseminated disease. Overall, this advocates for patients with disseminated GCT to be treated at, or in consultation with, high-volume centers. Early involvement of a multidisciplinary team with a high level of expertise in management of disseminated GCT allows for optimal adherence to guidelines-based treatment.

Maintaining dose density and achieving the target cumulative chemotherapy dose have also been shown to improve outcomes. This Principle was demonstrated for different regimens, such as PVB[9] and BEP,[10] and is further discussed below.

RISK STRATIFICATION

The treatment of disseminated GCT in the first-line setting is based on risk stratification by prognostic groups, which were developed by the International Germ Cell Cancer Collaborative Group (IGCCCG).[11] The IGCCCG classification is informed by histology (seminoma vs nonseminoma or mixed), extent of disease (presence or absence of nonpulmonary visceral metastases), tumor marker levels (α-fetoprotein [AFP], β-human choriogonadotropin hormone [β -human chorionic gonadotropin (HCG)], and lactate dehydrogenase [LDH]); location of the primary tumor (testicular or retroperitoneal vs mediastinal) is also used for nonseminomatous GCT (NSGCT). Patients are categorized into the good-, intermediate-, or poor-prognostic group, as shown in **Table 2**.

In the initial cohort of patients treated between 1975 and 1990, good-, intermediate-, and poor-prognosis groups were associated with a 5-year overall survival (OS) of 91%, 79%, and 48%, respectively. A meta-analysis of patients treated between 1989 and 2004 reported improved 5-year survival rates of 94%, 83%, and 71% for the same prognostic groups.[12] This improvement is driven by adherence to guidelines, delivery of cisplatin-containing standard chemotherapy across different geographies, and consequent utilization of postchemotherapy surgery in nonseminoma.

GOOD PROGNOSIS DISSEMINATED GERM CELL TUMORS

Patients with good-risk disease constitute approximately 56% of patients presenting with disseminated disease. The standard treatment of patients with good-prognosis disseminated GCT is 3 cycles of BEP chemotherapy. Consecutive randomized trials of deescalating therapy while maintaining cure rates have resulted in 3 cycles of BEP as today's optimal standard regimen for good-risk disease. A phase 3 clinical trial validated this approach in 2001[13]: 812 patients with good-prognosis disease were randomized to 3 or 4 cycles of BEP, and 681 of these were also randomized along a 2 × 2 factorial design to a 3-day or 5-day per cycle administration regimen for cisplatin and etoposide. There was no difference between 3 and 4 cycles of chemotherapy

Table 2
International Germ Cell Cancer Collaborative Group prognostic groups

Prognosis	Nonseminoma	Seminoma
Good	Testis or primary extragonadal retroperitoneal tumor *and* low markers: AFP <1000 ng/mL *and* β-HCG <5000 IU/L (<1000 ng/mL) *and* LDH <1.5 × normal level *and* no nonpulmonary visceral metastases	Any primary location Any marker level *and* no nonpulmonary visceral metastases
Intermediate	Testis or primary extragonadal retroperitoneal tumor *and* intermediate tumor markers AFP 1000–10000 ng/mL *and/or* β-HCG 5000–50000 IU/L (1000–10000 ng/mL) *and/or* LDH 1.5–10 × normal level *and* no presence of nonpulmonary visceral metastases	Any primary localization *and* presence of nonpulmonary visceral metastases (liver, CNS, bone, intestinum) Any marker level
Poor	Primary mediastinal germ cell tumor (any marker level) *Or* testis or primary extragonadal retroperitoneal tumor *and* presence of nonpulmonary visceral metastases (liver, CNS, bone, intestinum) *and/or* high tumor markers AFP >10,000 ng/mL, *and/or* β -HCG >50,000 IU/L (10,000 ng/mL) *and/or* LDH >10 × normal level	

(2-year progression-free survival [PFS] of 90.4% and 89.4%, respectively), but patients who received 3 cycles had better maintenance of quality of life. There was no difference in survival between a 3-day and 5-day administration schedule either (2-year PFS 89.7% and 88.8%, respectively); however, the 3-day regimen was associated with increased long-term toxicity, including ototoxicity, peripheral neurotoxicity, or Raynaud syndrome, particularly when 4 cycles are given.

If contraindications to bleomycin exist, 4 cycles of EP chemotherapy (described in **Table 1**) can be used. The omission of bleomycin can reduce toxicity, in particular, acute and delayed pulmonary toxicities. A French study[14] compared 3 cycles of BEP (BEP × 3) to 4 cycles of EP (EP × 4), with 500 mg/m^2 per cycle of etoposide in both arms. The study included 257 patients with NSGCT who were predicted to have a good prognosis based on the Institut Gustave Roussy prognostic model (most of these met the IGCCCG criteria for good prognosis). The study was designed to demonstrate equivalence of the primary endpoint of rate of favorable response, defined as one of the following:

- Clinical complete response (normal levels of serum tumor markers, no clinical or radiological evidence of residual disease);
- Pathologic complete response (normal levels of serum tumor markers and complete

resection of residual masses with pathologic analysis revealing necrotic debris, fibrosis, or mature or immature teratoma);
- Surgical complete response (normal levels of serum tumor markers and complete resection of residual masses with pathologic analysis revealing persistent viable cancer cells); or
- Partial responses (normal levels of serum tumor markers and infracentrimetric residual masses)

This primary endpoint was met, with 124 and 122 patients having a favorable response in the BEP × 3 and EP × 4 arms, respectively (P = .34). At the 4-year mark, event-free survival was 91% for BEP × 3 and 86% for EP × 4 (P = .135). Events were defined as incomplete responses, relapses from favorable responses, or deaths; pure teratoma relapses were not defined as events. The study was underpowered to evaluate survival outcomes; however, double the number of GCT-related deaths was observed on the EP arm as compared with the BEP arm.

Further deescalation of treatment has led to inferior outcomes. The Australian and New Zealand Germ Cell Trials Group conducted a study on 166 patients with good prognosis GCT (defined using a modified Memorial Sloan Kettering scale). They were randomized to 3 cycles of standard BEP versus 4 cycles of reduced-dose BEP (30 units of bleomycin and 360 mg/m^2 of etoposide per cycle). After a median follow-up of 8.5 years,

OS was superior in patients who received 3 cycles of BEP (8-year OS 92% vs 83%; hazard ratio [HR] = 0.38, P = .037), despite a lower cumulative dose of cisplatin. These data supports the notion of delivering chemotherapy with a sufficient dose density to achieve a cure. Based on the results of these randomized studies, 3 cycles of BEP according to the Indiana University system protocol represent the standard of care for patients with IGCCCG good prognosis criteria. EP × 4 is a reasonable option for patients with contraindications to bleomycin[15] (**Box 1**). Carboplatin should not be substituted for cisplatin, and EP alone for 3 cycles should also not be used.

INTERMEDIATE- AND POOR-PROGNOSIS DISSEMINATED GERM CELL TUMORS

The standard treatment of patients with intermediate-/poor-prognosis disseminated GTC is 4 cycles of BEP chemotherapy. Williams and colleagues[6] showed that 4 cycles of BEP were associated with less toxicity than 4 cycles of PVB as well as higher response rates (P<.05) and OS in patients with high-volume disease (P = .048). Despite 30 years of subsequent clinical trials, BEP × 4 remains the standard of care.

For patients with contraindications to bleomycin, 4 cycles of chemotherapy with ifosfamide, etoposide, and cisplatin (VIP; described in **Table 1**) are an accepted alternative. An intergroup trial[16] randomized 304 patients with advanced stage disseminated GCT (defined according to the Indiana University system[17]) to BEP × 4 or VIP × 4. In the final analysis, 283 patients were reclassified

using the IGCCCG system (37 as good prognosis, 65 as intermediate prognosis, and 181 as poor prognosis). At a median follow-up of 7.3 years, the PFS and OS rates were equivalent between the treatment arms. There were more grade 3 to 5 adverse events overall with VIP (93% vs 79%; P = .0002), including more grade 3 to 5 hematologic toxicity (90% vs 76%; P = .003). However, VIP avoids bleomycin toxicity. Granulocyte colony-stimulating factor prophylaxis should be given to patients with poor-risk criteria and/or receiving VIP chemotherapy.

Clinical trials have explored other regimens in order to improve outcomes. Combination regimens using the following were studied:

- Cisplatin, etoposide, bleomycin, vincristine, and ifosfamide[18]
- Cisplatin, bleomycin, cyclophosphamide, doxorubicin, and vinblastine[19]
- Cisplatin, etoposide, bleomycin, carboplatin, and vincristine[20]

None of these studies showed superiority to BEP × 4. Studies of high-dose chemotherapy with stem cell rescue (HDC/SCR) were similarly negative when compared with BEP × 4.[21,22] More recently, the GETUG-13 trial explored an individualized approach based on marker decline. Patients received an initial cycle of BEP; those with an expected decline in tumor markers continued on to receive a total of 4 cycles of BEP. Patients with an unfavorable decline were randomized to either the same BEP × 4 regimen or an intensified approach combining BEP with paclitaxel and oxaliplatin. The study randomized 203 patients (80% of patients treated) because of an unfavorable decline in tumor markers. An initial report showed these patients had an improved 3-year PFS with the intensified approach (59% vs 48%; HR = 0.66, P = .05).[23] An update with a median follow-up of 5.6 years showed an ongoing significant benefit for PFS. The difference in OS was not significant (70.4% vs 60.8%; HR = 0.69, P = .12), although this was not the primary endpoint.[24] Based on this study, a marker decline–based approach can be justified, but the optimal intensification regimen has yet to be defined.

STAGE II DISEASE

Patients with clinical stage II testicular cancer (only with retroperitoneal lymphadenopathy) can be treated with the same clinical paradigm as those with more widespread disease. Most of these cases will fit the definition of good prognosis by IGCCCG classification.[11] However, other treatment modalities can be used, including primary

---

Box 1
Contraindications to administration of bleomycin

Absolute

  Previous hypersensitivity to bleomycin

Relative

  Age >40

  Compromised pulmonary function (diffusing capacity for carbon monoxide (DLCO) <40%) or smoking

  Impaired renal function

  Concomitant chest radiotherapy

  Cumulative dose >450 units

  Requirement for future thoracic surgery (bilateral lung metastases or primary mediastinal GCT)

retroperitoneal lymph node dissection (for NSGCT) and radiotherapy (for seminoma). In addition, a trial of retroperitoneal lymph node dissection for seminoma is currently underway (NCT02537548). The management of patients with stage 2 testicular cancer is discussed in greater detail in Alireza Ghoreifi and Hooman Djaladat's article, "Management of Primary Testicular Tumor," in this issue.

PREDOMINANT OR PURE CHORIOCARCINOMA

A small subset of patients with poor-prognosis disseminated GCT presents with "choriocarcinoma syndrome."[25,26] These patients have rapidly progressive widespread disease and often markedly elevated β-HCG levels (>100,000). Predominant or pure choriocarcinoma is a highly aggressive and rapidly progressing disease requiring immediate transfer to an expert center and initiation of chemotherapy under close supervision. Treatment should not be delayed to obtain a pathologic diagnosis.

Choriocarcinoma syndrome was initially described as patients with high-volume lung metastases who developed acute respiratory distress syndrome (ARDS) due to pulmonary hemorrhage at presentation or during initial chemotherapy.[27] Patients can be treated with an attenuated cycle of chemotherapy, such as 3 days of EP, as described in **Table 1**.[28] Massard and colleagues[29] described a series of 10 cases of patients with poor prognosis and respiratory failure who were initially treated with attenuated EP. Three of the 10 patients developed ARDS, which was fatal in 2 cases. They compared this with a series of 15 cases treated before the introduction of the attenuated EP protocol, when 13/15 patients developed ARDS, which was fatal in 10 cases. After an attenuated chemotherapy cycle, treatment should proceed with full-dose chemotherapy delivered on time and for 4 cycles. In most cases, this will be done with VIP due to the preexisting burden of lung disease and potential need for post-chemotherapy resection.

Of note, patients with very elevated β-HCG levels at baseline may not experience a complete normalization of their tumor marker after 4 cycles of chemotherapy; they may have some level of detectable β-HCG for weeks or even months after completing treatment despite no residual disease. These patients should be monitored and proceed with planned resection of residual masses. Only if HCG level starts to increase again should salvage chemotherapy be initiated.

CENTRAL NERVOUS SYSTEM METASTASES

Patients with disseminated GCT may present with brain metastases either initially or at the time of relapse.[30] Initial presentation with brain involvement is rare, and most of these patients have NSGCT, especially poor-prognosis choriocarcinoma. Baseline central nervous system (CNS) imaging is not necessary in asymptomatic good-risk patients but should always be obtained in patients with poor-risk or intermediate-risk and high-volume pulmonary metastases.

Even in the presence of CNS involvement, patients with disseminated GCT may be cured.[31] They should always be treated in an expert center. Patients with brain metastases will generally require multimodality treatment. Asymptomatic brain metastases may be treated upfront with chemotherapy, followed by either resection or consolidative radiotherapy. They should be closely monitored due to the risk of intracranial hemorrhage, especially during the first cycle of chemotherapy. Observation may be a viable option for patients with a complete response to chemotherapy, but large retrospective reviews[12] have shown that patients treated with a multimodality approach have better outcomes. For patients who present with solitary symptomatic brain metastases, especially in the context of intracranial hemorrhage, upfront resection followed by standard chemotherapy is an option.

Patients who develop brain metastases as a site of relapse after chemotherapy have a worse prognosis than those who presented with brain metastases upfront.[30] In a series of 523 men with brain metastases,[12] patients with CNS involvement at relapse had a 3-year OS of 27% versus 48% for those with upfront brain metastases (P<.01). Patients with multiple brain metastases or other factors generally associated with the IGCCCG poor-prognostic category (elevated tumor markers, liver or bone involvement, or primary mediastinal NSGCT) also had worse outcomes.

FOLLOW-UP AFTER CHEMOTHERAPY

After completion of chemotherapy, patients should be followed for relapse as well as delayed complications and late toxicity from chemotherapy.

Scenarios whereby patients have a complete radiological response, or residual masses but no evidence of progression, are outlined.

PATIENTS WITH COMPLETE RESPONSE

Some patients with disseminated GCT achieve a complete response to chemotherapy, including normalization of imaging and serum tumor markers. No standard follow-up schedule exists.[1] Follow-up is a combination of physical examination, serum tumor markers, and imaging. Patients are followed for at least 5 years, with more frequent investigations early on when the risk of relapse is highest.[11,32] The vast majority of relapses occurs within 2 years after completion of first-line chemotherapy.

MANAGEMENT OF RESIDUAL MASSES

The management of residual masses after chemotherapy varies depending on histology. It is a complex issue that is covered in greater detail in Saum Ghodoussipour and Siamak Daneshmand's article, "Post-chemotherapy Resection of Residual Mass in Non Seminomatous Germ Cell Tumor," in this issue.

For pure seminoma, observation is generally acceptable. Patients with residual masses less than 3 cm are followed with the same guidelines as patients with complete response, unless they had intrathoracic disease, in which case computed tomography of the chest is integrated in their follow-up. The SEMPET trial explored the added value of functional imaging with PET with fluorodeoxyglucose F 18 (FDG) in this setting.[33] The initial report in a cohort of 51 patients found 8 lesions to be PET positive; all were confirmed to contain viable seminoma either histologically (resection) or clinically (with response to further chemotherapy); there were 2 false negative lesions, both less than 3 cm. Subsequent studies identified considerable rates of false positivity with the use of FDG-PET; a multicenter retrospective study of 125 cases treated between 2008 and 2010 showed a negative predictive value of 91%, but a positive predictive value of only 25%.[34] Scans performed less than 6 weeks from day 21 of the last cycle of chemotherapy were more likely to be false positive. A retrospective review of the Global Germ Cell Cancer Group Registry identified 90 patients with positive FDG-PET imaging between 2003 and 2016.[35] In this cohort, 35 patients underwent resection or biopsy. Only 5 of these cases were found to have viable seminoma. The positive predictive value was only 23%.

Salvage therapy should only be initiated in patients with clear evidence of radiological progression. Given the potential added morbidity of resection or radiotherapy, FDG avidity alone is not an indication for salvage treatment. Serial FDG-PET imaging is unnecessary.

For NSGCT, residual masses are routinely resected. All patients with residual masses greater than 1 cm in size should be considered for surgery. In patients with post-chemotherapy marker normalization, resections can be expected to yield necrotic tissue only in 50% of cases, mature teratoma in 35% of cases, and viable germ cell elements (nonteratoma) in 15% of cases.[36,37] Both viable germ cell elements and teratomas should be fully resected; although composed of mature elements, teratomas have the potential to metastasize and transform into highly aggressive malignancies.[38,39] The management of patients with viable germ cell elements at resection is controversial. Patients with incomplete resection, greater than 10% viable germ cell elements in the resected specimen, or intermediate/poor prognosis at baseline according to the IGCCCG classification[11] have worse outcomes.[40] A retrospective case series showed improved PFS, but not OS, for patients who received additional chemotherapy after resection showing viable germ cell elements. The authors' approach is to use postsurgery surveillance in all cases of completely resected disease. Patients with incompletely resected disease should be managed in a multidisciplinary setting.

In cases whereby retroperitoneal and extraperitoneal residual masses are present, a staged approach first addressing the retroperitoneum can be used. Hartmann and colleagues[41] demonstrated that in 70% of cases, the histology of the residual masses will be concordant. Furthermore, Besse and colleagues[42] found that although there can be discordance between the retroperitoneum and lung masses in 25% of cases, patients with bilateral lung disease will have concordant intrathoracic histology in 95% of cases. Given the potentially high morbidity attached to bilateral lung resections, patients with only necrosis found on retroperitoneal lymph node dissection(RPLND) and at resection of the dominant lung mass may be adequately treated with active surveillance. In all cases, the potential morbidity has to be balanced with the potential advantage of early surgical intervention over close surveillance.

LATE TOXICITY FROM CHEMOTHERAPY

Acute side effects from chemotherapy are well known. However, because patients with disseminated GCT are diagnosed relatively early in life, and most of them will achieve a cure, concerns arise around late side effects from chemotherapy.

Cardiovascular side effects related to cisplatin exposure include a higher incidence of metabolic syndrome[43] (particularly hypertension and dyslipidemia), but patients appear to have a higher rate of cardiovascular events even after adjusting for these risk factors.[44] Patients who received subdiaphragmatic radiotherapy were also found to have an increased incidence of diabetes; a case series also showed an independent association between subdiaphragmatic radiotherapy and cardiovascular events.[45] These data support aggressive management of risk factors related to the metabolic syndrome, counseling on avoidance of smoking, and a low index of suspicion for the development of early coronary disease even in patients without those additional risk factors. If they are not followed up in specialty clinics, patients should be counseled to have regular follow-up with their primary care provider, including screening for hypertension, dyslipidemia, and diabetes.

Fertility can be affected by treatment of disseminated GCT. At baseline, patients presenting with disseminated testicular cancer have a 50% rate of impaired spermatogenesis after orchiectomy, and before any other treatment is given.[46] The addition of 3 or 4 cycles of cisplatin-containing chemotherapy has been shown to further affect spermatogenesis, although for most patients this effect is transient. A series of 178 patients with serial sperm count showed that impaired pre-chemotherapy spermatogenesis was an important risk factor.[47] Patients received a wide range of treatments in this series; for patients who received up to 4 cycles of cisplatin-based chemotherapy, recovery occurred between 1 and 5 years after completion of chemotherapy. In the long term, patients with baseline azoospermia (classified as "poor chance" for recovery of spermatogenesis) had an approximately 30% chance of recovery, whereas those with normo/oligospermia (classified as "medium chance") had a recovery rate greater than 90%. Men with testicular cancer who underwent abdominal radiotherapy or received cisplatin-based chemotherapy are also at higher risk of developing low testosterone levels.[48] Patients who may wish to conceive in the future should be routinely referred for sperm banking before initiation of treatment, whether chemotherapy, radiotherapy, or RPLND. In addition, serum testosterone should be checked longitudinally in patients who underwent treatment with either chemotherapy or radiotherapy, because they may need replacement.

Pulmonary complications have been described in patients with prior exposure to bleomycin and/or cisplatin. Bleomycin is known to potentially cause acute hypersensitivity pneumonitis during treatment, or a subacute form with pulmonary fibrosis that can occur during, or in the months following, treatment; factors that increase the risk of bleomycin-induced lung injury are relative contraindications to its use, as listed in **Box 1**. In addition, patients with previous exposure to bleomycin are at risk of developing ARDS during major

surgeries. It has been suggested that this is related to exposure to high concentrations of oxygen, but data are inconsistent, and it has also been suggested that this complication may be due to intraoperative fluid shifts.[49] Irrespective of the cause, patients must be taught to inform their health care providers of previous exposure to bleomycin. A study of 1049 long-term survivors of GCT found decreased pulmonary function in patients who had received a high cumulative dose of cisplatin (>850 mg) as well as in those who received cisplatin and required lung resections.[50] With respect to follow-up, health care providers should keep a low index of suspicion for the development of respiratory disease in long-term survivors of disseminated GCT. Smoking cessation is highly recommended.

Other side effects of cisplatin include ototoxicity and peripheral neuropathy. Along with renal impairment, these complications most often develop during treatment administration and may resolve afterward. Despite this, they remain by far the most frequent adverse events reported by patients with prior exposure to chemotherapy.[6,51] Efforts are underway to better characterize these patients, including possible genetic markers that could indicate a higher risk of adverse event.[52] It is important to question patients regarding these issues, and if necessary, to provide the appropriate support to address their symptoms.

Second malignancies occur at an increased rate in patients treated with chemotherapy as well as radiotherapy. In a cohort of 40,576 survivors of testicular cancer, 2285 second solid cancers were reported.[53] Patients had a 1.9 times higher risk of developing a second cancer 10 years after their diagnosis of GCT, and this relative risk increase was noted as far as 35 years after diagnosis. There was a significantly higher risk of developing a new primary cancer in lung, colon, bladder, pancreas, stomach, esophagus, and pleura (mesothelioma). The relative risk decreased as the age of diagnosis of GCT increased. The authors' current guidelines focus on adherence to age-appropriate population-based screening investigations.[1]

RELAPSED GERM CELL TUMORS AFTER FIRST-LINE CHEMOTHERAPY

Although first-line platinum-based chemotherapy is curative for a large number of patients with disseminated GCT, some will unfortunately relapse. Relapses can be classified as platinum sensitive (occurring >1 month after completion of first-line chemotherapy) or platinum refractory (occurring during or within 1 month of completing first-line chemotherapy). Relapses after 2 lines of cisplatin-based chemotherapy are also considered cisplatin refractory.

Similar to the IGCCCG prognostic groups for untreated disseminated GCT, the International Prognostic Factors Study Group has developed a scoring system for patients with relapsed GCT, as detailed in **Table 3**.[54] It uses histology, location of the primary tumor, response to first-line chemotherapy, progression-free interval (PFI), tumor markers at the time of relapse (AFP and β-HCG), and the presence or absence of liver, bone, or brain metastases to assign 1 of 5 risk categories to patients. The categories range from very low (3-year OS of 77%) to very high (3-year OS of 6.1%).

PLATINUM-SENSITIVE RELAPSE

The preferred approach for patients with platinum-sensitive relapsed GCT is tandem high-dose chemotherapy with stem cell rescue (tHDC/SCR). The usefulness of HDC/SCR with high-dose etoposide and carboplatin was initially demonstrated by Nichols and colleagues[55] in the second-line setting. After the initial proof of concept, clinical trials compared standard salvage regimen with induction chemotherapy and 1 cycle of HDC/SCR. The largest trial, IT-94, randomized 280 patients with relapsed GCT to either 4 cycles of standard chemotherapy or 3 cycles of chemotherapy and 1 cycle of HDC/SCR.[56] The standard chemotherapy was cisplatin, ifosfamide, and etoposide (or vinblastine), and the high-dose regimen contained carboplatin, etoposide, and cyclophosphamide. The study showed no benefit from the addition of 1 cycle of HDC/SCR; at a median follow-up of 45 months, 53% of patients had died in both arms. On the other hand, a retrospective cohort of 1594 patients with relapsed GCT showed significantly superior outcomes for patients treated with HDC/SCR when compared with standard chemotherapy, in terms of both PFS (HR = 0.44) and PFS (HR = 0.65).[3] When compared with IT-94, this population had a higher-risk profile; 50% of patients treated with HDC/SCR received at least 2 cycles of this regimen (tandem approach, tHDC/SCR). A study attempting to answer whether multiple cycles of HDC/SCR are beneficial over a single cycle had to close early due to excessive toxicity in the standard arm (3 cycles of VIP followed by a cycle of

Table 3
Prognostic categories for patients with relapsed germ cell tumors

Parameter	Primary Score Value			
	0	1	2	3
Primary site	Gonadal	Extragonadal	—	Mediastinal nonseminoma
Prior response	CR/PRm−	PRm+/SD	PD	—
PFI, mo	>3	≤3	—	—
AFP salvage	Normal	≤1000	>1000	—
HCG salvage	≤1000	>1000	—	—
LBB	No	Yes	—	—
Step 1: Primary score sum (values from 0 to 10, from 6 factors above)				
Step 2: Regroup score sum into categories: (0) = 0; (1 or 2) = 1; (3 or 4) = 2; (5 or more) = 3				
Step 3: Add histology score point to category value: pure seminoma = −1; nonseminoma or mixed = 0				

Final Prognostic Score (ranges from −1 to +3):		
Score	Risk Category	3-y OS (%)
−1	Very low	77.0
0	Low	65.6
1	Intermediate	58.3
2	High	27.1
3	Very high	6.1

Abbreviations: CR, complete remission; LBB, liver, bone, brain metastases; PD, progressive disease; PRm−, partial remission, negative markers; PRm+, partial remission, positive markers; SD, stable disease.

Adapted from International Prognostic Factors Study Group, Lorch A, Beyer J, Bascoul-Mollevi C, Kramar A, Einhorn LH, et al. Prognostic factors in patients with metastatic germ cell tumors who experienced treatment failure with cisplatin-based first-line chemotherapy. J Clin Oncol. 2010 Nov 20;28(33):4909; with permission.

HDC/SCR with carboplatin, etoposide, and cyclophosphamide).[57,60,61]

PLATINUM-REFRACTORY RELAPSE

It is important to distinguish growing teratoma syndrome from platinum-refractory GCT. Some patients with NSGCT may develop radiological progression during treatment. In cases whereby baseline tumor markers were elevated and are decreasing as expected, the elements that are progressing are more likely to be chemoresistant mature teratoma.[58] These patients should complete their first-line treatment and have the residual masses resected. On the other hand, patients with rising tumor markers, marker-negative pure embryonal cancer, or pure seminoma are more likely to have true platinum refractory disease. These rare cases should always be managed in expert centers. If they have not been exposed to it, HDC/SCR is a viable salvage option. Otherwise, non-cisplatin-based combinations can be used, such as gemcitabine and paclitaxel,[59] possibly with the addition of oxaliplatin.[60] However, the likelihood of achieving a durable cure is low, and participation in clinical trials should be encouraged.

LATE RELAPSE

Relapses that occur more than 2 years after completion of first chemotherapy are considered "late." These rare cases should be managed in a multidisciplinary context, and metastatectomy plays an important role for the management of NSGCT in this setting. In a retrospective review[61] of 80 patients with late relapses of NSGCT, those treated with surgery had been rendered free of disease in most cases, whereas only 15% of those treated with chemotherapy alone were free of disease. Pure seminoma can still be salvaged with chemotherapy,[62] and depending on the pattern of relapse, radiotherapy can also be used.

SUMMARY

Disseminated GCTs are a highly curable group of malignancies. Three or 4 cycles of BEP remain the cornerstone of treatment, allowing for alternative regimen in patients at increased risk of toxicity from bleomycin. Treatment is best carried out in a high-volume expert center with a multidisciplinary team. First-line treatment should be delivered without unnecessary delays or dose reductions.

After initial treatment, all patients need close follow-up. Patients with pure seminoma and residual masses can generally be managed with surveillance, whereas patients with NSGCTs should undergo resection of all residual disease, if possible. Long-term survivors of GCT who have received chemotherapy or radiotherapy will need lifelong medical care for the management of late complications of chemotherapy.

Relapses after initial chemotherapy may still be cured with salvage tHDC/SCR. Nevertheless, even with aggressive guideline-based management in high-volume centers, disseminated GCT can still be a fatal disease. Given the rarity of this situation within testicular cancer, and the rarity of testicular cancer itself, large collaborative efforts are necessary to develop new treatments.

REFERENCES

1. Wood L, Kollmannsberger C, Jewett M, et al. Canadian consensus guidelines for the management of testicular germ cell cancer. Can Urol Assoc J 2010;4(2):e19–38.
2. Albers P, Albrecht W, Algaba F, et al. Guidelines on testicular cancer: 2015 update. Eur Urol 2015;68(6): 1054–68.
3. Lorch A, Bascoul-Mollevi C, Kramar A, et al. Conventional-dose versus high-dose chemotherapy as first salvage treatment in male patients with metastatic germ cell tumors: evidence from a large international database. J Clin Oncol 2011;29(16):2178–84.
4. Einhorn LH, Donohue J. Cis-diamminedichloroplatinum, vinblastine, and bleomycin combination chemotherapy in disseminated testicular cancer. Ann Intern Med 1977;87(3):293–8.
5. Einhorn LH. Treatment of testicular cancer: a new and improved model. J Clin Oncol 1990;8(11): 1777–81.
6. Williams SD, Birch R, Einhorn LH, et al. Treatment of disseminated germ-cell tumors with cisplatin, bleomycin, and either vinblastine or etoposide. N Engl J Med 1987;316(23):1435–40.
7. Paffenholz P, Heidegger IM, Kuhr K, et al. Non-guideline-concordant treatment of testicular cancer is associated with reduced relapse-free survival. Clin Genitourin Cancer 2017. https://doi.org/10.1016/j.clgc.2017.08.018.
8. Woldu SL, Matulay JT, Clinton TN, et al. Impact of hospital case volume on testicular cancer outcomes and practice patterns. Urol Oncol 2018; 36(1):14.e7-15.
9. Miyanaga N, Akaza H, Hattori K, et al. The importance of dose intensity in chemotherapy of advanced testicular cancer. Urol Int 1995;54(4): 220–5.
10. Grimison PS, Stockler MR, Thomson DB, et al. Comparison of two standard chemotherapy regimens for good-prognosis germ cell tumors: updated analysis of a randomized trial. J Natl Cancer Inst 2010;102(16):1253–62.

11. International germ cell consensus classification: a prognostic factor-based staging system for metastatic germ cell cancers. International Germ Cell Cancer Collaborative Group. J Clin Oncol 1997;15(2): 594–603.

12. Feldman DR, Lorch A, Kramar A, et al. Brain metastases in patients with germ cell tumors: prognostic factors and treatment options—an analysis from the Global Germ Cell Cancer Group. J Clin Oncol 2016;34(4):345–51.

13. de Wit R, Roberts JT, Wilkinson PM, et al. Equivalence of three or four cycles of bleomycin, etoposide, and cisplatin chemotherapy and of a 3- or 5-day schedule in good-prognosis germ cell cancer: a randomized study of the European Organization for Research and Treatment of Cancer Genitourinary Tract Cancer Cooperative Group and the Medical Research Council. J Clin Oncol 2001;19(6):1629–40.

14. Culine S, Kerbrat P, Kramar A, et al. Refining the optimal chemotherapy regimen for good-risk metastatic nonseminomatous germ-cell tumors: a randomized trial of the Genito-Urinary Group of the French Federation of Cancer Centers (GETUG T93BP). Ann Oncol 2007;18(5):917–24.

15. O'Sullivan JM, Huddart RA, Norman AR, et al. Predicting the risk of bleomycin lung toxicity in patients with germ-cell tumours. Ann Oncol 2003;14(1):91–6.

16. Hinton S, Catalano PJ, Einhorn LH, et al. Cisplatin, etoposide and either bleomycin or ifosfamide in the treatment of disseminated germ cell tumors: final analysis of an intergroup trial. Cancer 2003;97(8): 1869–75.

17. Birch R, Williams S, Cone A, et al. Prognostic factors for favorable outcome in disseminated germ cell tumors. J Clin Oncol 1986;4(3):400–7.

18. Culine S, Kramar A, Theodore C, et al. Randomized trial comparing bleomycin/etoposide/cisplatin with alternating cisplatin/cyclophosphamide/doxorubicin and vinblastine/bleomycin regimens of chemotherapy for patients with intermediate- and poor-risk metastatic nonseminomatous germ cell tumors: Genito-Urinary Group of the French Federation of Cancer Centers Trial T93MP. J Clin Oncol 2008; 26(3):421–7.

19. Kaye SB, Mead GM, Fossa S, et al. Intensive induction-sequential chemotherapy with BOP/VIP-B compared with treatment with BEP/EP for poor-prognosis metastatic nonseminomatous germ cell tumor: a Randomized Medical Research Council/European Organization for Research and Treatment of Cancer study. J Clin Oncol 1998;16(2):692–701.

20. Fossa SD, Paluchowska B, Horwich A, et al. Intensive induction chemotherapy with C-BOP/BEP for intermediate- and poor-risk metastatic germ cell tumours (EORTC trial 30948). Br J Cancer 2005; 93(11):1209–14.

21. Daugaard G, Skoneczna I, Aass N, et al. A randomized phase III study comparing standard dose BEP with sequential high-dose cisplatin, etoposide, and ifosfamide (VIP) plus stem-cell support in males with poor-prognosis germ-cell cancer. An intergroup study of EORTC, GTCSG, and Grupo Germinal (EORTC 30974). Ann Oncol 2011;22(5): 1054–61.

22. Motzer RJ, Nichols CJ, Margolin KA, et al. Phase III randomized trial of conventional-dose chemotherapy with or without high-dose chemotherapy and autologous hematopoietic stem-cell rescue as first-line treatment for patients with poor-prognosis metastatic germ cell tumors. J Clin Oncol 2007; 25(3):247–56.

23. Fizazi K, Pagliaro L, Laplanche A, et al. Personalised chemotherapy based on tumour marker decline in poor prognosis germ-cell tumours (GETUG 13): a phase 3, multicentre, randomised trial. Lancet Oncol 2014;15(13):1442–50.

24. Fizazi K, Flechon A, Le Teuff G, et al. Mature results of the GETUG 13 phase III trial in poor-prognosis germ-cell tumors (GCT). JCO 2016; 34(Suppl 15):4504.

25. Moran-Ribon A, Droz JP, Kattan J, et al. Super-high-risk germ-cell tumors: a clinical entity. Report of eleven cases. Support Care Cancer 1994;2(4): 253–8.

26. Zon RT, Nichols C, Einhorn LH. Management strategies and outcomes of germ cell tumor patients with very high human chorionic gonadotropin levels. J Clin Oncol 1998;16(4):1294–7.

27. McGowan MP, Pratter MR, Nash G. Primary testicular choriocarcinoma with pulmonary metastases presenting as ARDS. Chest 1990;97(5): 1258–9.

28. Honecker F, Bokemeyer C. Patients with advanced non-seminomatous germ-cell tumour: the art of the start. Ann Oncol 2010;21(8):1569–71.

29. Massard C, Plantade A, Gross-Goupil M, et al. Poor prognosis nonseminomatous germ-cell tumours (NSGCTs): should chemotherapy doses be reduced at first cycle to prevent acute respiratory distress syndrome in patients with multiple lung metastases? Ann Oncol 2010;21(8):1585–8.

30. Bokemeyer C, Nowak P, Haupt A, et al. Treatment of brain metastases in patients with testicular cancer. J Clin Oncol 1997;15(4):1449–54.

31. Fossa SD, Bokemeyer C, Gerl A, et al. Treatment outcome of patients with brain metastases from malignant germ cell tumors. Cancer 1999;85(4):988–97.

32. Kollmannsberger C, Tandstad T, Bedard PL, et al. Patterns of relapse in patients with clinical stage I testicular cancer managed with active surveillance. J Clin Oncol 2015;33(1):51–7.

33. De Santis M, Becherer A, Bokemeyer C, et al. 2-18fluoro-deoxy-D-glucose positron emission

tomography is a reliable predictor for viable tumor in postchemotherapy seminoma: an update of the prospective multicentric SEMPET trial. J Clin Oncol 2004;22(6):1034–9.

34. Bachner M, Loriot Y, Gross-Goupil M, et al. 2-(1)(8) fluoro-deoxy-D-glucose positron emission tomography (FDG-PET) for postchemotherapy seminoma residual lesions: a retrospective validation of the SEMPET trial. Ann Oncol 2012;23(1):59–64.

35. Cathomas R, Klingbiel D, Bernard B, et al. Questioning the value of fluorodeoxyglucose positron emission tomography for residual lesions after chemotherapy for metastatic seminoma: results of an international global germ cell cancer group registry. J Clin Oncol 2018;JCO1800210. https://doi.org/10.1200/JCO.18.00210.

36. Fossa SD, Qvist H, Stenwig AE, et al. Is postchemotherapy retroperitoneal surgery necessary in patients with nonseminomatous testicular cancer and minimal residual tumor masses? J Clin Oncol 1992;10(4):569–73.

37. Stenning SP, Parkinson MC, Fisher C, et al. Postchemotherapy residual masses in germ cell tumor patients: content, clinical features, and prognosis. Medical Research Council Testicular Tumour Working Party. Cancer 1998;83(7):1409–19.

38. Comiter CV, Kibel AS, Richie JP, et al. Prognostic features of teratomas with malignant transformation: a clinicopathological study of 21 cases. J Urol 1998;159(3):859–63.

39. Carver BS, Shayegan B, Serio A, et al. Long-term clinical outcome after postchemotherapy retroperitoneal lymph node dissection in men with residual teratoma. J Clin Oncol 2007;25(9):1033–7.

40. Fizazi K, Tjulandin S, Salvioni R, et al. Viable malignant cells after primary chemotherapy for disseminated nonseminomatous germ cell tumors: prognostic factors and role of postsurgery chemotherapy–results from an international study group. J Clin Oncol 2001;19(10):2647–57.

41. Hartmann JT, Candelaria M, Kuczyk MA, et al. Comparison of histological results from the resection of residual masses at different sites after chemotherapy for metastatic non-seminomatous germ cell tumours. Eur J Cancer 1997;33(6):843–7.

42. Besse B, Grunenwald D, Flechon A, et al. Nonseminomatous germ cell tumors: assessing the need for postchemotherapy contralateral pulmonary resection in patients with ipsilateral complete necrosis. J Thorac Cardiovasc Surg 2009;137(2):448–52.

43. van den Belt-Dusebout AW, de Wit R, Gietema JA, et al. Treatment-specific risks of second malignancies and cardiovascular disease in 5-year survivors of testicular cancer. J Clin Oncol 2007;25(28):4370–8.

44. Huddart RA, Norman A, Shahidi M, et al. Cardiovascular disease as a long-term complication of treatment for testicular cancer. J Clin Oncol 2003;21(8):1513–23.

45. Haugnes HS, Wethal T, Aass N, et al. Cardiovascular risk factors and morbidity in long-term survivors of testicular cancer: a 20-year follow-up study. J Clin Oncol 2010;28(30):4649–57.

46. Fossa SD, Abyholm T, Aakvaag A. Spermatogenesis and hormonal status after orchiectomy for cancer and before supplementary treatment. Eur Urol 1984;10(3):173–7.

47. Lampe H, Horwich A, Norman A, et al. Fertility after chemotherapy for testicular germ cell cancers. J Clin Oncol 1997;15(1):239–45.

48. Sprauten M, Brydoy M, Haugnes HS, et al. Longitudinal serum testosterone, luteinizing hormone, and follicle-stimulating hormone levels in a population-based sample of long-term testicular cancer survivors. J Clin Oncol 2014;32(6):571–8.

49. Donat SM, Levy DA. Bleomycin associated pulmonary toxicity: is perioperative oxygen restriction necessary? J Urol 1998;160(4):1347–52.

50. Haugnes HS, Aass N, Fossa SD, et al. Pulmonary function in long-term survivors of testicular cancer. J Clin Oncol 2009;27(17):2779–86.

51. Fung C, Sesso HD, Williams AM, et al. Multi-institutional assessment of adverse health outcomes among North American Testicular Cancer Survivors after modern cisplatin-based chemotherapy. J Clin Oncol 2017;35(11):1211–22.

52. Dolan ME, El Charif O, Wheeler HE, et al. Clinical and genome-wide analysis of cisplatin-induced peripheral neuropathy in survivors of adult-onset cancer. Clin Cancer Res 2017;23(19):5757–68.

53. Travis LB, Fossa SD, Schonfeld SJ, et al. Second cancers among 40,576 testicular cancer patients: focus on long-term survivors. J Natl Cancer Inst 2005;97(18):1354–65.

54. International Prognostic Factors Study Group, Lorch A, Beyer J, Bascoul-Mollevi C, et al. Prognostic factors in patients with metastatic germ cell tumors who experienced treatment failure with cisplatin-based first-line chemotherapy. J Clin Oncol 2010;28(33):4906–11.

55. Nichols CR, Tricot G, Williams SD, et al. Dose-intensive chemotherapy in refractory germ cell cancer—a phase I/II trial of high-dose carboplatin and etoposide with autologous bone marrow transplantation. J Clin Oncol 1989;7(7):932–9.

56. Pico JL, Rosti G, Kramar A, et al. A randomised trial of high-dose chemotherapy in the salvage treatment of patients failing first-line platinum chemotherapy for advanced germ cell tumours. Ann Oncol 2005;16(7):1152–9.

57. Lorch A, Kollmannsberger C, Hartmann JT, et al. Single versus sequential high-dose chemotherapy

in patients with relapsed or refractory germ cell tumors: a prospective randomized multicenter trial of the German Testicular Cancer Study Group. J Clin Oncol 2007;25(19):2778–84.

58. Spiess PE, Kassouf W, Brown GA, et al. Surgical management of growing teratoma syndrome: the M. D. Anderson cancer center experience. J Urol 2007;177(4):1330–4 [discussion: 1334].

59. Hinton S, Catalano P, Einhorn LH, et al. Phase II study of paclitaxel plus gemcitabine in refractory germ cell tumors (E9897): a trial of the Eastern Cooperative Oncology Group. J Clin Oncol 2002; 20(7):1859–63.

60. Bokemeyer C, Oechsle K, Honecker F, et al. Combination chemotherapy with gemcitabine, oxaliplatin, and paclitaxel in patients with cisplatin-refractory or multiply relapsed germ-cell tumors: a study of the German Testicular Cancer Study Group. Ann Oncol 2008;19(3):448–53.

61. George DW, Foster RS, Hromas RA, et al. Update on late relapse of germ cell tumor: a clinical and molecular analysis. J Clin Oncol 2003;21(1): 113–22.

62. Dieckmann KP, Albers P, Classen J, et al. Late relapse of testicular germ cell neoplasms: a descriptive analysis of 122 cases. J Urol 2005; 173(3):824–9.

Postchemotherapy Resection of Residual Mass in Nonseminomatous Germ Cell Tumor

Saum Ghodoussipour, MD, Siamak Daneshmand, MD*

KEYWORDS

- Germ cell tumor • Testicular cancer • Nonseminomatous • Retroperitoneal lymph node dissection

KEY POINTS

- Although a majority of patients with disseminated nonseminomatous germ cell tumors are cured with cisplatin-based chemotherapy alone, up to one-third will have a residual mass.
- Surgical resection after chemotherapy is indicated in patients with a mass greater than 1 cm, after salvage chemotherapy, in certain cases with elevated markers, after late relapse, and growing teratoma syndrome.
- Postchemotherapy resection in nonseminomatous germ cell tumors is an often-challenging procedure with the need for adjunctive procedures and extraretroperitoneal resections.
- Modern techniques to minimize morbidity include laparoscopic, robotic, and midline extraperitoneal approaches.

INTRODUCTION

Retroperitoneal lymph node dissection (RPLND) has been an important component in the management of testicular cancer since its description in the early 1900s.[1] The introduction of cisplatin-based chemotherapy has revolutionized the care of patients with testicular germ cell tumors such that cure is now achieved in more than 95% of all patients.[2] Although the majority will have a complete response after chemotherapy for disseminated disease, RPLND still has a role because one-third of all patients will have a residual mass after chemotherapy.[3] In this article, we review the current indications for surgery in patients with nonseminomatous germ cell tumors (NSGCT) and residual mass after chemotherapy and highlight important technical considerations of this often-challenging operation.

INDICATIONS FOR RESECTION
Residual Mass Greater Than 1 cm After Primary Chemotherapy

The rationale for postchemotherapy RPLND (PC-RPLND) in patients with NSGCT is to remove residual teratoma or active disease. Although the size of a residual mass after chemotherapy is an independent predictor of relapse,[4] it is the histopathologic findings of residual lesions that determine the need for further treatments or surveillance. Unfortunately, modern imaging techniques poorly differentiate residual necrosis/fibrosis, teratoma, or viable cancer after chemotherapy.[5] The false-negative rate for NSGCT with PET scan is up to 40% and particularly poor with teratoma.[6] Thus, consensus on the need for PC-RPLND of residual masses greater than 1 cm is universal and attributable to the 40% to 45%

Disclosure Statement: The authors have nothing to disclose.
Norris Comprehensive Cancer Center, USC Institute of Urology, 1441 Eastlake Avenue, Suite 7416, Los Angeles, CA 90033, USA
* Corresponding author.
E-mail address: daneshma@med.usc.edu

Urol Clin N Am 46 (2019) 389–398
https://doi.org/10.1016/j.ucl.2019.04.004

risk of teratoma and 10% to 15% risk of viable malignancy found in patients with marker negative disease.[3–5,7] Teratoma is a chemotherapy-resistant histology with the potential for growth and malignant transformation, but cure rates of greater than 90% are achieved with complete resection.[8] When completely resected at PC-RPLND, the 5-year overall survival (OS) rates for patients with viable NSGCT are 70%.[9]

Some have proposed a role for PC-RPLND in patients with subcentimeter retroperitoneal nodes owing to an estimated 24% risk of teratoma and 4% risk of viable tumor.[10] However, the safety of surveillance in these patients has been demonstrated in several large series. Ehrlich and colleagues[11] observed a cohort of 141 patients with complete response after chemotherapy and found a recurrence rate of only 9% at a median of 11 months. The only predictor of relapse was the International Germ Cell Consensus Classification risk classification. Kollmannsberger and colleagues[12] similarly studied 276 patients who had chemotherapy for NSGCT and found 161 with complete response and 46 with a partial response (lymph node <1 cm). These patients were observed and at a median follow-up of 52 months, 10 patients (6%) recurred with 100% disease-specific survival after a median follow-up of 64 months from recurrence. Thus, surveillance of patients with subcentimeter nodes seems to be a safe option that minimizes overtreatment.

Residual Mass After Salvage Chemotherapy

Surgical resection is imperative in patients with residual disease after salvage chemotherapy because the risk of viable carcinoma increases to 50%.[13] Resection of such masses can be challenging. Aside from greater rates of viable tumor, such operations are fraught with greater rates of incomplete resection and recurrence when compared with PC-RPLND after induction chemotherapy.[14] However, aggressive resection does improve survival. Cary and colleagues[15] reported on 92 patients who received high-dose chemotherapy with stem cell transplantation before RPLND. Seventy patients (76%) were treated as first-line salvage and 21 (23%) as second-line salvage. The final pathology for the 48 patients with marker negative disease before surgery was necrosis in 39%, teratoma in 41%, and viable cancer in 20%. At a median follow-up of 80 months, the 5-year OS for these patients with normal tumor markers was 83%. The high survival rate in this series, despite a greater proportion of active disease compared with those undergoing PC-RPLND after induction chemotherapy,

underscores the importance of surgical management. Moreover, a complete resection may obviate the need for further therapy in patients with viable cancer at PC-RPLND after salvage chemotherapy. Donohue and colleagues[16] reported on 53 patients who underwent complete resection after salvage chemotherapy with persistent NSGCT. Repeat salvage chemotherapy was administered to 25 patients and 28 were observed. Survival was equivalent with 12 patients dying in each group.

Resection with Elevated Tumor Markers

Surgical resection in patients with residual disease and elevated markers after chemotherapy is often termed "desperation" PC-RPLND. Resection should be considered in patients with elevated but plateaued markers after induction chemotherapy and in those not responding to salvage chemotherapy, but with resectable disease.

Of the 30% of patients with residual disease after induction chemotherapy, 10% to 15% will have elevated markers.[17,18] After ruling out disease in sanctuary sites (brain, contralateral testicle), options for patients include salvage high-dose chemotherapy or complete surgical resection. Although surgery in this setting is controversial, it can spare patients from the morbidity of high-dose chemotherapy, especially in those with chemoresistant disease, and surgery can avoid the risk of tumor progression that may compromise resection.[19]

Resection with elevated markers after salvage chemotherapy is a more accepted indication for RPLND. A series by Beck and colleagues[17] studied 114 patients who underwent desperation PC-RPLND between 1977 and 2000. Surgery was performed after first-line chemotherapy in 50 patients and after second-line chemotherapy in 64 patients. Germ cell cancer was identified in 53.5% of all patients, but in 28% of those undergoing surgery after first-line chemotherapy and in 75% of those receiving second-line chemotherapy. Despite the elevated markers, pathology showed teratoma in 34.2% and fibrosis in 12.3%. Declining markers at the time of surgery, beta-human chorionic gonadotropin of less than 100 and first-line chemotherapy only were associated with finding teratoma or fibrosis on final pathology. The 5-year OS was 31.4% in those with viable tumor, 77.5% with teratoma, and 85.7% in those with necrosis and fibrosis. A plausible explanation for the benign pathology found in almost one-half of the patients despite elevated markers is a slow leakage of alpha fetoprotein and beta-human chorionic gonadotropin that may come from cystic teratomas.[20] In the previously mentioned study examining the outcomes of RPLND after high-dose chemotherapy by Cary and colleagues,[15] the subset of patients with elevated markers had a final pathology of necrosis in 26% and teratoma in 34%. Such pathology must be considered in this subset of patients with elevated markers but resectable disease, because surgery may be curative while avoiding unnecessary second-line chemotherapy.

Late Relapse

Late relapse is defined as any recurrence, most commonly a retroperitoneal mass, that occurs 2 or more years after curative treatment. A majority of these patients will have relapse more than 5 years after initial treatment.[21,22] Although the true incidence is unknown, estimates suggest a 3.2% risk of late relapse in patients with NSGCT.[23] Surgical resection is the gold standard in this situation; the most common pathology found in relapsed masses is teratoma.[24] In a series by Baniel and colleagues,[25] 81 patients were treated for late relapse and then followed for a median of 4.8 years. Twenty-one patients (25%) were disease free at the final follow-up and all but 2 underwent surgical resection. Of the 65 patients treated initially with chemotherapy for their relapse, only 17 (26%) had a complete response and only 2 were continuously disease free without surgery. A later series by Sharp and colleagues[22] examined 75 patients with late relapse. Primary management was not surgical in 93% of the patients and the median time to relapse was 6.9 years. The 5-year cancer-specific survival for the entire cohort was 60%, but 79% with complete resection versus 36% without. In sum, both studies showed only modest success with chemotherapy but greatly improved survival with complete surgical resection for masses with late relapse.

Growing Teratoma Syndrome

The presence of a residual mass that continues to grow after chemotherapy despite normalization of markers should alert physicians to the possibility of growing teratoma syndrome (GTS). This is an often-challenging surgical problem defined as a mass in a patient with NSGCT with: normal markers, growth during or after chemotherapy, and final surgical histology of mature teratoma.[26] Again, mild elevations of tumor markers may be seen owing to sequestration within large cystic teratomas.[20] GTS is a rare phenomenon with various reports, suggesting a prevalence of 3% in all patients treated for NSGCT.[27] Given the rarity of cases and absence of teratoma in up to 60% of

orchiectomy specimens in patients with GTS, no reliable predictors exist.[28] Cystic features are often see on computed tomography scans and, despite an often manageable size at diagnosis (median, 6–7 cm) and relatively slow growth (0.5–0.7 cm per month),[27–29] early surgical management is necessary because these tumors are chemoresistant and may grow to invade surrounding structures, ultimately leading to death.[30] A recent report of 22 patients treated with surgical resection showed an OS of 95.5% at 25 months. These surgeries were not without consequence; 23% experienced postoperative complications and 18% required adjunctive procedures, including resection of the aorta, vena cava, or intestine, or nephrectomy.[27]

Another rare entity that is tied to GTS is the unknown potential of otherwise benign teratomas to undergo malignant transformation, often into a somatic-type malignancy. Rice and colleagues[31] reported on 121 patients with germ cell tumors and somatic-type malignancy at orchiectomy or subsequent resection. Only 32 of the patients had somatic-type malignancy at the original diagnosis and the median time to diagnosis for those with delayed presentation was 33 months. The most prevalent histologies identified were sarcoma in 49%, carcinoma in 26% and sarcomatoid yolk sac tumor in 14%. There were no factors predictive of prognosis, but the 5-year cancer-specific survival was 64% in those undergoing resection. Given an unknown response to chemotherapy, the management of tumors with malignant transformation should include complete surgical resection.

TECHNICAL CONSIDERATIONS

PC-RPLND is a technically demanding surgery that requires intimate familiarity with abdominal and retroperitoneal anatomy, as well as expertise in vascular techniques. As in all aspects of testicular germ cell tumor management, outcomes are directly correlated with experience.[2] A recent query of the National Cancer Database showed that the use of RPLND for NSGCT is significantly more common in academic centers.[32] A separate query found that, despite worse disease characteristics at high-volume hospitals, patients with NSGCT had significantly worse OS when treated at low-volume hospitals (81% vs 90% 5-year OS at low-volume hospitals vs high-volume hospitals, respectively).[33] Experienced surgeons may have a greater understanding of and ability to perform adjunctive procedures when needed, extraretroperitoneal resections when indicated, and a greater emphasis on methods to minimize morbidity of the operation.

Need for Adjunctive Procedures

When faced with residual disease after chemotherapy, oncologic outcomes depend on complete resection. This factor, coupled with demanding dissections, makes the need for adjunctive procedures a reality in PC-RPLND (**Fig. 1**). Such procedures are required in more than 20% of all patients undergoing PC-RPLND.[34–38] The most common adjunctive procedure in contemporary series is nephrectomy at around 10%, followed by vascular resection or reconstruction in less than 10% of patients.[37] Teratomas have been shown to invade the vena cava and, when they do, resection of the mass, tumor thrombectomy, and even resection of the vena cava may be indicated. Reconstruction of the vena cava is rarely needed in patients with large retroperitoneal masses because most patients have well-established collaterals owing to preexisting caval obstruction.[39]

Other procedures occur at less frequent rates. We have avoided nephrectomy with partial ureteral resection and appendiceal substitution (**Fig. 2**).[38] Jacob and colleagues[40] presented 39 patients who underwent partial duodenectomy for duodenal involvement during PC-RPLND. The median tumor size was 8.95 cm, 50% of the cases were standard PC-RPLND, and the rest were redo, desperation, or late relapse cases. Duodenectomy with primary duodenorrhaphy was performed safely in all patients, but with a 45% rate of postoperative ileus and a 3% rate of duodenal fistula. Despite the aggressive nature of such procedures, acceptable morbidity and excellent oncologic outcomes with complete resection validates their use.

Several factors have been shown to predict the need for an adjunctive procedure, including elevated markers, final retroperitoneal pathology, and risk group, but residual tumor size is the most important predictor. Cary and colleagues[36] found a tumor size of greater than 10 cm to have an odds ratio of 7.2 (95% confidence interval, 2.6–19.5) in predicting the need for any adjunctive procedure. A recent report by Johnson and colleagues[41] studied 97 patients with complete preoperative imaging available and found 16 who underwent inferior vena cava or abdominal aortic resection. Dominant mass size and degree of circumferential vessel involvement (>135° for the vena cava and >330° for the aorta) predicted resection or reconstruction.

Extraretroperitoneal Resection

Although the retroperitoneum is the most common site of metastatic spread, 40% of patients with disseminated disease will have a residual mass in extraretroperitoneal sites after chemotherapy.[42] The retroperitoneum should be addressed first, because patients with viable disease may need salvage therapy regardless of the histology at other sites. Even so, pathology at other sites may be discordant 30% of the time.[43] Thus, the decision to resect extraretroperitoneal sites should not rely on findings of PC-RPLND alone. With the exception of the lung, where necrosis at PC-RPLND is associated with a 90% chance of concordance,[44] all residual lesions should be removed if feasible.

Concurrent resection is often feasible at the time of PC-RPLND for disease in the lower mediastinum, neck, abdomen, and pelvis. Many advocate for such resections with a midline approach, but bulkier and suprahilar tumors may require a thoracoabdominal incision.[45] This incision is useful for disease in the lower thorax, but is not without morbidity.[46] Other investigators have endorsed a transabdominal transdiaphragmatic approach to resect mediastinal masses.[47] We prefer a transabdominal approach via a midline incision and division of the ipsilateral crus for access to residual masses in the lower posterior mediastinum (**Fig. 3**).

Abdominal involvement is possible with the liver and mesentery serving as potential landing sites for NSGCT. We prefer to defer liver resection at the time of PC-RPLND and allow retroperitoneal pathology to dictate further chemotherapy, which can make subsequent resections easier and less morbid. We have rarely, but effectively, performed mesenteric lymphadenectomy for NSGCT (**Fig. 4**).[48]

Although pelvic metastases are rare, several groups have reported outcomes after pelvic lymphadenectomy at the time of RPLND. Jacob and colleagues[49] reported on 134 patients with pelvic disease. Almost all (98%) were in a postchemotherapy setting and 24% presented as late relapse. Final pathology revealed necrosis in 16.5%, viable NSGCT in 21%, teratoma in 55%, and sarcoma in 6%. A higher stage at presentation and prior history of groin surgery predicted the presence of pelvic metastases. Alanee and colleagues[50] examined all PC-RPLNDs at their institution from 1981 to 2011 and found that 1.7% of patients underwent pelvic lymphadenectomy for residual mass on preoperative imaging. The median size of the mass was 5 cm and final pathology showed teratoma in 33% and mixed teratoma with yolk sac tumors in 10%. After a median follow-up of 58 months, only one patient had a recurrence.

Minimizing Morbidity

Early series on PC-RPLND quoted complication rates that ranged from 30% to 36%.[51,52]

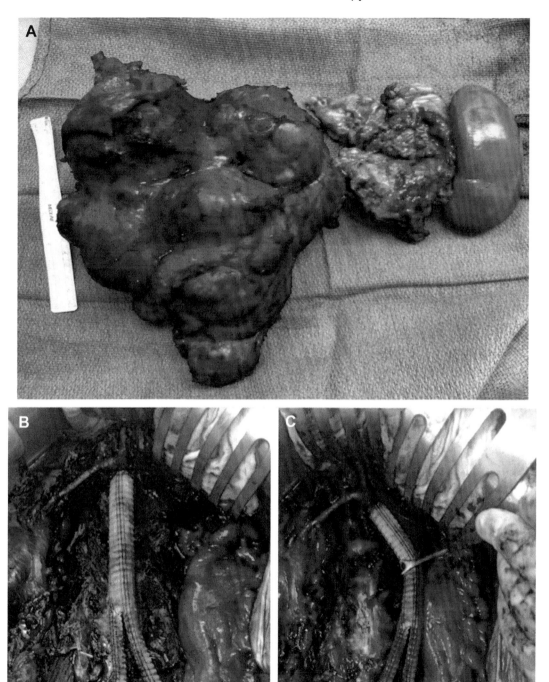

Fig. 1. (*A*) Postchemotherapy resection of residual mass with left nephrectomy, (*B, C*) as well as resection of vena cava and aorta with reconstruction using aortic graft.

PC-RPLND as compared with primary RPLND is associated with worse outcomes and longer hospital stay (odds ratio, 3.75).[37,53] Complications seemed to have improved in the modern era, with the most common complication still being wound infection, postoperative ileus, and deep venous thrombosis.[36] Improvements over time are owed to surgeons' modernizing surgical

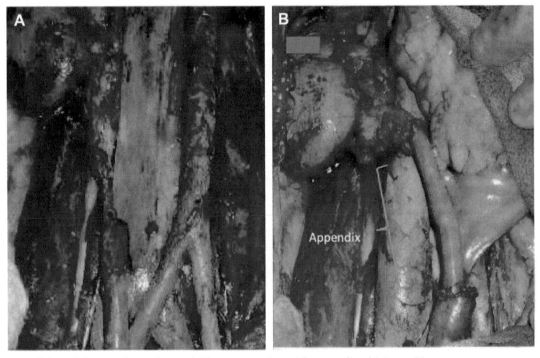

Fig. 2. (*A*) Partial ureteral resection and (*B*) reconstruction with appendiceal interposition.

techniques with the aim of minimizing the morbidity of PC-RPLND. One such example is the use of nerve sparing procedures, which can preserve antegrade ejaculation in more than 80% of patients undergoing PC-RPLND without compromise of oncologic outcomes.[54]

Several series have reported on the feasibility of laparoscopic approaches to PC-RPLND. The presumed benefit of such cases being decreased pain, blood loss, and hospital stay. Faria and colleagues[55] presented 25 patients treated with laparoscopic PC-RPLND between 2008 and 2015. The median size of residual mass was 3.3 cm and 1 patient required conversion to an open surgery. The median operative time was 213 minutes and the estimated blood loss 260 mL. Final pathology

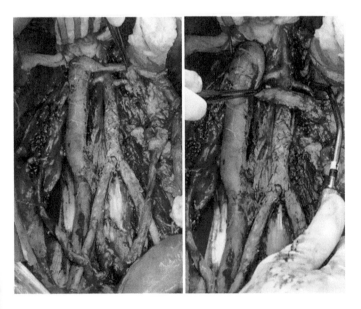

Fig. 3. Suprahilar dissection at the time of PC-RPLND.

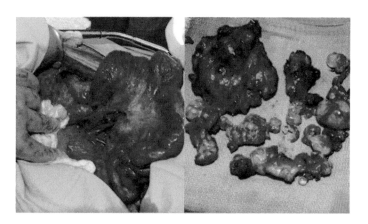

Fig. 4. Mesenteric lymphadenopathy performed concurrently with retroperitoneal lymphadenectomy.

was necrosis in 36%, teratoma in 36%, and viable tumor in 24%. All patients had preserved antegrade ejaculation and, at a median follow-up of 30 months, 2 patients with viable disease recurred. One recurrence was in the mediastinum and one was suprahilar. Both recurrences were successfully treated with salvage chemotherapy. The largest series of laparoscopic PC-RPLND came from Steiner and colleagues,[56] who performed resection in 100 patients with a median residual mass of 1.4 cm. They included patients with stage II NSGCT and excluded those with bulky disease that encased the retroperitoneal vessels. The median operative time was 343 minutes for bilateral dissections, estimated blood loss was 84 mL, and the median hospital stay was 3.9 days. Antegrade ejaculation was preserved in 95.2% of patients. There was 1 conversion to open surgery and 1 recurrence. The final pathology showed teratoma in 38% of patients and viable disease in 2%.

Small series have reported on the use of robotic assisted laparoscopic PC-RPLND. Cheney and colleagues[57] performed robotic RPLND on 18 patients, 9 of whom had residual masses after chemotherapy. There was no significant difference in lymph node yield (22 vs 18 nodes), blood loss (100 mL vs 313 mL) or length of stay (2.75 days vs 2.2 days) between the patients undergoing primary RPLND and PC-RPLND, respectively. Those with PC-RPLND did have significantly longer operations (369 minutes vs 311 minutes) and 2 (22%) were converted to an open procedure. Kamel and colleagues[58] reported on 12 PC-RPLNDs performed robotically from 2011 to 2015. Nine procedures (75%) were for NSGCT. One patient required conversion to an open operation. The mean blood loss was 475 mL, the mean operative time 312 minutes, and the mean hospital stay was 3.2 days. The final pathology

was teratoma in 45.5%, viable tumor in 9%, and necrosis in 45.5%. Antegrade ejaculation was preserved in 67% of patients and after a median follow-up of 31 months, and there were no recurrences. In sum, the literature on minimally invasive PC-RPLND demonstrates feasibility of the procedure, but is not robust enough as of yet to make conclusions regarding oncologic efficacy or to replace the open technique as the standard of care.

We have developed a novel approach to RPLND with a midline extraperitoneal incision that aims to minimize the morbidity associated with entering the peritoneal cavity. The procedure involves a midline abdominal incision from several centimeters below the xiphoid process to 4 to 5 cm below the umbilicus. Beginning in the infraumbulical portion of the incision, the extraperitoneal space between the peritoneum and transversalis fascia is developed until the peritoneal sac can be mobilized freely and medialized off the dissection field. A self-retaining retractor is placed to retract the abdominal wall and the peritoneal sac (**Fig. 5**). From 2010 to 2015, we performed 68 extraperitoneal RPLNDs, including 37 PC-RPLNDs for NSGCT. The median mass size was 2.2 cm, but 46% of residual masses after chemotherapy were greater than 10 cm. Median estimated blood loss was 325 mL and the median number of nodes removed was 36. Patients had a median time to flatus of 2 days and no patients experienced postoperative ileus. The median length of stay was 3 days and antegrade ejaculation was achieved in 96.8% of patients undergoing PC-RPLND. One patient had a recurrence after PC-RPLND and this was a patient who had surgery performed after salvage chemotherapy with high-volume teratoma and 2% viable disease found on surgical pathology.[59]

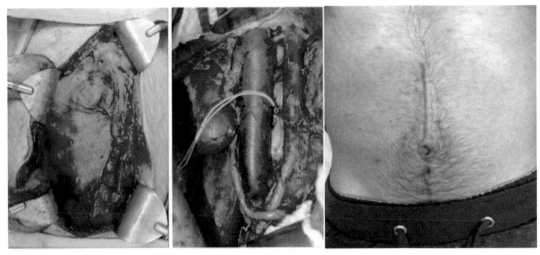

Fig. 5. A midline extraperitoneal approach to PC-RPLND.

SUMMARY

Surgical resection of residual masses after chemotherapy remains a vital component of the management of patients with NSGCT. There are clear indications for surgical resection, which remains challenging, especially in cases of advanced disease. Surgeons caring for patients in the postchemotherapy setting must be familiar with techniques and indications for adjunctive procedures, extraperitoneal resections and methods to minimize morbidity for their patients.

REFERENCES

1. Chevassu, M. Tumeurs du testicule. These, Paris, 1906.
2. Tandstad T, Kollmannsberger CK, Roth BJ, et al. Practice makes perfect: the rest of the story in testicular cancer as a model curable neoplasm. J Clin Oncol 2017;35(31):3525–8.
3. Daneshmand S, Albers P, Fossa SD, et al. Contemporary management of postchemotherapy testis cancer. Eur Urol 2012;62(5):867–76.
4. Shayegan B, Carver BS, Stasi J, et al. Clinical outcome following post-chemotherapy retroperitoneal lymph node dissection in men with intermediate- and poor-risk nonseminomatous germ cell tumour. BJU Int 2007;99(5):993–7.
5. Daneshmand S, Djaladat H, Nichols C. Management of residual mass in nonseminomatous germ cell tumors following chemotherapy. Ther Adv Urol 2011; 3(4):163–71.
6. Pfannenberg AC, Oechsle K, Bokemeyer C, et al. The role of [(18)F] FDG-PET, CT/MRI and tumor marker kinetics in the evaluation of post chemotherapy residual masses in metastatic germ cell tumors–prospects for management. World J Urol 2004;22(2):132–9.
7. Mano R, Di Natale R, Sheinfeld J. Current controversies on the role of retroperitoneal lymphadenectomy for testicular cancer. Urol Oncol 2018;37(3): 209–21.
8. Carver BS, Shayegan B, Serio A, et al. Long-term clinical outcome after postchemotherapy retroperitoneal lymph node dissection in men with residual teratoma. J Clin Oncol 2007;25(9):1033–7.
9. Fizazi K, Oldenburg J, Dunant A, et al. Assessing prognosis and optimizing treatment in patients with postchemotherapy viable nonseminomatous germcell tumors (NSGCT): results of the sCR2 international study. Ann Oncol 2008;19(2):259–64.
10. Ravi P, Gray KP, O'Donnell EK, et al. A meta-analysis of patient outcomes with subcentimeter disease after chemotherapy for metastatic nonseminomatous germ cell tumor. Ann Oncol 2014; 25(2):331–8.
11. Ehrlich Y, Brames MJ, Beck SD, et al. Long-term follow-up of Cisplatin combination chemotherapy in patients with disseminated nonseminomatous germ cell tumors: is a postchemotherapy retroperitoneal lymph node dissection needed after complete remission? J Clin Oncol 2010;28(4):531–6.
12. Kollmannsberger C, Daneshmand S, So A, et al. Management of disseminated nonseminomatous germ cell tumors with risk-based chemotherapy followed by response-guided postchemotherapy surgery. J Clin Oncol 2010;28(4):537–42.
13. Fox EP, Weathers TD, Williams SD, et al. Outcome analysis for patients with persistent nonteratomatous germ cell tumor in postchemotherapy retroperitoneal lymph node dissections. J Clin Oncol 1993; 11(7):1294–9.

14. Heidenreich A, Pfister D. Retroperitoneal lymphade-nectomy and resection for testicular cancer: an up-date on best practice. Ther Adv Urol 2012;4(4):187–205.

15. Cary C, Pedrosa JA, Jacob J, et al. Outcomes of postchemotherapy retroperitoneal lymph node dissection following high-dose chemotherapy with stem cell transplantation. Cancer 2015;121(24):4369–75.

16. Donohue JP, Fox EP, Williams SD, et al. Persistent cancer in postchemotherapy retroperitoneal lymph-node dissection: outcome analysis. World J Urol 1994;12(4):190–5.

17. Beck SD, Foster RS, Bihrle R, et al. Outcome anal-ysis for patients with elevated serum tumor markers at postchemotherapy retroperitoneal lymph node dissection. J Clin Oncol 2005;23(25):6149–56.

18. Ong TA, Winkler MH, Savage PM, et al. Retroperito-neal lymph node dissection after chemotherapy in patients with elevated tumour markers: indications, histopathology and outcome. BJU Int 2008;102(2):198–202.

19. Daneshmand S. Role of surgical resection for refrac-tory germ cell tumors. Urol Oncol 2015;33(8):370–8.

20. Beck SD, Patel MI, Sheinfeld J. Tumor marker levels in post-chemotherapy cystic masses: clinical impli-cations for patients with germ cell tumors. J Urol 2004;171(1):168–71.

21. Baniel J, Foster RS, Gonin R, et al. Late relapse of testicular cancer. J Clin Oncol 1995;13(5):1170–6.

22. Sharp DS, Carver BS, Eggener SE, et al. Clinical outcome and predictors of survival in late relapse of germ cell tumor. J Clin Oncol 2008;26(34):5524–9.

23. Oldenburg J, Martin JM, Fossa SD. Late relapses of germ cell malignancies: incidence, management, and prognosis. J Clin Oncol 2006;24(35):5503–11.

24. Michael H, Lucia J, Foster RS, et al. The pathology of late recurrence of testicular germ cell tumors. Am J Surg Pathol 2000;24(2):257–73.

25. Baniel J, Foster RS, Rowland RG, et al. Complica-tions of primary retroperitoneal lymph node dissec-tion. J Urol 1994;152(2 Pt 1):424–7.

26. Logothetis CJ, Samuels ML, Trindade A, et al. The growing teratoma syndrome. Cancer 1982;50(8):1629–35.

27. Paffenholz P, Pfister D, Matveev V, et al. Diagnosis and management of the growing teratoma syn-drome: a single-center experience and review of the literature. Urol Oncol 2018;36(12):529.e23-30.

28. Lee DJ, Djaladat H, Tadros NN, et al. Growing tera-toma syndrome: clinical and radiographic character-istics. Int J Urol 2014;21(9):905–8.

29. Spiess PE, Kassouf W, Brown GA, et al. Surgical management of growing teratoma syndrome: the M. D. Anderson cancer center experience. J Urol 2007;177(4):1330–4 [discussion: 4].

30. Karam JA, Raj GV. Growing teratoma syndrome. Urology 2009;74(4):783–4.

31. Rice KR, Magers MJ, Beck SD, et al. Manage-ment of germ cell tumors with somatic type malignancy: pathological features, prognostic fac-tors and survival outcomes. J Urol 2014;192(5):1403–9.

32. Hugen CM, Hu B, Jeldres C, et al. Utilization of retro-peritoneal lymph node dissection for testicular can-cer in the United States: results from the National Cancer Database (1998-2011). Urol Oncol 2016;34(11):487.e7-11.

33. Woldu SL, Matulay JT, Clinton TN, et al. Impact of hospital case volume on testicular cancer out-comes and practice patterns. Urol Oncol 2018;36(1):14.e7-15.

34. Stephenson AJ, Tal R, Sheinfeld J. Adjunctive ne-phrectomy at post-chemotherapy retroperitoneal lymph node dissection for nonseminomatous germ cell testicular cancer. J Urol 2006;176(5):1996–9 [discussion: 1999].

35. Winter C, Pfister D, Busch J, et al. Residual tumor size and IGCCCG risk classification predict addi-tional vascular procedures in patients with germ cell tumors and residual tumor resection: a multi-center analysis of the German Testicular Cancer Study Group. Eur Urol 2012;61(2):403–9.

36. Cary C, Masterson TA, Bihrle R, et al. Contemporary trends in postchemotherapy retroperitoneal lymph node dissection: additional procedures and periop-erative complications. Urol Oncol 2015;33(9):389.e15-21.

37. Macleod LC, Rajanahally S, Nayak JG, et al. Char-acterizing the morbidity of postchemotherapy retro-peritoneal lymph node dissection for testis cancer in a national cohort of privately insured patients. Urology 2016;91:70–6.

38. Djaladat H, Nichols C, Daneshmand S. Adjuvant surgery in testicular cancer patients un-dergoing postchemotherapy retroperitoneal lymph node dissection. Ann Surg Oncol 2012;19(7):2388–93.

39. Duty B, Daneshmand S. Resection of the inferior vena cava without reconstruction for urologic malig-nancies. Urology 2009;74(6):1257–62.

40. Jacob JM, Cary C, Jiang S, et al. Management of duodenal involvement during retroperitoneal lymph node dissection for germ cell tumors. Urology 2017;99:169–73.

41. Johnson SC, Smith ZL, Nottingham C, et al. Clinical and radiographic predictors of great vessel resec-tion or reconstruction during retroperitoneal lymph node dissection for testicular cancer. Urology 2018;123:186–90.

42. Hu B, Daneshmand S. Role of extraretroperitoneal surgery in patients with metastatic germ cell tumors. Urol Clin North Am 2015;42(3):369–80.

43. Hartmann JT, Candelaria M, Kuczyk MA, et al. Comparison of histological results from the resection of residual masses at different sites after chemotherapy for metastatic non-seminomatous germ cell tumours. Eur J Cancer 1997;33(6):843–7.

44. Steyerberg EW, Donohue JP, Gerl A, et al. Residual masses after chemotherapy for metastatic testicular cancer: the clinical implications of the association between retroperitoneal and pulmonary histology. Re-analysis of Histology in Testicular Cancer (ReHiT) Study Group. J Urol 1997;158(2):474–8.

45. Albers P, Holtl W, Heidenreich A, et al. Thoracoabdominal resection of retrocrural residual tumors. Aktuelle Urol 2004;35(2):141–50 [quiz: 151–2]. [in German].

46. Skinner DG, Melamud A, Lieskovsky G. Complications of thoracoabdominal retroperitoneal lymph node dissection. J Urol 1982;127(6):1107–10.

47. Fadel E, Court B, Chapelier AR, et al. One-stage approach for retroperitoneal and mediastinal metastatic testicular tumor resection. Ann Thorac Surg 2000;69(6):1717–21.

48. Djaladat H, Movassaghi K, Ahmadi H, et al. Mesenteric lymphadenopathy in testicular germ cell tumor. Urology 2014;83(3):e7–8.

49. Jacob JM, Mehan R, Beck SD, et al. Management of pelvic metastases in patients with testicular cancer. Urology 2017;102:159–63.

50. Alanee SR, Carver BS, Feldman DR, et al. Pelvic lymph node dissection in patients treated for testis cancer: the Memorial Sloan Kettering Cancer Center experience. Urology 2016;95:128–31.

51. Sago AL, Ball TP, Novicki DE. Complications of retroperitoneal lymphadenectomy. Urology 1979;13(3):241–3.

52. Staubitz WJ, Early KS, Magoss IV, et al. Surgical management of testis tumor. J Urol 1974;111(2):205–9.

53. Subramanian VS, Nguyen CT, Stephenson AJ, et al. Complications of open primary and post-chemotherapy retroperitoneal lymph node dissection for testicular cancer. Urol Oncol 2010;28(5):504–9.

54. Pettus JA, Carver BS, Masterson T, et al. Preservation of ejaculation in patients undergoing nerve-sparing postchemotherapy retroperitoneal lymph node dissection for metastatic testicular cancer. Urology 2009;73(2):328–31 [discussion: 331–2].

55. Faria EF, Neves HS, Dauster B, et al. Laparoscopic retroperitoneal lymph node dissection as a safe procedure for postchemotherapy residual mass in testicular cancer. J Laparoendosc Adv Surg Tech A 2018;28(2):168–73.

56. Steiner H, Leonhartsberger N, Stoehr B, et al. Postchemotherapy laparoscopic retroperitoneal lymph node dissection for low-volume, stage II, nonseminomatous germ cell tumor: first 100 patients. Eur Urol 2013;63(6):1013–7.

57. Cheney SM, Andrews PE, Leibovich BC, et al. Robot-assisted retroperitoneal lymph node dissection: technique and initial case series of 18 patients. BJU Int 2015;115(1):114–20.

58. Kamel MH, Littlejohn N, Cox M, et al. Post-chemotherapy robotic retroperitoneal lymph node dissection: institutional experience. J Endourol 2016;30(5):510–9.

59. Syan-Bhanvadia S, Bazargani ST, Clifford TG, et al. Midline extraperitoneal approach to retroperitoneal lymph node dissection in testicular cancer: minimizing surgical morbidity. Eur Urol 2017;72(5):814–20.

Indications for Surgery in Disseminated Seminoma

Phillip Martin Pierorazio, MD, Michael Janney Biles, MD

KEYWORDS

• Seminoma • RPLND • Radiotherapy

KEY POINTS

• Seminoma is commonly diagnosed in young men, and it has therefore become a disease of long-term survivors.
• As the late toxic effects of radiation and chemotherapy are better understood, it is becoming imperative to focus management advancements on reducing exposure to toxic agents.
• Retroperitoneal lymph node dissection (RPLND) currently is indicated as a salvage procedure in postchemotherapy patients with residual masses.
• Primary RPLND currently being is explored further in patients with clinical stage (CS) IIA and CSIIB disease in 2 prospective studies, Surgery in Early Metastatic Seminoma and Trial to Evaluate Progression Free Survival with Primary Retroperitoneal Lymph-Node Dissection (pRPLND) Only in Patients with Seminomatous Testicular Germ Cell Tumors with Clinical Stage IIA/B, which are expected to conclude in 2020 and 2021, respectively.

INTRODUCTION

Testicular cancer is the most common malignancy of young men aged 15 to 44 years old in the United States. Seminoma accounts for approximately 52% to 56% of germ cell tumors, of which there were an estimated 9000 new cases in the United States in 2018.[1,2] In general, seminoma has a favorable course and pathophysiology. Men with seminoma typically present at an early stage with 85% of patients presenting with clinical stage (CS) I disease, 10% with CSII disease, and 5% with CSIII disease. Men with CSI seminoma have a low incidence of occult metastasis (10%–20%), particularly in comparison to men with CSI nonseminomatous germ cell tumor (NSGCT) (15%–50%).[3] Patterns for metastasis in seminoma are reliable and reproducible, initially traveling via lymphatic systems to the retroperitoneum prior to hematogenous dissemination to the lungs or other viscera. Seminoma is sensitive to both platin-based chemotherapy and radiotherapy

(RT). The combination of a predictable metastatic progression and radiation sensitivity results in a 1% to 4% risk of systemic relapse after treatment of the retroperitoneum with RT, highlighting the effectiveness of treating early-stage (CSI and CSIIA/B) seminoma with locoregional therapy.[1] Most men with early-stage disease who recur on surveillance or after RT are cured with salvage chemotherapy.[4] Therefore, seminoma can be treated successfully with extirpative surgery, radiation, or chemotherapy, offering numerous options for oncologic control. As multidisciplinary treatments for testicular cancer have advanced and most men are cured of their disease, greater emphasis is placed on survivorship, which is particularly important in this young patient population. New efforts are being explored to develop progressive risk stratification models to optimize management approaches, thereby minimizing treatment related side effects and long-term toxicity, while not compromising cancer survival outcomes.

Disclosure Statement: The author has nothing to disclose.
Department of Urology, Brady Urological Institute, Johns Hopkins Hospital, 600 North Wolfe Street, Park 217, Baltimore, MD 21287-0005, USA
E-mail address: philpierorazio@jhmi.edu

CLINICAL STAGE I

Most patients with seminoma (85%) present with CSI local disease, with no evidence of metastases. Per National Comprehensive Cancer Network (NCCN) guidelines, management options for CSI disease include surveillance, single-agent carboplatin, or RT (20 Gy), although surveillance is the preferred recommendation for most patients.[5] Nevertheless, each treatment paradigm has unique benefits and risks.

Surveillance is the preferred treatment option for patients with CSI seminoma according to NCCN and European Association of Urology guidelines.[5,6] The supporting evidence demonstrates that a majority of men with CSI are cured with orchiectomy alone, and patients who relapse with good risk disease are able to be salvaged with chemotherapy. This practice minimizes unnecessary treatments (70%–80% of patients currently are overtreated), reducing treatment-related morbidity, while maintaining a 5-year cancer-specific survival approaching 100%. The major limitation of surveillance is that it has the highest risk of relapse, with associated anxiety for some patients. The 5-year disease-free survival (DFS) in surveillance is 88%, compared with 98% in patients receiving single-agent carboplatinum or RT.[7] Relapses occur in the retroperitoneum in 84% to 100% of recurrences.[8] The median time to recurrence is 14 months, although late recurrences are not uncommon, with 5% of patients recurring after 5 years.[9,10] Lastly, when relapses do occur, treatment requires more intensive salvage therapies than what is used during adjuvant treatment.

RT also has excellent oncologic outcomes, with a less than 1% in field recurrence rate and a 1% to 6% overall recurrence rate. In a randomized phase III trial comparing carboplatinum to RT, the 4-year relapse-free survival (RFS) rates were comparable (RT RFS 96.7% vs carboplatinum RFS 97.7%).[11]

Risk-stratified approaches have been developed to better determine patient populations that are appropriate for either surveillance or adjuvant treatments in an effort to minimize overtreating patients. Identified factors associated with increased risk include

- Tumor size greater than 4 cm (13.6% 5-year risk of recurrence)
- Rete testis invasion (20% 5-year risk of recurrence)

Patients without either risk factor have a decreased risk of recurrence with a 4.8% 5-year risk of recurrence.[7] Utilizing risk stratification may better identify appropriate candidates for surveillance instead of adjuvant treatments to reduce

toxic side effects; however, the risk-adapted approach to the management of stage I seminoma has yet to be validated or widely accepted outside the Spanish Germ Cell Cancer Group experience.[7]

CLINICAL STAGE IIA AND CLINICAL STAGE IIB

Patients with CSIIA or CSIIB disease, who comprise approximately 15% to 20% of seminoma patients, traditionally have been treated with either RT to the para-aortic and ipsilateral iliac lymph nodes or primary chemotherapy (3 cycles bleomycin/etoposide/cisplatin [BEP] or 4 cycles etoposide/cisplatin). RT has excellent outcomes with long-term DFS in CSIIA of 92% to 100% and 87% to 90% in CSIIB. Almost all relapses are cured with chemotherapy, leading to a disease-specific survival approaching 100%.[1,12,13] Induction chemotherapy is equally effective, with a 5-year RFS of 90% and overall survival of 90% to 95%.[1,14,15] Chemotherapy typically is recommended over RT for patients with bulky masses greater than 3 cm or multiple retroperitoneal masses, given the lower efficacy of RT in these patients.

CLINICAL STAGE IIC AND CLINICAL STAGE III

Patients with CSIIC and CSIII are considered to have systemic disease and receive induction chemotherapy per NCCN guidelines, with the specific regimen and number of cycles determined by risk status. As previously mentioned, seminoma is particularly chemosensitive. In good-risk patients, which includes all metastatic patients except those with nonpulmonary visceral metastases, complete radiographic responses range from 70% to 90%, and the 5-year overall survival is 91% after 3 cycles of BEP chemotherapy.[16,17] In intermediate-risk patients, 4 cycles of BEP or etoposide (VP-16)/ifosfamide/cisplatin are used to achieve a progression-free survival of 75% and 5-year overall survival of 79%.[1]

SURGERY FOR ADVANCED SEMINOMA

As discussed previously, men with advanced seminoma (CSIIC and CSIII) are treated for systemic disease with induction chemotherapy. Residual masses commonly are found after treatment of disseminated seminoma with primary chemotherapy. Approximately 60% to 80% of patients have postchemotherapy masses detected on imaging.[18] Most of these residual masses (60%), however, resolve spontaneously in the following 12 months to 18 months. Histologic examination of masses that do not resolve reveals that 90% are composed of necrotic tissue and only 10% represent viable malignancy. In total, approximately 15% to 20% of patients with advanced seminoma relapse after induction chemotherapy, including 10% of patients who initially had a complete response.[1,18–20] Men who have persistent disease or who recur after treatment of advanced disease have a guarded prognosis and can be challenging to manage.

The management of residual masses in this setting is controversial. In the short term, most patients undergo surveillance, given the low likelihood of residual malignancy, relatively high salvage rate with second-line chemotherapy, and high morbidity of postchemotherapy retroperitoneal lymph node dissection (RPLND) in seminomatous disease. The size of the mass, tumor markers, and fludeoxyglucose-PET scans are used to predict which residual masses harbor viable malignancy and need further treatment. Rising tumor markers or a growing mass on serial imaging is indicative of progressive disease and managed with salvage chemotherapy or RPLND. In its absence, tumor size generally guides recommendations, although the data analyzing size as a predictor of malignancy are controversial. Masses less than 3 cm with normal serum markers have a 0% to 4% risk of containing malignancy, and surveillance typically is recommended.[5,18,20,21] Per NCCN guidelines, masses greater than 3 cm with normal serum markers require a PET scan. If the scan is negative, surveillance is recommended. If the scan is positive, surgical resection of the residual mass or second-line chemotherapy is recommended.[5] This recommendation is based on the SEMPET trial, which demonstrated that PET scans were more accurate than CT scans in distinguishing between residual masses harboring persistent seminoma versus fibrosis. In this study, PET had an 80% sensitivity, 100% specificity, 100% positive predictive value, and 96% negative predictive value. In masses greater than 3 cm, the sensitivity improved to 100%.[21] A follow-up study, however, revealed promising but imperfect results. In this study, the sensitivity and negative predictive value were 100%, but the positive predictive value was only 67%. This suggests that one-third of patients who have a positive PET scan will undergo unnecessary surgical resections.[22]

Within the first 6 months to 12 months after induction chemotherapy for advanced seminoma, the authors favors a cautious surveillance protocol with tumor markers and PET imaging. Although tumor markers normalize rapidly with chemotherapy, imaging findings evolve over a longer duration. Initial PET CT imaging after chemotherapy may indicate a large and/or PET-avid mass. Over subsequent images, the mass may continue to decrease in size and decrease in PET avidity. Therefore, with normal serum tumor markers, an initial PET CT with a residual mass that has decreased in size should not trigger reflex additional therapy because the mass may continue to decrease in size with subsequent imaging. The author makes similar recommendations for masses that are PET avid but decreased in size in the setting of negative tumor markers. PET avidity will evolve and likely decrease over time. Present but decreasing PET avidity is a sign of response to chemotherapy. Multidisciplinary review of imaging and discussion among providers with germ cell tumor experience can determine findings suspicious for viable malignancy. Elevated and/or rising serum tumor markers, growing masses, and increasing PET avidity are indicative of viable germ cell tumor.

For residual masses indicative of viable germ cell tumor on imaging, the decision regarding salvage chemotherapy or RPLND involves a nuanced discussion of risks and benefits. Postchemotherapy RPLND in patients with disseminated seminoma is technically challenging due to the intense desmoplastic reaction associated with chemotherapy. Dense fibrosis and obliterated tissue planes can result in grossly incomplete resections or retroperitoneal recurrences due to microscopic disease left behind despite resection of all visible disease. Complete surgical resections after chemotherapy are achieved in only 60% to 74% of patients.[18–20] Small, older studies have demonstrated favorable survival in postchemotherapy patients with residual retroperitoneal disease managed with RPLND.[19,23] A more recent study, however, evaluating the largest group of postchemotherapy patients with viable seminoma managed with RPLND was less optimistic. It found the 5-year cancer-specific survival significantly lower, at 54%, with a mean post-RPLND survival of 7 months. The RFS was only 25%, and of these patients half required additional chemotherapy. In this study, 75% of patients experienced either an incomplete resection or post-RPLND recurrence, of which 70% recurred in the retroperitoneum.[24] The data suggest that viable chemorefractory seminoma is particularly difficult to control with local treatment. Postchemotherapy RPLND is technically demanding, and a minority of patients achieve a durable cure, likely due to microscopically incomplete resections.

The technical challenges of performing postchemotherapy RPLND also lead to increased morbidity, although it is acceptable in carefully selected patients. Mosharafa and colleagues[25] found that 38% of patients undergoing postchemotherapy RPLND for seminoma required additional intraoperative procedures. These procedures most commonly included nephrectomies (26%), inferior vena caval resections (9%), arterial grafts (5%), small bowel resections (5%), and hepatic resections (3%). Postoperative complications also are common, occurring in 25% of patients. The most common complications were of pulmonary origin, such as atelectasis, acute respiratory distress syndrome, and pleural effusion, but other common complications included ascites and wound infections.

If a resected residual mass specimen is positive for viable seminoma, second-line chemotherapy is recommended, although small volume of viable tumor also may be observed.[5] If the mass is negative for seminoma, the patient may undergo surveillance. Rarely, teratoma can be discovered in the retroperitoneum of men with pure seminoma at orchiectomy indicating a burned-out nonseminomatous component of their primary. These patients should subsequently be managed as an NSGCT. Also, men who relapse or fail to respond to chemotherapy or radiation are at higher risk of harboring a nonseminomatous element in their metastatic sites.[26]

Salvage chemotherapy is an alternative to RPLND. In patients treated with second-line vinblastine/ifosfamide/cisplatin, 83% achieved an initial complete response, although 40% of those patients developed a recurrence, with a long-term survival of 54%.[27] High-dose chemotherapy (HDCT) also has been evaluated for salvage therapy. Studies have shown that 90% of patients receiving HDCT as second-line treatment achieved a durable RFS. If used as third-line or fourth-line therapy, however, the complete response rate decreases to 67%.[28]

Given the effectiveness of second-line chemotherapy or HDCT for refractory or recurrent setting, the author favors RPLND only in select settings. In general, isolated masses that do not circumferentially involve great vessels or renal vasculature may be resected with reasonable risk of morbidity. Circumferential vessel involvement is predictive of vascular reconstruction, and loss of a renal unit may preclude future chemotherapy due to decreases in glomerular filtration rate.[29,30] RPLND, in general, is technically easier in smaller masses (especially when a plane is visible between the mass and vasculature) and oncologically more effective in smaller masses. RPLND is less effective in men with elevated tumor markers, and salvage RPLND should be used only cautiously in men with low-level human chorionic gonadotropin elevations.[23,31] Resection of other distant sites of disease (lung, liver, mediastinum, and so forth) should be considered only when an oncologic plan is clear (biopsy-proved viable malignancy) and surgical

resection poses little risk of major morbidity. Therefore, the author recommends the indications for these surgeries be reviewed in multidisciplinary settings with referral to or consultation with germ cell tumor centers of excellence.

SURGERY IN CLINICAL STAGE IIA AND CLINICAL STAGE IIB SEMINOMA

The modern approach of multimodal therapy in managing patients with seminoma resulted in excellent oncologic outcomes. Understanding testicular cancer as a disease of young survivors with increasing knowledge regarding the burden of morbidity for men receiving chemotherapy and/or radiation, strategies continue to develop to reduce treatment-related morbidity without compromising survival. Efforts include increasing utilization of surveillance in CSI disease, decreasing radiation dosage, limiting the fields of radiation, and single-agent chemotherapy regimens. Additionally, RPLND is reconsidered primary treatment of low-volume metastatic seminoma to the retroperitoneum.[32]

CONSIDERATIONS OF LONG-TERM TOXICITY

This article does not focus on the toxicities associated with chemotherapy and radiation; however, they are discussed briefly to better understand the rationale for re-evaluating extirpative surgery in early-stage (CSIIA and CSIIB), disseminated seminoma.

External beam radiation treatment (RT) and systemic chemotherapy are the standard of care for patients with seminoma and limited retroperitoneal lymphadenopathy, with excellent oncologic outcomes. There is growing evidence, however, that these treatment modalities are associated with significant toxicity and cumulative burden of morbidity.[33] The short-term side effects can include alopecia, bowel irritability, fatigue, nausea, vomiting, mucositis, myelosuppression, or sleep disorders.[34] The late toxicities of chemotherapy and radiation are of growing concern to both patients and providers. Patients with seminoma treated with chemotherapy and/or RT are at increased risk of developing secondary solid malignancies, hematologic malignancies, and cardiovascular disease, particularly when treated at a younger age.[35–37] Additionally, there are higher rates of pulmonary disease, nephrotoxicity, ototoxicity, infertility, and peripheral neuropathy.[38–42]

In patients diagnosed with seminoma and treated by age 35 years, the cumulative risk of developing a solid malignancy within the next

40 years is 36%, in comparison to 23% for the general population (relative risk = 1.9; 95% CI, 1.8–2.1). In long-term survivors of testicular cancer, patients who received chemotherapy were also at increased risk of coronary artery disease (5.7-fold; 95% CI, 1.9–17.1), myocardial infarction (3.1-fold; 95% CI, 1.2–7.7), and atherosclerotic disease (hazard ratio [HR] 2.6; 95% CI, 1.1–5.9) in comparison to patients treated with surgery alone.[43] RT as monotherapy is associated with increased prevalence of diabetes (odds ratio 2.3; 95% CI, 1.5–3.7) as well as atherosclerotic disease (HR 2.3; 95% CI, 1.04–5.3), and combination RT with chemotherapy has been shown to have additive or synergistic effects.[43] The combination of chemotherapy and RT leads to a cumulative risk of both secondary cancer and cardiovascular disease in comparison to either modality alone.[44] Most importantly, late toxicities from these treatment modalities have been linked to decreased overall survival.[45,46]

RATIONALE FOR RETROPERITONEAL LYMPH NODE DISSECTION IN EARLY-STAGE SEMINOMA

RPLND is a well-established, effective treatment of early-stage and advanced NSGCT, and this experience may be translatable to seminoma management. NCCN NSGCT guidelines recommend RPLND as possible primary treatment of CSI and CSII disease, as postchemotherapy management of patients with CSII or CSIII disease with a complete response, or as salvage therapy in patients with a residual mass after primary chemotherapy.[5] In particular, RPLND has been an effective primary treatment strategy in patients with CSII NSGCT. It is curative in most patients, and relapses can be salvaged with chemotherapy, resulting in overall survival rates approaching 100%. Although data are limited, RPLND may offer a similarly effective approach for men with limited volume CSII seminoma as an alternative to chemotherapy or radiation.

The rationale for RPLND in the management of low-volume CSII seminoma is based on several established observations. First, seminoma metastasizes in a reliable pattern via the lymphatic system to the retroperitoneum. Therefore, RPLND may offer more accurate staging for men with early-stage seminoma than in NSGCT, where there is a higher likelihood of hematogenous dissemination to the lung or viscera without retroperitoneal lymphadenopathy. In NSGCT, pathologic stage often is different from CS. In men with CSI NSCGT undergoing surveillance, approximately 20% to 30% of patients are found to have occult metastases to the retroperitoneum at RPLND, and in CSII disease, approximately 6% to 35% of patients are down-staged to CSI at RPLND.[47,48] RPLND provides accurate staging, which is pivotal for developing appropriate surveillance and treatment strategies.

Second, early-stage seminoma is effectively managed by retroperitoneal control. Numerous studies demonstrate the efficacy of primary RT for the treatment of CSI and CSII seminoma. Dog-leg RT to the retroperitoneum and ipsilateral pelvis previously was considered the standard of care in CSI seminoma. In this population, progression-free probability after primary RT is 95% to 97%, with an in-field recurrence of less than 1%.[1,49,50] Primary RT also is effective in CSII disease. Long-term DRF ranges from 92% to 100% in CSIIA disease, and 87% to 90% in CSIIB disease, with in-field recurrences of 0% to 2% and 0% to 7%, respectively.[12–14,51] Relapses in both CSI and CSII disease almost always are cured with chemotherapy, with disease-specific survival approaching 100%.[1] Although data are limited, a study by Warszawski and Schmücking[48] indicates that in-field, retroperitoneal recurrences were similar for men undergoing RPLND or RT.

Lastly, the risks of primary RPLND are realized in the perioperative period and the long-term complications are minimal in comparison to chemotherapy or radiation. The best data regarding complications associated with RPLND indicate an overall complication rate of 10% to 24% for primary RPLND and 20% to 30% for postchemotherapy RPLND and a major complication rate of 5% at centers of excellence.[52] Complications include symptomatic lymphocele (1% to 2%), chylous ascites (2%), ileus (2% to 20%), small bowel obstruction (2%), wound infection (4%), postoperative hemorrhage (0% to 1%), and pulmonary embolism (<1% in chemotherapy-naïve patients).[52,53] Advancements in surgical technique, particularly at high-volume centers, such as template dissections, nerve-sparing operations, and laparoscopic or robotic approaches, have led to decreased morbidity associated with the procedure, such as prevention of retrograde ejaculation (antegrade ejaculation preserved in almost 100% of patients), decreased blood loss, and shorter hospitalization.[54,55]

RPLND for early-stage seminoma may offer effective retroperitoneal control, minimizing patient exposure to radiation and chemotherapy and reducing long-term toxicity. In comparison to RPLND for early-stage NSGCT, it provides better staging (less skip metastases), comparable locoregional control, and similar short-term toxicity profiles.

DATA SUPPORTING RETROPERITONEAL LYMPH NODE DISSECTION FOR EARLY-STAGE SEMINOMA

There have been several retrospective studies evaluating RPLND as primary treatment of seminoma. In 1997, Warszawski and Schmücking[48] reported the first study, which included 63 patients with CSI or CSII disease who underwent RPLND. In patients with CSI, 17.5% were found to have occult retroperitoneal disease, and 6.3% of patients with CSII were down-staged. Furthermore, RPLND provided excellent local control, comparable RT, but with decreasing effectiveness with increased nodal disease. The recurrence rates for CSI, CSIIA, DSIIB, and CSIIC were 7%, 0%, 67%, and 40%, respectively. There were also no in-field recurrences for CSI and CSIIA disease after RPLND.[48] A second, small retrospective study reported by Mezvrishvili and Managadze[56] evaluated 10 patients with CSI and 4 patients with CSIIA disease who underwent RPLND. At a mean follow-up of 56 months, there were no recurrences. A third study of 4 patients, 3 with CSIIA seminoma and 1 with CSIIC, who underwent RPLND, also found no recurrences at a median follow-up of 25 months.[57] Lastly, the fourth study, evaluating 11 patients with CSIIA or CSIIB seminoma who underwent RPLND, reported a 36% recurrence rate at 18 months. All were salvaged with RT and/or chemotherapy.[58] In total, 92 patients with CSI to CSIIC were treated primarily with RPLND, with a 14% recurrence rate.

More recent population-based studies also have demonstrated RPLND has similar efficacy in comparison to RT as a form of regional control. Analyzing the Surveillance, Epidemiology, and End Results Program registries of 17,681 patients with CSI or CSII disease, it has been demonstrated that RPLND is used in 1.3% of patients with CSI disease and 10.6% in CSII disease and that RPLND has a overall survival and cancer-specific survival comparable to RT.[30]

ONGOING CLINICAL TRIALS

Recent efforts to reduce the long-term toxicity of chemotherapy and RT resulted in a resurgence in the use of RPLND as primary treatment of patients with disseminated seminoma to the retroperitoneum. Currently, there are 2 active prospective trials evaluating RPLND in metastatic seminoma, which may change the future treatment paradigm.

The Surgery in Early Metastatic Seminoma (SEMS) trial is a multi-institutional phase II trial in the United States, evaluating primary RPLND for patients with seminoma with retroperitoneal metastases. Inclusion criteria include 1 to 2 retroperitoneal lymph nodes between 1 cm and 3 cm in size that were present at diagnosis or the result of recurrence. The trial was started in August 2015 and currently is still recruiting patients, with a completion date set for August 2020. The primary outcome is RFS at 2 years. Secondary outcomes include RFS at 5 years, percent of patients who can avoid RT or chemotherapy, and RPLND complication rates.[32,59] This trial hopes to demonstrate that RPLND has a high cure rate in patients with nonbulky retroperitoneal lymphadenopathy and can lead to the avoidance of adjuvant treatments with chemotherapy or RT.

The Trial to Evaluate Progression Free Survival with Primary Retroperitoneal Lymph-Node Dissection (pRPLND) Only in Patients with Seminomatous Testicular Germ Cell Tumors with Clinical Stage IIA/B (PRIMETEST) is a promising trial out of Germany. Patients with CSIIA/B disease or patients with recurrence after single-dose carboplatin chemotherapy will undergo either an open or robotically assisted laparoscopic modified template RPLND. The primary endpoint is progression-free survival at 3 years. Secondary endpoints include overall survival, complication rates, quality-of-life metrics, and retrograde ejaculation rate. The study will be completed in June 2021. PRIMETEST evaluates RPLND in patients with bulkier lymphadenopathy than the SEMS trial and hypothesizes that surgery with a single dose of chemotherapy for systemic control will lead to good oncologic control and reduce exposure to full-course chemotherapy regimens, thereby minimizing long-term toxicity.[32,58]

Primary RPLND is an effective treatment strategy in treating seminoma patients with retroperitoneal disease based on retrospective studies. The SEMS and PRIMETEST trials are the first prospective trials to evaluate this strategy and may be pivotal in expanding the role of RPLND in patients with disseminated seminoma.

SUMMARY

Seminoma is a highly curable disease given its sensitivity to both chemotherapy and RT. It is commonly diagnosed in young men, and it has therefore become a disease of long-term survivors. As the late toxic effects of radiation and chemotherapy are better understood, it is becoming imperative to focus management advancements on reducing exposure to toxic agents. RPLND currently is indicated as a salvage procedure in postchemotherapy patients with residual masses. In this population, oncologic control is difficult to achieve with either

RPLND or chemotherapy, and RPLND is technically challenging with significant morbidity. Based on promising retrospective data, the role of RPLND may be expanded in seminoma treatment to include primary treatment of patients with limited retroperitoneal disease. Primary RPLND currently is being further explored in patients with CSIIA and CSIIB disease in 2 prospective studies, SEMS and PRIMETEST, which are expected to still accurate, conclude in 2020 and 2021, respectively. The results of these trials may be paramount in changing the current treatment paradigm of patients with disseminated seminoma, with the primary goal of minimizing toxicity associated with chemotherapy and RT, while preserving oncologic outcomes.

REFERENCES

1. Wein AJ, Kavoussi LR, Partin AW, et al. Campbell-walsh urology. Philadelphia: Elsevier; 2016. https://doi.org/10.1007/s13398-014-0173-7.2.

2. SEER Database Cancer Statistics - Testicular Cancer.

3. Powles TB, Bhardwa J, Shamash J, et al. The changing presentation of germ cell tumours of the testis between 1983 and 2002. BJU Int 2005. https://doi.org/10.1111/j.1464-410X.2005.05504.x.

4. Kollmannsberger C, Tandstad T, Bedard PL, et al. Patterns of relapse in patients with clinical stage I testicular cancer managed with active surveillance. J Clin Oncol 2015. https://doi.org/10.1200/JCO.2014.56.2116.

5. NCCN Guidelines - Testicular Cancer. NCCN Guidelines (2018).

6. Albers P, Albrecht W, Algaba F, et al. EAU guidelines on testicular cancer: 2011 update. Eur Urol 2011. https://doi.org/10.1016/j.eururo.2011.05.038.

7. Aparicio J, Maroto P, del Muro XG, et al. Risk-adapted treatment in clinical stage I testicular seminoma: The third Spanish Germ Cell Cancer Group study. J Clin Oncol 2011. https://doi.org/10.1200/JCO.2011.36.0503.

8. Choo R, Thomas G, Woo T, et al. Long-term outcome of postorchiectomy surveillance for Stage I testicular seminoma. Int J Radiat Oncol Biol Phys 2005. https://doi.org/10.1016/j.ijrobp.2004.06.209.

9. Mortensen MS, Lauritsen J, Kier MG, et al. Late relapses in stage I testicular cancer patients on surveillance. Eur Urol 2016. https://doi.org/10.1016/j.eururo.2016.03.016.

10. Chung P, Parker C, Panzarella T, et al. Surveillance in stage I testicular seminoma—risk of late relapse. Can J Urol 2002;9:1637–40.

11. Oliver RTD, Mason MD, Mead GM, et al. Radiotherapy versus single-dose carboplatin in adjuvant treatment of stage I seminoma: a randomised trial. Lancet 2005. https://doi.org/10.1016/S0140-6736(05)66984-X.

12. Zagars GK, Pollack A. Radiotherapy for stage II testicular seminoma. Int J Radiat Oncol Biol Phys 2001. https://doi.org/10.1016/S0360-3016(01)01701-1.

13. Classen J, Schmidberger H, Meisner C, et al. Radiotherapy for stages IIA/B testicular seminoma: final report of a prospective multicenter clinical trial. J Clin Oncol 2003. https://doi.org/10.1200/JCO.2003.06.065.

14. Chung PW, Gospodarowicz MK, Panzarella T, et al. Stage II testicular seminoma: patterns of recurrence and outcome of treatment. Eur Urol 2004. https://doi.org/10.1063/1.88185.

15. Garcia-del-Muro X, Maroto P, Gumà J, et al. Chemotherapy as an alternative to radiotherapy in the treatment of stage IIA and IIB testicular seminoma: a Spanish germ cell cancer group study. J Clin Oncol 2008. https://doi.org/10.1200/JCO.2007.15.9103.

16. Mencel PJ, Motzer RJ, Mazumdar M, et al. Advanced seminoma: treatment results, survival, and prognostic factors in 142 patients. J Clin Oncol 1994. https://doi.org/10.1200/JCO.1994.12.1.120.

17. Gholam D, Fizazi K, Terrier-Lacombe MJ, et al. Advanced seminoma - treatment results and prognostic factors for survival after first-line, cisplatin-based chemotherapy and for patients with recurrent disease: a single-institution experience in 145 patients. Cancer 2003. https://doi.org/10.1002/cncr.11574.

18. Fléchon A, Bompas E, Biron P, et al. Management of post-chemotherapy residual masses in advanced seminoma. J Urol 2002. https://doi.org/10.1016/S0022-5347(05)64275-9.

19. Ravi R, Ong J, Oliver RT, et al. The management of residual masses after chemotherapy in metastatic seminoma. BJU Int 1999. https://doi.org/10.1046/j.1464-410X.1999.00974.x.

20. Herr HW, Sheinfeld J, Puc HS, et al. Surgery for a post-chemotherapy residual mass in seminoma. J Urol 1997. https://doi.org/10.1016/S0022-5347(01)65065-1.

21. De Santis M, Becherer A, Bokemeyer C, et al. 2-18fluoro-deoxy-D-glucose positron emission tomography is a reliable predictor for viable tumor in postchemotherapy seminoma: an update of the prospective multicentric SEMPET trial. J Clin Oncol 2004. https://doi.org/10.1200/JCO.2004.07.188.

22. Lewis DA, Tann M, Kesler K, et al. Positron emission tomography scans in postchemotherapy seminoma patients with residual masses: a retrospective review from Indiana University Hospital. J Clin Oncol 2006. https://doi.org/10.1200/JCO.2006.08.1737.

23. Puc HS, Heelan R, Mazumdar M, et al. Management of residual mass in advanced seminoma: results and recommendations from the Memorial

Sloan-Kettering Cancer Center. J Clin Oncol 1996. https://doi.org/10.1200/JCO.1996.14.2.454.

24. Rice KR, Beck SD, Bihrle R, et al. Survival analysis of pure seminoma at post-chemotherapy retroperitoneal lymph node dissection. J Urol 2014. https://doi.org/10.1016/j.juro.2014.04.097.

25. Mosharafa AA, Foster RS, Leibovich BC, et al. Is post-chemotherapy resection of seminomatous elements associated with higher acute morbidity? J Urol 2003. https://doi.org/10.1097/01.ju.0000060121.33899.4b.

26. Bredael JJ, Vugrin D, Whitmore WF. Autopsy findings in 154 patients with germ cell tumors of the testis. Cancer 1982;50(3):548.

27. Miller KD, Loehrer PJ, Gonin R, et al. Salvage chemotherapy with vinblastine, ifosfamide, and cisplatin in recurrent seminoma. J Clin Oncol 1997. https://doi.org/10.1200/JCO.1997.15.4.1427.

28. Agarwala AK, Perkins SM, Abonour R, et al. Salvage chemotherapy with high-dose carboplatin and etoposide with peripheral blood stem cell transplant in patients with relapsed pure seminoma. Am J Clin Oncol 2011. https://doi.org/10.1097/COC.0b013e3181d6b518.

29. Johnson SC, Smith ZL, Nottingham C, et al. Clinical and radiographic predictors of great vessel resection or reconstruction during retroperitoneal lymph node dissection for testicular cancer. Urology 2019. https://doi.org/10.1016/j.urology.2018.08.028.

30. Patel HD, Joice GA, Schwen ZR, et al. Retroperitoneal lymph node dissection for testicular seminomas: population-based practice and survival outcomes. World J Urol 2018. https://doi.org/10.1007/s00345-017-2099-0.

31. Cary C, Pedrosa JA, Jacob J, et al. Outcomes of postchemotherapy retroperitoneal lymph node dissection following high-dose chemotherapy with stem cell transplantation. Cancer 2015. https://doi.org/10.1002/cncr.29678.

32. Hu B, Daneshmand S. Retroperitoneal lymph node dissection as primary treatment for metastatic seminoma. Adv Urol 2018. https://doi.org/10.1155/2018/7978958.

33. Kerns SL, Fung C, Monahan PO, et al. Cumulative burden of morbidity among testicular cancer survivors after standard cisplatin-based chemotherapy: a multi-institutional study. J Clin Oncol 2018. https://doi.org/10.1200/JCO.2017.77.0735.

34. Gil T, Sideris S, Aoun F, et al. Testicular germ cell tumor: short and long-term side effects of treatment among survivors. Mol Clin Oncol 2016;5(3):258–64.

35. Travis LB, Fosså SD, Schonfeld SJ, et al. Second cancers among 40 576 testicular cancer patients: focus on long-term survivors. J Natl Cancer Inst 2005. https://doi.org/10.1093/jnci/dji278.

36. Kollmannsberger C, Hartmann JT, Kanz L, et al. Therapy-related malignancies following treatment of germ cell cancer. Int J Cancer 1999;83(6):860–3.

37. Travis LB, Andersson M, Gospodarowicz M, et al. Treatment-associated leukemia following testicular cancer. J Natl Cancer Inst 2000. https://doi.org/10.1136/BMJ.J4859.

38. Vogelzang NJ, Torkelson JL, Kennedy BJ. Hypomagnesemia, renal dysfunction, and Raynaud's phenomenon in patients treated with cisplatin, vinblastine, and bleomycin. Cancer 1985;56(12):2765–70.

39. Fosså SD, Gilbert E, Dores GM, et al. Noncancer causes of death in survivors of testicular cancer. J Natl Cancer Inst 2007. https://doi.org/10.1093/jnci/djk111.

40. Haugnes HS, Bosl GJ, Boer H, et al. Long-term and late effects of germ cell testicular cancer treatment and implications for follow-up. J Clin Oncol 2012. https://doi.org/10.1200/JCO.2012.43.4431.

41. Nord C, Bjøro T, Ellingsen D, et al. Gonadal hormones in long-term survivors 10 years after treatment for unilateral testicular cancer. Eur Urol 2003. https://doi.org/10.1016/S0302-2838(03)00263-X.

42. Brydøy M, Fosså SD, Klepp O, et al. Paternity following treatment for testicular cancer. J Natl Cancer Inst 2005. https://doi.org/10.1093/jnci/dji339.

43. Haugnes HS, Wethal T, Aass N, et al. Cardiovascular risk factors and morbidity in long-term survivors of testicular cancer: a 20-year follow-up study. J Clin Oncol 2010. https://doi.org/10.1200/JCO.2010.29.9362.

44. Van Den Belt-Dusebout AW, de Wit R, Gietema JA, et al. Treatment-specific risks of second malignancies and cardiovascular disease in 5-year survivors of testicular cancer. J Clin Oncol 2007. https://doi.org/10.1200/JCO.2006.10.5296.

45. Zagars GK, Ballo MT, Lee AK, et al. Mortality after cure of testicular seminoma. J Clin Oncol 2004. https://doi.org/10.1200/JCO.2004.05.205.

46. Hanks GE, Peters T, Owen J. Seminoma of the testis: long term beneficial and deleterious results of radiation. Int J Radiat Oncol Biol Phys 1992. https://doi.org/10.1016/0360-3016(92)90475-W.

47. Yadav K. Retroperitoneal lymph node dissection: an update in testicular malignancies. Clin Transl Oncol 2017. https://doi.org/10.1007/s12094-017-1622-5.

48. Warszawski N, Schmücking M. Relapses in early-stage testicular seminoma: radiation therapy versus retroperitoneal lymphadenectomy. Scand J Urol Nephrol 1997. https://doi.org/10.3109/00365599709030619.

49. Warde P, Gospodarowicz MK, Panzarella T, et al. Stage I testicular seminoma: results of adjuvant irradiation and surveillance. J Clin Oncol 1995. https://doi.org/10.1200/JCO.1995.13.9.2255.

50. Tandstad T, Smaaland R, Solberg A, et al. Management of seminomatous testicular cancer: a

binational prospective population-based study from the Swedish Norwegian Testicular Cancer Study Group. J Clin Oncol 2011. https://doi.org/10.1200/JCO.2010.30.1044.

51. Chung PW, Warde PR, Panzarella T, et al. Appropriate radiation volume for stage IIA/B testicular seminoma. Int J Radiat Oncol Biol Phys 2003. https://doi.org/10.1016/S0360-3016(03)00011-7.

52. Subramanian VS, Nguyen CT, Stephenson AJ, et al. Complications of open primary and post-chemotherapy retroperitoneal lymph node dissection for testicular cancer. Urol Oncol 2010. https://doi.org/10.1016/j.urolonc.2008.10.026.

53. Heidenreich A, Albers P, Hartmann M, et al. Complications of primary nerve sparing retroperitoneal lymph node dissection for clinical stage I nonseminomatous germ cell tumors of the testis: experience of the German Testicular Cancer Study Group. J Urol 2003. https://doi.org/10.1097/01.ju.0000060960.18092.54.

54. Donohue JP, Thornhill JA, Foster RS, et al. Clinical stage B non-seminomatous germ cell testis cancer: The Indiana University experience (1965-1989) using routine primary retroperitoneal lymph node dissection. Eur J Cancer 1995. https://doi.org/10.1016/0959-8049(95)00330-L.

55. Pearce SM, Golan S, Gorin MA, et al. Safety and early oncologic effectiveness of primary robotic retroperitoneal lymph node dissection for nonseminomatous germ cell testicular cancer. Eur Urol 2017. https://doi.org/10.1016/j.eururo.2016.05.017.

56. Mezvrishvili Z, Managadze L. Retroperitoneal lymph node dissection for high-risk stage I and stage IIA seminoma. Int Urol Nephrol 2006. https://doi.org/10.1007/s11255-005-4793-x.

57. Hu B, Shah S, Shojaei S, et al. Retroperitoneal lymph node dissection as first-line treatment of node-positive seminoma. Clin Genitourin Cancer 2015. https://doi.org/10.1016/j.clgc.2015.01.002.

58. Lusch A, Gerbaulet L, Winter C, et al. Primary retroperitoneal lymph node dissection (RPLND) in stage IIA/B seminoma patients without adjuvant treatment: a phase II trial (PRIMETEST). J Urol 2017;197(4): e1044–5.

59. Retroperitoneal lymph node dissection in treating patients with testicular seminoma. Natl Libr Med 2017. Available at: ClinicalTrials.gov.

The Role of Robotic Retroperitoneal Lymph Node Dissection for Testis Cancer

Zachary Klaassen, MD, MSc[a,b],
Robert J. Hamilton, MD, MPH, FRCSC[c,d],*

KEYWORDS

- RPLND • Retroperitoneal lymph node dissection • Robotic • da Vinci • Testis cancer
- Testicular cancer

KEY POINTS

- Initial series of robotic retroperitoneal lymph node dissection (RPLND) have shown improved cosmesis, less blood loss, and decreased length of stay compared with historical open RPLND; however, long-term oncologic outcomes are still necessary.
- Our preference for performing robotic RPLND is via a transperitoneal approach with the patient in the supine position, thus facilitating a bilateral template dissection identical to that used in all our open procedures.
- Robotic RPLND should only be attempted by surgeons fluent in evidence-based testis cancer management algorithms, who have high-volume experience with open RPLND, a nuanced understanding of the retroperitoneum and its anatomic variance, and experience with dealing with intraoperative and postoperative complications.

INTRODUCTION

Retroperitoneal lymph node dissection (RPLND) for testicular germ cell malignancy remains a complex and potentially morbid procedure, particularly in the postchemotherapy setting. As supported by several guidelines, primary RPLND remains a treatment option for patients with high-risk clinical stage I[1] and clinical stage IIA nonseminomatous germ cell tumor (NSGCT).[2] RPLND has also been used in IIB disease but with increased relapse rates.[3] There is also a role for RPLND in patients relapsed on surveillance with retroperitoneal nodal disease only (stage IIA/B equivalent),[4] and in postchemotherapy residual masses greater than or equal to 1 cm. In seminoma, RPLND has traditionally been reserved for postchemotherapy residual retroperitoneal masses that are larger than 3 cm and PET avid; however, increasingly small case series have shown that primary RPLND may also have a role in stage II A/B seminoma.[5]

In an attempt to decrease morbidity and recovery after open RPLND, laparoscopic and more recently robotic RPLND series have been reported in the literature. This article discusses the current role of robotic RPLND, highlighting advantages

---

Disclosure: The authors have nothing to disclose.
a Division of Urology, Medical College of Georgia, Augusta University, 1120 15th Street, BA-8414, Augusta, GA 30912, USA; b Georgia Cancer Center, Augusta, GA, USA; c Division of Urology, University Health Network, 610 University Avenue – Suite 3-130, Toronto, Ontario M5G 2M9, Canada; d Princess Margaret Cancer Centre, Toronto, Ontario, Canada
* Corresponding author. 610 University Avenue – Suite 3-130, Toronto, Ontario M5G 2M9, Canada.
E-mail address: rob.hamilton@uhn.ca

Urol Clin N Am 46 (2019) 409–417
https://doi.org/10.1016/j.ucl.2019.04.009
0094-0143/19/© 2019 Elsevier Inc. All rights reserved.

and disadvantages of the procedure and appropriate indications for a minimally invasive approach.

EVOLUTION OF MINIMALLY INVASIVE RETROPERITONEAL LYMPH NODE DISSECTION

Laparoscopic RPLND was developed to provide staging information comparable with the open approach but with less morbidity and increased recovery time for the patient.[6] However, with experience, it evolved from a diagnostic procedure to one with therapeutic benefit in that patients with low-volume retroperitoneal disease were able to avoid adjuvant chemotherapy.

The first laparoscopic RPLND was described in 1992 by Rukstalis and Chodak[7] at the University of Chicago. They performed a laparoscopic modified bilateral RPLND for clinical stage I NSGCT, which took 510 minutes with minimal blood loss and a length of stay of 5 days. The lymph node yield was 28 (all negative) and the patient retained antegrade ejaculation; at 2-month follow-up he was without disease recurrence.

Over the next several years, subsequent case reports/series were published describing laparoscopic RPLND.[8–10] In 1994, Gerber and colleagues[11] published a multi-institutional series of 20 patients with NSGCT, noting an operative time of 6 hours, estimated blood loss of 250 mL, median lymph node yield of 14.5 lymph nodes, with most patients staying in hospital less than 3 days. Subsequently, Janetschek and colleagues[12] compared 29 consecutive patients undergoing laparoscopic (1992–1995) with 30 patients undergoing open RPLND (1988–1992) for clinical stage I NSGCT. Open RPLND was associated with more blood loss (38%), longer postoperative stay (10.6 days vs 4.0 days), and more complications. Since these initial reports, several centers have published durable long-term oncologic results[13–15] and described laparoscopic nerve-sparing techniques.[16] However, the widespread adoption of laparoscopic RPLND has been limited by several factors: (1) the complexity of the operation, with most series originating from centers of excellence with advanced laparoscopic surgeons[17,18]; (2) the liberal use of adjuvant chemotherapy for any positive lymph nodes found, thus rendering the view of the laparoscopic procedure more as staging rather than curative intent; (3) the uncertain oncologic efficacy of the procedure, because many series are populated with clinical stage I patients who may not harbor disease in their retroperitoneum.

With the adoption of the da Vinci robotic platform in the early 2000s for radical prostatectomy and partial nephrectomy, the same platform over the past decade has been used for robotic RPLND. The robotic approach has allowed greater dissemination of a minimally invasive approach secondary to several advantages, including enhanced vision with three-dimensional optics, magnification, improved dexterity and instrument precision, and ergonomic advantages allowing a more controlled and delicate dissection crucial for an RPLND. Specific advantages to robotic RPLND include (1) circumferential dissection around structures secondary to the wristed flexible instruments, (2) enhanced ability to control bleeding (ie, from lumbar vessels or the great vessels), and (3) access to nodal tissue posterior to the great vessels, which may be challenging with conventional laparoscopy.[6]

The first robotic RPLND was performed in 2006[19] at Geisinger Medical Center on an 18-year-old with a clinical stage IA NSGCT. The patient underwent a bilateral template robotic RPLND in 169 minutes of console time, with just 125 mL of estimated blood loss and was discharged in less than 48 hours. Since this time several additional reports have been published (**Table 1**),[6,20–25] including 1 multicenter cohort of 47 patients.[20]

In this study, 42 patients had clinical stage I disease and 5 clinical stage II. There was a median follow-up of 16 months (interquartile range, 9–23 months) with two-thirds of patients having more than 1 year of follow-up. The 2-year recurrence-free survival rate was 97% and, among 8 pathologic stage II patients, 5 received adjuvant chemotherapy and 3 were managed with surveillance. Among the 3 that did not receive adjuvant chemotherapy post-RPLND, no recurrence was noted at a median follow-up of 6 months. With the advent of the da Vinci Xi platform, there is additional feasibility to performing robotic RPLND, including performing the retroperitoneal and spermatic cord dissection without robot repositioning, as well as additional space for the bedside assistant secondary to the improved robotic arm reach with the Xi system.[6]

ROBOTIC RETROPERITONEAL LYMPH NODE DISSECTION TECHNIQUE

The authors believe strongly that, in adopting a robotic platform, open oncologic principles should not be compromised. That is, whatever the clinician's personal or institutional policy is regarding patient selection, template selection, nerve sparing, or use of adjuvant chemotherapy, none

Table 1
Clinical, demographic and outcomes data from case series/studies evaluating robotic retroperitoneal lymph node dissection

Variable	Cheney et al,[21] 2015	Harris et al,[22] 2015	Kamel et al,[24] 2016	Pearce et al,[20] 2017	Stepanian et al,[6] 2016	Singh et al,[25] 2017	Overs et al,[23] 2018
Sample size (n)	18	16	12	47	20	13	11
Mean age (y)	32	30 (median)	38	30 (median)	31	26 (median)	33 (median)
TNM Stage (n)							
I	10	14	0	42	11	0	0
II	7	2	6	5	6	3	10
III	1	0	6	0	3	10	1
Prior chemotherapy (n)	8	0	12	0	4	13	11
Mean operative time (min)	337	271 (median)	321	235 (median)	288	200 (median)	153 (median)
Mean EBL (mL)	172	75 (median)	893	50 (median)	125	120 (median)	120 (median)
Clavien-Dindo grade ≥ III complication	0	1	1	0	1	2	0
Mean LOS (d)	3.1	NR	3.5	1 (median)	1.5	4 (median)	3
Conversion (n)	3	1	1	1	0	0	0
Mean node yield	20	30 (median)	8	26 (median)	19.5 (median)	20 (median)	7 (median)
Mean follow-up (mo)	22	13.5 (median)	27	16 (median)	49 (median)	23 (median)	4
Retroperitoneal recurrence (n)	0	0	0	0	0	0	0

Abbreviations: EBL, estimated blood loss; LOS, length of stay; TNM, tumor-node-metastasis.
Adapted from Pal RP, Koupparis AJ. Expanding the indications of robotic surgery in urology: a systematic review of the literature. Arab J Urol 2018;16(3):275; with permission.

of these principles should be altered to allow a patient or surgeon to use the robot.

Our preference for performing robotic RPLND is via a transperitoneal approach with the patient in the supine position, thus facilitating a bilateral template dissection identical to that used in all our open procedures. Our technique closely mimics that of Dr James Porter and his team.[6] As noted in **Fig. 1**, port placement includes a 12-mm midline camera port, 3 8-mm robotic ports, a single 12-mm assistant port, and a 5-mm port in the right upper quadrant used mostly for retraction/elevation of the inferior vena cava (IVC) and aorta with vessel loops (see **Fig. 1**).

Following port placement, the patient is placed in a slight Trendelenburg position (~30°) to allow cephalad mobilization of the bowel, and laparoscopic bowel graspers are used to facilitate bowel mobilization and exposure of the root of the bowel mesentery and retroperitoneum; the robot is then docked over the patient's head. In order to prepare the retroperitoneum for dissection, we start by lifting the small bowel mesentery with the fourth arm and incise the peritoneum to the level of the appendix and cephalad medial to the duodenum up to the crossing point of the inferior mesenteric vein, at the level of the renal veins. The bowel is then anchored ventrally to the abdominal wall by placing 4 2-0 Biosyn sutures (2 on each side of the midline) through the cut edge of the peritoneum, tenting the posterior peritoneum upward. The fourth arm provides ventral retraction cephalad to finalize our cephalad exposure to the full retroperitoneum. The lymphadenectomy then commences along the left renal vein using serial Hem-o-lok clips to secure lymphatics until the level of the IVC. We start the lymphadenectomy with the paracaval nodes, rolling the IVC medially and dissecting as far as the sympathetic chain. IVC retraction is facilitated through 1 or 2 vessel loops held by the right upper quadrant assistant port. Dissection is carried down to the mid common iliac where the ureter crosses. We then commence dissection of the interaoartocaval region where the IVC is rolled right-laterally to allow removal of all tissue behind the IVC and medial to the sympathetic chain. Small vessels off the IVC are controlled with bipolar cautery, larger lumbar vessels are secured with green Hem-o-lok or metal clips. Lumbar arteries are preserved unless involved with disease. It is at this point that nerve sparing is accomplished by identifying the sympathetic chain, the right-sided postganglionic sympathetic fibers, and the hypogastric plexus. Care is taken to minimize cautery use near the nerves. The dissection continues up to the left renal vein and right renal artery. Dissection continues proximally to control the distal aspect of the cisterna chyli underneath the aortic crus. During interaortocaval dissection the aorta is rolled left laterally with vessel loops, similar to the IVC.

Subsequently, the dissection moves to include the para-aortic nodes both above and below the inferior mesenteric artery (IMA), which is preserved. The aorta is retracted medially and all tissue underneath the aorta is excised. Again, left-sided lumbar arteries are preserved unless involved with disease. The left sympathetic chain is identified and left-sided postganglionic sympathetic fibers coursing under the IMA are identified and preserved down to the hypogastric plexus. The dissection carries on to the point where the ureter crosses the left common iliac artery.

The procedure concludes by dissecting and removing the ipsilateral spermatic cord down to

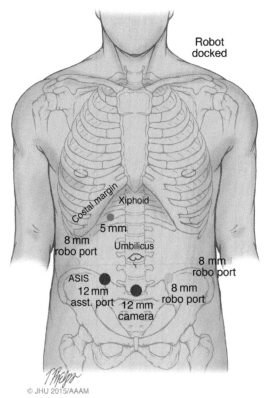

© JHU 2015/AAAM

Fig. 1. Port placement for robotic RPLND in the supine position. This positioning facilitates full bilateral template dissection. Port placement includes a 12-mm midline camera port, 3 8-mm robotic ports, a single 12-mm assistant (asst.) port, and a 5-mm port in the right upper quadrant. The robot is docked over the patient's head. (*From* Pearce SM, Golan S, Gorin MA, et al. Safety and early oncologic effectiveness of primary robotic retroperitoneal lymph node dissection for nonseminomatous germ cell testicular cancer. Eur Urol 2017;71(3):478; with permission.)

the level of ligation at the time of orchiectomy (typically a silk stitch). With the da Vinci Si system, this necessitates undocking and redocking from the ipsilateral side. With the Xi system, no undocking is needed and the arms can be repurposed for pelvic-oriented dissection.

THE CASE FOR AND AGAINST ROBOTIC PRIMARY RETROPERITONEAL LYMPH NODE DISSECTION
For

There are several arguments for performing an RPLND using a robotic platform. First, in an otherwise young, healthy male population, robotic surgery provides a superior cosmetic result to the large midline laparotomy-style incision from xiphisternum to below the umbilicus and sometimes to the pubic symphysis (although smaller incisions are made in some centers) associated with open RPLND. In a single-center, multidisciplinary, randomized prospective study of 62 patients undergoing cardiac surgery, those undergoing robotic surgery (n = 33) had superior self-esteem, body image, overall Observer Scar Assessment Scale scores, and overall Patient Scar Assessment Scale scores compared with the conventional open surgery cohort.[26] In patients with testis cancer, who may still be having difficulty processing their cancer diagnosis and treatment side effects, these psychological benefits cannot be overstated.

Second, in the primary RPLND setting, the robotic approach results in less blood loss and shorter length of stay compared with open surgery, although most of these series are not comparing with contemporary series.[6,20–22,27–29]

In a series of primary robotic RPLND reports, the median estimated blood loss was consistently less than 100 mL (range, 50–100 mL; **Table 2**), whereas several open studies report ~200 mL (range, 150–207 mL). Similarly, robotic cases series report a much shorter length of stay (range, 1–3 days) compared with the historic open experience (range, 3–8 days; see **Table 2**) with primary RPLND. A smaller incisional burden with the robotic approach has likely decreased length of stay in this cohort, in conjunction with greater acceptance of enhanced recovery after surgery protocols across abdominal oncologic operations[30] (see **Table 2**).

Although it has not been studied specifically in patients undergoing robotic RPLND, compared with open approaches, patients undergoing robotic procedures have less pain, faster recovery and return to work, and a much lower risk of incisional hernia. In a study of 142 patients undergoing either robotic or open laparotomy for endometrial cancer, patients undergoing robotic surgery had decreased 24-hour opioid consumption as well as an increased perception of recovery based on Quality of Recovery Questionnaire scores compared with the open approach.[32] Among 2571 men undergoing radical prostatectomy in Sweden, patients undergoing robotic surgery returned to work after a median 35 days compared with 48 days for open radical prostatectomy ($P<.001$), showing shorter convalescence.[33] Furthermore, within the first month, patients having a robotic prostatectomy returned to work nearly 4 times quicker. A systematic review of patients undergoing minimally invasive versus open techniques for kidney transplant

Table 2
Comparison of robotic and open primary retroperitoneal lymph node dissection

	Median Estimated Blood Loss (mL)	Median Operative Time (min)	Median Length of Stay (d)
Robotic Series			
Harris et al,[22] 2015 (JHH)	75	271	NR
Pearce et al,[20] 2017 (Multicenter)	50	235	1
Stepanian et al,[6] 2016 (Swedish)	50	293	1
Cheney et al,[21] 2015 (Mayo)	100	330	3
Open Series			
Beck et al,[27] 2007 (Indiana)	207	132	3
Williams et al,[28] 2010 (Brigham)	194	206	4
Masterson et al,[31] 2012 (MSKCC)	200	NR	7
Heidenreich et al,[29] 2003 (GTCSG)	150	214	8

Abbreviations: GTCSG, German Testicular Cancer Study Group; JHH, Johns Hopkins Hospital; MSKCC, Memorial Sloan Kettering Cancer Center.

Table 3
Oncologic efficacy among patients undergoing primary robotic retroperitoneal lymph node dissection

	Cases (n)	Median Follow-up (mo)	N+ Disease (n)	Receipt of Chemotherapy (n)	Recurrence and Location
Harris et al,[22] 2015 (JHH)	16	13.5	2 (13%)	NR	NR
Pearce et al,[20] 2017 (Multicenter)	47	16	8 (17%)	5, adjuvant	1, pelvic
Stepanian et al,[6] 2016 (Swedish)	16	49	6 (38%)	1, adjuvant 1, recurrence	1, lung
Cheney et al,[21] 2015 (Mayo)	10	11.5	3 (30%)	2, recurrence	2, thorax

Abbreviation: NR, not reported.

found incisional hernia rates of 0% to 6% for minimally invasive surgery compared with 4% to 16% for open approaches.[34] Given the sizable difference in incisional burden for robotic versus open RPLND and based on our clinical experience, it is reasonable to extrapolate the aforementioned benefits to patients undergoing primary robotic RPLND.

Against

There are several potential disadvantages to performing primary robotic RPLND. First, a robotic approach is associated with a longer operative time compared with open RPLND. Contemporary robotic studies report a median operative time range of 235 to 330 minutes compared with 132 to 214 minutes for open primary RPLND.[6,20–22,27–29] Longer operating times lead to increased anesthesia cost.[35] Combined with instrument expenditures associated with robotic surgery, robotic RPLND is more expensive than an open approach. With refinement of the learning curve, perhaps a cost-neutral margin is attainable, but this has yet to be achieved among more commonly performed robotic procedures (eg, robotic prostatectomy).[36]

Second, advocates of open RPLND may suggest that the surgeon's remote console may be dangerous in the setting of a vascular injury, necessitating open conversion. Although this complication in the current series is rare, it highlights the necessity of having an experienced bedside assistant for robotic RPLND procedures, including having a laparoscopic Satinsky clamp and 5-0 polypropylene suture readily available, and, in cases of catastrophic hemorrhage, having a hand or Gelport available to facilitate vessel

compression while a laparotomy is being performed.

Arguably, the most important detraction for robotic RPLND is the dogma among seasoned urologic oncologists that the procedure is an inferior oncologic operation compared with open RPLND.[37] Strict adherence to the oncologic principles of an RPLND must be followed regardless of the operative approach. At present, equivalent oncologic efficacy is difficult to assess for several reasons.

First, too many patients with clinical stage IA disease were included in studies thus far and arguably should have never undergone surgery but should have been on active surveillance.[38–41] It is difficult to assess the oncologic efficacy of a surgical procedure when the patient was already cancer free.

Second, too many patients with clinical stage IB disease were also included in these studies and an argument can also be made that they too should never have undergone a primary RPLND.[38–41] For example, the 3 largest series reported pN0 rates (all clinical stages) of 63% to 83%,[6,20,22] thus making an assessment of oncologic efficacy challenging.

Third, there is overuse of adjuvant (post-RPLND) chemotherapy. In the published series reporting such outcomes,[6,22] of the patients with pN+ disease, 40% to 62% received adjuvant chemotherapy, making it difficult to discern the independent contribution of the robotic RPLND to oncologic control.

In addition, there is a lack of long-term oncologic follow-up, considering that initial series have only been published in the last several years (**Table 3**). Stepanian and colleagues[6] have the longest follow-up at 49 months (n = 16 patients), but most primary RPLND series are ~1 year of follow-up.

ROBOTIC POSTCHEMOTHERAPY RETROPERITONEAL LYMPH NODE DISSECTION

Although most robotic RPLND studies have been reported in the primary setting, several groups have reported cases series of patients undergoing postchemotherapy RPLND in select patients. Not surprisingly, these series have noted the same challenges encountered in an open RPLND; namely increased desmoplastic reaction after chemotherapy, increased tumor complexity, and increased complication rates.[42]

There are 3 published series assessing postchemotherapy RPLND (see **Table 1**). In the first reported series, Kamel and colleagues[24] performed 12 procedures with a mean operative time of 321 minutes, mean estimated blood loss of 893 mL, and mean hospital stay of 3.5 days. The mean number of lymph nodes removed was 8, with 6 patients having masses greater than 5 cm. Antegrade ejaculation was preserved in 8 patients after a mean 27 months of follow-up, and there were no recurrences. Overs and colleagues[23] performed 11 postchemotherapy robotic RPLNDs using a single-docking technique in the lateral decubitus position. The median size of residual mass was 20 mm, median operative time was 153 minutes, median estimated blood loss was 120 mL, and there were no intraoperative complications. However, the median node count was only 7 (range, 1–24). The investigators reported a 72.7% antegrade ejaculation rate at 1 month from surgery and a median clinical recurrence-free survival of 100% for 6 patients 2 years from surgery.[23] At the 2018 American Urological Association annual meeting, Singh and colleagues[25] from India provided an update of their initial single-center experience, reporting 18 patients undergoing postchemotherapy robotic RPLND from 2011 to 2017.[43] The mean console time was 181 minutes and mean estimated blood loss was 208 mL, with a mean lymph node yield of 20. There were 12 patients (67%) that had antegrade ejaculation at last follow-up; however, 6 patients developed a chyle leak, 2 of whom required an exploratory laparotomy and ligation of the cisterna chlyi. After a mean follow-up of 19.5 months, no patients had recurred.

Although postchemotherapy robotic RPLND may be technically feasible, based on several of the published series having suboptimal lymph node yield compared with the open series, it is important to not compromise an oncologic operation for a minimally invasive approach. These lower lymph node yields are likely in part secondary to modified template dissections.[23,25] A modified versus bilateral template dissection in the postchemotherapy setting has been widely debated[44,45]; the authors advocate bilateral template with nerve sparing when technically feasible. Particularly in the postchemotherapy setting, it is of paramount importance to adhere to strict oncologic principles, because postchemotherapy robotic RPLNDs should only be performed by surgeons already comfortable with the open approach.

THE PRINCESS MARGARET CANCER CENTRE PHILOSOPHY

Our philosophy for performing robotic RPLND is to replicate the open approach at every point in the operation, with no change from the current multidisciplinary clinical algorithm. Given that we are proponents of non–risk-adapted surveillance for clinical stage I germ cell tumors,[38,39,41] our case selection includes (1) primary RPLND for clinical stage IIA disease; (2) primary RPLND for patients who have progressed on surveillance to a clinical stage IIA equivalent; and (3) postchemotherapy RPLND for patients with residual masses less than 3 cm without large (>70%) tumor volume reduction from the prechemotherapy volume.[46] In addition, we perform full bilateral template robotic RPLNDs with bilateral nerve sparing when feasible.

Who Should Be Performing Robotic Retroperitoneal Lymph Node Dissection?

Given the pros and cons described earlier and the complex nature of robotic RPLND, the authors think that robotic RPLND should only be attempted by surgeons fluent in evidence-based testis cancer management algorithms who have high-volume experience with open RPLND, a nuanced understanding of the retroperitoneum and its anatomic variance, and experience with dealing with intraoperative and postoperative complications. The stakes are high for these young men, who will experience any complications for decades after surgery, including the need to receive chemotherapy when a properly executed open operation may have avoided such need. Fluidity with robotic kidney and prostate surgery does not automatically translate into a well-executed robotic RPLND. Thus, the authors think that, while the appropriate data on robotic RPLND are gathered, that these surgeries should be done by high-volume centers and ideally on a research protocol with informed patient consent.

SUMMARY

RPLND should be performed with a goal of cure and minimal morbidity. Procedures that are performed robotically should unquestionably mimic the open approach with regard to oncologic principles. Initial series reporting their experience with robotic RPLND are encouraging, including less blood loss, shorter length of hospitalization, and decreased morbidity; however, existing oncologic comparative efficacy data to the open series are lacking.[47]

Ultimately, the authors think that robotic RPLND will prove efficacious and have a role in the care of select patients at centers of excellence, but, until such long-term efficacy and safety data are reported, the procedure should be used with caution in the setting of a protocol.

REFERENCES

1. Motzer RJ, Agarwal N, Beard C, et al. NCCN clinical practice guidelines in oncology: testicular cancer. J Natl Compr Canc Netw 2009;7(6):672–93.

2. Albers P, Albrecht W, Algaba F, et al. Guidelines on testicular cancer: 2015 update. Eur Urol 2015;68(6):1054–68.

3. Stephenson AJ, Bosl GJ, Motzer RJ, et al. Non-randomized comparison of primary chemotherapy and retroperitoneal lymph node dissection for clinical stage IIA and IIB nonseminomatous germ cell testicular cancer. J Clin Oncol 2007;25(35):5597–602.

4. Hamilton RJ, Nayan M, Anson-Cartwright L, et al. Treatment of Relapse of Clinical Stage I Nonseminomatous Germ Cell Tumors on Surveillance. J Clin Oncol 2019. [Epub ahead of print].

5. Hu B, Shah S, Shojaei S, et al. Retroperitoneal lymph node dissection as first-line treatment of node-positive seminoma. Clin Genitourin Cancer 2015;13(4):e265–9.

6. Stepanian S, Patel M, Porter J. Robot-assisted laparoscopic retroperitoneal lymph node dissection for testicular cancer: evolution of the technique. Eur Urol 2016;70(4):661–7.

7. Rukstalis DB, Chodak GW. Laparoscopic retroperitoneal lymph node dissection in a patient with stage 1 testicular carcinoma. J Urol 1992;148(6):1907–9.

8. Stone NN, Schlussel RN, Waterhouse RL, et al. Laparoscopic retroperitoneal lymph node dissection in stage A nonseminomatous testis cancer. Urology 1993;42(5):610–4.

9. Janetschek G, Reissigl A, Peschel R, et al. Laparoscopic retroperitoneal lymph node dissection for clinical stage I nonseminomatous testicular tumor. Urology 1994;44(3):382–91.

10. Klotz L. Laparoscopic retroperitoneal lymphadenectomy for high-risk stage 1 nonseminomatous germ cell tumor: report of four cases. Urology 1994;43(5):752–6.

11. Gerber GS, Bissada NK, Hulbert JC, et al. Laparoscopic retroperitoneal lymphadenectomy: multi-institutional analysis. J Urol 1994;152(4):1188–91.

12. Janetschek G, Hobisch A, Holtl L, et al. Retroperitoneal lymphadenectomy for clinical stage I nonseminomatous testicular tumor: laparoscopy versus open surgery and impact of learning curve. J Urol 1996;156(1):89–93.

13. Rassweiler JJ, Frede T, Lenz E, et al. Long-term experience with laparoscopic retroperitoneal lymph node dissection in the management of low-stage testis cancer. Eur Urol 2000;37(3):251–60.

14. Janetschek G, Hobisch A, Peschel R, et al. Laparoscopic retroperitoneal lymph node dissection for clinical stage I nonseminomatous testicular carcinoma: long-term outcome. J Urol 2000;163(6):1793–6.

15. Bhayani SB, Ong A, Oh WK, et al. Laparoscopic retroperitoneal lymph node dissection for clinical stage I germ cell testicular cancer: a long-term update. Urology 2003;62(2):324–7.

16. Peschel R, Gettman MT, Neururer R, et al. Laparoscopic retroperitoneal lymph node dissection: description of the nerve-sparing technique. Urology 2002;60(2):339–43.

17. Finelli A. Laparoscopic retroperitoneal lymph node dissection for nonseminomatous germ cell tumors: long-term oncologic outcomes. Curr Opin Urol 2008;18(2):180–4.

18. Hamilton RJ, Finelli A. Laparoscopic retroperitoneal lymph node dissection for nonseminomatous germ-cell tumors: current status. Urol Clin North Am 2007;34(2):159–69.

19. Davol P, Sumfest J, Rukstalis D. Robotic-assisted laparoscopic retroperitoneal lymph node dissection. Urology 2006;67(1):199.

20. Pearce SM, Golan S, Gorin MA, et al. Safety and early oncologic effectiveness of primary robotic retroperitoneal lymph node dissection for nonseminomatous germ cell testicular cancer. Eur Urol 2017;71(3):476–82.

21. Cheney SM, Andrews PE, Leibovich BC, et al. Robot-assisted retroperitoneal lymph node dissection: technique and initial case series of 18 patients. BJU Int 2015;115(1):114–20.

22. Harris KT, Gorin MA, Ball MW, et al. A comparative analysis of robotic vs laparoscopic retroperitoneal lymph node dissection for testicular cancer. BJU Int 2015;116(6):920–3.

23. Overs C, Beauval JB, Mourey L, et al. Robot-assisted post-chemotherapy retroperitoneal lymph node dissection in germ cell tumor: is the single-docking with lateral approach relevant? World J Urol 2018;36(4):655–61.

24. Kamel MH, Littlejohn N, Cox M, et al. Post-chemo-therapy robotic retroperitoneal lymph node dissec-tion: institutional experience. J Endourol 2016; 30(5):510–9.

25. Singh A, Chatterjee S, Bansal P, et al. Robot-assis-ted retroperitoneal lymph node dissection: Feasi-bility and outcome in postchemotherapy residual mass in testicular cancer. Indian J Urol 2017;33(4): 304–9.

26. Iyigun T, Kaya M, Gulbeyaz SO, et al. Patient body image, self-esteem, and cosmetic results of mini-mally invasive robotic cardiac surgery. Int J Surg 2017;39:88–94.

27. Beck SD, Peterson MD, Bihrle R, et al. Short-term morbidity of primary retroperitoneal lymph node dissection in a contemporary group of patients. J Urol 2007;178(2):504–6.

28. Williams SB, McDermott DW, Winston D, et al. Morbidity of open retroperitoneal lymph node dissection for testicular cancer: contemporary peri-operative data. BJU Int 2010;105(7):918–21.

29. Heidenreich A, Albers P, Hartmann M, et al. Compli-cations of primary nerve sparing retroperitoneal lymph node dissection for clinical stage I nonsemi-nomatous germ cell tumors of the testis: experience of the German Testicular Cancer Study Group. J Urol 2003;169(5):1710–4.

30. Azhar RA, Bochner B, Catto J, et al. Enhanced re-covery after urological surgery: a contemporary sys-tematic review of outcomes, key elements, and research needs. Eur Urol 2016;70(1):176–87.

31. Masterson TA, Carver BS, Abel EJ, et al. Impact of age on clinicopathological outcomes and recurrence-free survival after the surgical manage-ment of nonseminomatous germ cell tumour. BJU Int 2012;110(7):950–5.

32. Cohn DE, Castellon-Larios K, Huffman L, et al. A prospective, comparative study for the evaluation of postoperative pain and quality of recovery in pa-tients undergoing robotic versus open hysterectomy for staging of endometrial cancer. J Minim Invasive Gynecol 2016;23(3):429–34.

33. Plym A, Chiesa F, Voss M, et al. Work disability after robot-assisted or open radical prostatectomy: a nationwide, population-based study. Eur Urol 2016; 70(1):64–71.

34. Wagenaar S, Nederhoed JH, Hoksbergen AWJ, et al. Minimally invasive, laparoscopic, and robotic-assisted techniques versus open techniques for kid-ney transplant recipients: a systematic review. Eur Urol 2017;72(2):205–17.

35. Avondstondt AM, Wallenstein M, D'Adamo CR, et al. Change in cost after 5 years of experience with

robotic-assisted hysterectomy for the treatment of endometrial cancer. J Robot Surg 2018;12(1):93–6.

36. Shih YT, Shen C, Hu JC. Do robotic surgical systems improve profit margins? A cross-sectional analysis of California Hospitals. Value Health 2017;20(8): 1221–5.

37. Mottet N. Editorial comment on: laparoscopic retro-peritoneal lymph node dissection: does it still have a role in the management of clinical stage I nonsemi-nomatous testis cancer? A European perspective. Eur Urol 2008;54(5):1018–9.

38. Goldberg H, Madhur N, Hamilton RJ. Conditional risk of relapse in patients with germ cell testicular tu-mors: personalizing surveillance in clinical stage 1 disease. Curr Opin Urol 2018;28(5):454–60.

39. Hamilton RJ. Active surveillance for stage I testicular cancer: a four-decade-old experiment proven cor-rect. Eur Urol 2018;73(6):908–9.

40. Pierorazio PM, Albers P, Black PC, et al. Non-risk-adapted surveillance for stage I testicular cancer: critical review and summary. Eur Urol 2018;73(6): 899–907.

41. Nayan M, Jewett MA, Hosni A, et al. Conditional risk of relapse in surveillance for clinical stage I testicular cancer. Eur Urol 2017;71(1):120–7.

42. Steiner H, Leonhartsberger N, Stoehr B, et al. Post-chemotherapy laparoscopic retroperitoneal lymph node dissection for low-volume, stage II, nonsemi-nomatous germ cell tumor: first 100 patients. Eur Urol 2013;63(6):1013–7.

43. Singh A, Jaipuria J, Baidya S, et al. MP26-14 robot assisted retroperitoneal lymph node dissection of post chemotherapy residual mass — a single center experience of 18 patients. J Urol 2018;199(4 Suppl): e342.

44. Cho JS, Kaimakliotis HZ, Cary C, et al. Modified retroperitoneal lymph node dissection for post-chemotherapy residual tumour: a long-term update. BJU Int 2017;120(1):104–8.

45. Carver BS, Shayegan B, Eggener S, et al. Incidence of metastatic nonseminomatous germ cell tumor outside the boundaries of a modified postchemo-therapy retroperitoneal lymph node dissection. J Clin Oncol 2007;25(28):4365–9.

46. Vergouwe Y, Steyerberg EW, Foster RS, et al. Pre-dicting retroperitoneal histology in postchemother-apy testicular germ cell cancer: a model update and multicentre validation with more than 1000 pa-tients. Eur Urol 2007;51(2):424–32.

47. Tselos A, Moris D, Tsilimigras DI, et al. Robot-as-sisted retroperitoneal lymphadenectomy in testic-ular cancer treatment: a systematic review. J Laparoendosc Adv Surg Tech A 2018;28(6): 682–9.

Management, Treatment, and Molecular Background of the Growing Teratoma Syndrome

Andreas Hiester, MD[a],*, Daniel Nettersheim, PhD[b], Alessandro Nini, MD[a], Achim Lusch, MD[a], Peter Albers, MD[a]

KEYWORDS

- Growing teratoma syndrome • Nonseminomatous germ cell cancer • Retroperitoneal tumor
- Residual tumor resection • Molecular development of growing teratoma syndrome

KEY POINTS

- Diagnosis: Increasing cystic tumor size with timely decreasing tumor markers during or directly after chemotherapy indicate a GTS.
- Therapeutic management: Completion of the initial stage-stratified number of chemotherapy courses is strictly recommended. In any case, a complete resection of the retroperitoneal tumor mass is recommended to reduce recurrence rates and avoid the development of a somatic malignant transformation of the postpubertal teratoma.
- Adjunctive surgery: For a complete resection, adjunctive procedures are necessary in 23% to 100%. This aspect has to be taken into consideration when planning surgical treatment of patients with GTS and patients should be treated in high-volume specialized centers.
- Molecular model of possible development of GTS: During therapy, embryonal carcinoma cells might develop/differentiate into transit amplifying cells of the germ layer lineages, which are able to self-renew or differentiate further into cells resembling tissues of all three germ layers (mesoderm, endoderm, ectoderm). This special cell type is termed teratoma forming–transit amplifying cells (TF-TAC).

INTRODUCTION AND CLINICAL BACKGROUND

Germ cell cancers are the most common solid tumors among men between 15 and 40 years. With a worldwide incidence of 70,000, germ cell cancers account for 1% of the male tumors.[1] In 2018, a total of 8720 patients with testis cancer have been registered in the United States with a mortality rate of 4.7% (410 patients).[2] During the last three decades the incidence of germ cell cancer increased in industrialized countries in the Northern hemisphere, whereas mortality decreased over time.[3,4] This decreasing mortality is because of more effective cisplatin-based chemotherapy leading to higher cure rates even in advanced stages,[5] whereas the increasing incidence of germ cell cancers cannot be entirely explained.

Disclosure Statement: There are no commercial or financial conflicts of interest for all authors regarding this work.
a Department of Urology, University of Duesseldorf, Medical Faculty, Heinrich-Heine-University, Moorenstr. 5, Duesseldorf 40225, Germany; b Department of Urology, Urological Research Lab, Translational Urooncology, University of Duesseldorf, Medical Faculty, Heinrich-Heine-University, Duesseldorf, Germany
* Corresponding author.
E-mail address: andreas.hiester@med.uni-duesseldorf.de

urologic.theclinics.com

In 1997, the International Germ Cell Cancer Collaborative Group (IGCCCG) published a classification of germ cell cancers defining three groups based on 5-year progression-free survival (PFS) and overall survival rates (OS).[6] In patients classified as good-risk, 5-year PFS was 88% and OS 91%. Intermediate-risk patients had 5-year PFS of 75% and OS of 79%. Patients described as poor-risk according to the IGCCCG presented with a 5-year PFS of 41% and an OS of 48%.[6,7] Besides the clinical features of the tumor, which were taken into account for the IGCCCG stratification, it was shown that the oncologic outcome was improved when patients were referred to high-volume centers.[8–10]

Treatment of patients with germ cell cancer often requires complex multidisciplinary management.[11] Depending on clinical stage and prognostic risk stratification (based on IGCCCG classification), the European Association of Urology and the National Comprehensive Cancer Network guidelines on testicular cancer recommend a stage-adapted treatment: surgery in localized stages or chemotherapy with or without subsequent surgery in advanced stages.[5,12] In advanced tumor stages with or without elevated serum tumor markers, a cisplatin-based chemotherapy is recommended.[5,12,13]

Success of treatment is monitored by decreasing serum tumor marker values (alpha fetoprotein [AFP], beta-human chorionic gonadotropin [hCG], lactate dehydrogenase [LDH]) and shrinking tumor size on imaging. The uncommon phenomenon that serum tumor markers normalize but tumor size increases on imaging under ongoing cisplatin-based chemotherapy has first been described by Logothetis and colleagues[14] in 1982 and has been named growing teratoma syndrome (GTS). Logothetis and colleagues[14] described six patients with mixed germ cell cancers who had been successfully treated with chemotherapy, all presenting with enlarging abdominal and/or pulmonary masses during chemotherapy. All patients were classified as chemorefractory, but after resection and assessment of histology only mature teratoma was found without evidence of malignant elements. GTS occurs mostly in the retroperitoneal anatomic region with an incidence of 2% to 8% in nonseminomatous germ cell cancers.[15–17]

A rare phenomenon in GTS are teratomas with malignant transformation with an incidence of 2% to 8%.[18] Teratomas with malignant transformations are defined as development of a somatic malignancy in formally pure germ cell cancer.[19] Histologically, mostly sarcomas (50%), primitive neuroectodermal tumors (25%), or adenocarcinomas (19%) are found.[20] Altogether, the clinical outcome of patients with malignant transformation is inferior to patients presenting with conventional GTS.[19]

BIOLOGIC BACKGROUND

Germ cell tumors are divided into two types of cancer:

- Type I
  - Pediatric, embryonal carcinoma/teratoma/yolk sac tumor
- Type II
  - Adult, seminoma/nonseminoma

All type II germ cell cancers derive from a common precursor lesion termed germ cell neoplasia in situ (GCNIS), which itself is thought to be the result of a defective (primordial) germ cell development.[21,22] Germ cell cancers are stratified into seminomas and nonseminomas.[21] Seminomas are highly similar to primordial germ cells and GCNIS cells with regard to histology, gene expression, and epigenetics, that is, they show a GCNIS-like morphology (roundish cells, with clear cytoplasm and a big nucleus) and express typical primordial germ cell/GCNIS markers, such as SOX17, OCT4, TFAP2C (AP2-gamma), PRDM1 (BLIMP1), PRAME, and cKIT. Additionally, the DNA of seminomas presents as hypomethylated.[21,23–28] Thus, the development of seminomas from GCNIS has been considered the default developmental pathway of germ cell cancer tumorigenesis.[21,29] In contrast, the stem cell population of the nonseminomas, the embryonal carcinoma, is often described as a malignant counterpart to embryonic stem cells. In line, embryonal carcinomas express embryonic stem cell and pluripotency factors, such as SOX2, NANOG, OCT4, GDF3, ZFP42 (REX1), DPPA2, DNMT3B, and NODAL.[21,24,29–32] Furthermore, the DNA of embryonal carcinoma cells is globally hypermethylated compared with GCNIS/seminomas.[25,28] Early during embryogenesis, at blastocyst stage, a distinct separation of cells of the inner cell mass (embryonic stem cells, giving rise to tissues of the developing embryo) from trophoblast cells (extraembryonic cells, giving rise to maternal tissues, such as the placenta) is crucial. Embryonal carcinomas are able to differentiate into cells of all three germ layers (mesoderm, endoderm, ectoderm), giving rise to teratomas and into extraembryonic tissues (yolk sac tumor, choriocarcinoma).[21] Thus, embryonal carcinomas are considered as totipotent and the ability to overcome the lineage barrier between embryonic and extraembryonic cell types is a unique feature of embryonal carcinomas.

Logothetis and coworkers[14] classified the germ cell cancers in context of GTS as mature teratomas. Mature teratomas mainly consist of terminally differentiated cells of all three germ layers. So, they should be strongly limited in their developmental potential and proliferative capacity. From a biologic point of view, a dedifferentiation of these terminally differentiated cells into a more aggressive, proliferative state seems unlikely. Thus, the driving force behind GTS has to be found elsewhere.

GTS is characterized by a growing nonseminomatous tumor mass after chemotherapy with serum markers (AFP, beta-hCG, and LDH) at normal levels. With regard to AFP and beta-hCG, absence of these markers in context of GTS is not unexpected, because AFP is a pathognomonic marker for yolk sac tumors and beta-hCG for choriocarcinomas, which consist of cytotrophoblast- and syncytiotrophoblast-like cells (extraembryonic tissue-like cells normally not present in mature teratoma histology). LDH is a general indicator of cell damage and has low specificity for germ cell cancers.[33] Additionally, LDH has been considered a trustworthy marker at levels greater than 2000 U/L.[34] In nonseminomas, elevated LDH levels may be the sole biochemical abnormality in only 10% of patients with persisting or recurring nonseminomatous germ cell cancers.[35] In light of these data and that mature teratomas do not grow invasively or cause severe cellular damage to the surrounding microenvironment, LDH might not be a reliable indicator for GTS.

Logothetis and coworkers[14] did not find any malignant histology in GTS tissues, suggesting that there are no (or too little) remaining embryonal carcinoma cells that fuel the growing tumor mass. A possible explanation of how tumor growth is driven, is the presence of a transiently amplifying cell pool derived from the embryonal carcinoma cells during differentiation and showing multipotency or unipotency. These cells could self-renew and continuously differentiate into the tissue they resemble (mesoderm, endoderm, ectoderm). Transiently amplifying cells have been described in the cornea, mammary glands, prostate epithelium, epidermis, gastrointestinal tract, different hair follicles, and the testis (in tissue types mimicked by teratomas and where germ cell cancers develop [testis]).[36–42] Based on their developmental and growth potential, different (stem) cell types are stratified as holoclones, paraclones, and meroclones. Holoclones (here, embryonal carcinomas) describe stem cell populations with a higher developmental potential than meroclones, whereas paraclones represent a differentiated cell population (here, the mature teratoma).

Meroclones show a lower developmental potential than holoclones and display a primed-to-differentiation-associated cell fate (here, our postulated transit amplifying cells [TAC]). Generally speaking, holoclones develop into meroclones that differentiate in paraclones. So, we postulate that GTS is the result of a development of embryonal carcinomas (holoclones) into TAC (meroclones) that resemble the stem cell pool of a germ layer tissue (**Fig. 1**). These TAC, which we term teratoma-forming TAC (TF-TAC), do not express germ cell cancer–related serum markers, are able to self-renew, and differentiate into the three germ layer lineages (mesoderm, ectoderm, endoderm) (paraclones). Additionally, these TF-TAC seem to be able to escape cisplatin-based chemotherapy or at least tolerate chemotherapy better than embryonal carcinomas. Thus, an embryonal carcinoma population dies under chemotherapy, which might explain the lack of malignant histology in GTS tissues and presence of the TF-TAC meroclone population that fuels the growth of a teratoma.

Of note, in in vitro cultivated teratoma cells, a previously unidentified epithelial cell population was found.[43] These epithelial cells grew rapidly only in the presence of fibroblasts, indicating that the microenvironment (ie, the extracellular matrix) may also have a considerable impact on the proliferative capacity of TF-TACs and progression of GTS.

CLINICAL EVIDENCE

Even though the initial definition of GTS by Logothetis and colleagues[14] was published more than 35 years ago, few reports are available. As Paffenholz and colleagues[44] recently published, only seven studies are available describing 9 to maximum 30 patients (**Table 1**). This small number of reports and patients makes it difficult to develop a standardized diagnostic and therapeutic work-up.

Diagnostic Work-up

The special challenge in diagnosis of GTS is the lack of unequivocal predictors of this syndrome before chemotherapy. Certainly, teratoma is often part of the histopathologic findings on primary orchiectomy but the predictive role of the histology of primary tumor of developing GTS is still unclear. Especially, the proportion of teratomas on primary orchiectomy histology does not correlate to developing GTS. As described in **Table 1**, the distribution and proportion of teratomas on primary histology of orchiectomy varies from 22% to 86% (see **Table 1**).[44–48] In several cases,

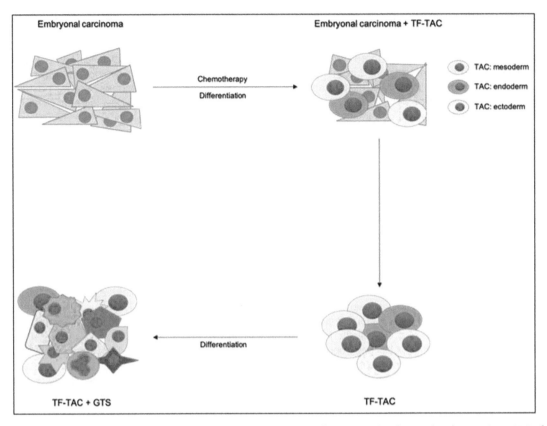

Fig. 1. Model of GTS development. Embryonal carcinoma cells differentiate/develop under therapy into TAC of the mesodermal/endodermal/ectodermal lineage. We hypothesize that these TAC are more resistant toward the cisplatin therapy than embryonal carcinoma cells. Thus, the embryonal carcinoma cell pool dies during therapy and the teratoma-forming TAC (TF-TAC) remain. TF-TACs are able to self-renew and differentiate further into the three germ layer lineages, thereby giving rise to a growing teratoma.

teratoma was not even the leading histology on orchiectomy specimen and therefore only of limited predictive value for developing a GTS. This is one reason why GTS is mostly diagnosed after completion of chemotherapy or by staging during chemotherapy. Growing teratoma is unpredictable in its growth rate. Lee and colleagues[48] published a series of 15 patients presenting a of linear growth was 0.5 cm/month (range, 0.03–2.9), and the increase in volume was 9.2 cm^3/month.

Fig. 2 shows a 29-year-old patient who initially presented with a clinical stage IIB nonseminomatous germ cell cancer (3% yolk sac, 2% teratoma, 95% embryonal carcinoma) classified as "good prognosis" according to IGCCCG (see **Fig. 2**). After three cycles of chemotherapy with bleomycin/etoposide/cisplatin, a computed tomography scan showed a retroperitoneal cystic tumor of 16 cm. After residual tumor resection, only teratoma was found on histopathologic findings.

Therapeutic Approach

The treatment of GTS is represented by a multidisciplinary approach, which includes chemotherapy and surgery. GTS is diagnosed during or after completion of chemotherapy. In cases where GTS is recognized during chemotherapy, such as with timely decreasing tumor markers and increasing tumor mass, the completion of the initially stage-stratified number of chemotherapy courses is strictly recommended. An interruption of chemotherapy is justified only with vital symptoms caused by increasing tumor size and thereby compression of neighboring organs (eg, bowel, lung, liver) with consecutive life-threatening organ failure. Only in these cases, earlier resection of the teratoma masses is reasonable.

In any case, a complete resection of the retroperitoneal tumor mass is recommended to reduce recurrence rates.[16,45] André and colleagues[45] described a series of 30 patients undergoing residual tumor resection for GTS. Twenty-four patients

Table 1
Overview of the literature available on the growing teratoma syndrome

	Patients (n)	Site of Primary Tumor	Histology of Primary Tumor	Complications (Clavien Dindo >III)	Adjunctive Surgery	Follow-up (mo)	Relapse	Outcome
Logothetis et al,[14] 1982	6	6/6 testicular primary tumor	Not available	Not available	Not available	18.5	0	6 patients are disease-free after median follow-up of 18.5 mo
Jeffery et al,[16] 1991	13		Not available	3	0	28	2	10 patients disease-free 2 relapses 1 death of other cause
Maroto et al,[49] 1997	11		Not available	Not available	4	110	8	5 patients with teratoma (stable disease) 6 patients disease-free
André et al,[45] 2000	30	28/30 testicular primary tumor site 2/30 mediastinal primary site	24/28 presented with mature teratoma on orchiectomy	Not available	4	54	GTS 6 NSGCC 5 Secondary malignancies 2	27 patients alive 20 patients disease-free 5 patients alive with GTS 2 patients alive with NSGCC
Spiess et al,[46] 2007	9	9/9 testicular primary tumor	8 mixed NSGCC 1 mature teratoma	4	2 (aortic repair, ureteral repair)	24	0	7 patients disease-free 1 death caused by sepsis 1 death caused by other cause
Stella et al,[47] 2012	12	12/12 testicular primary tumor	9 mixed NSGCC 1 embryonal carcinoma 2 choriocarcinoma	3	12	59	1	11 patients alive 1 lost to follow-up

(continued on next page)

Table 1
(continued)

	Patients (n)	Site of Primary Tumor	Histology of Primary Tumor	Complications (Clavien Dindo >III)	Adjunctive Surgery	Follow-up (mo)	Relapse	Outcome
Lee et al,[48] 2014	15	15/15 testicular primary tumor	12 NSGCC 2 seminoma 6 pure teratoma 6 pure yolk sac tumor	2	5 (nephrectomy, renal artery anastomosis, renal artery embolectomy, IVC tumor thrombectomy, resection of common iliac vein)	13.7	0	
Paffenholz et al,[44] 2018	22		16 mixed NSGCC 2 pure teratoma 2 pure embryonal carcinoma 2 pure yolk sac tumor	4	6 (2 aortal replacements, caval replacement, renal vein resection, nephrectomy)	25	2	1 patient death caused by relapsing disease 1 GTS stable disease

Abbreviations: IVC, inferior vena cava; NSGCC, non-seminomatous germ cell cancer (=NSGCT).

Modified from Paffenholz P, Pfister D, Matveev V, Heidenreich A. Diagnosis and management of the growing teratoma syndrome: a single-center experience and review of the literature. Urologic Oncology 2018;36(12):529.e528; with permission.

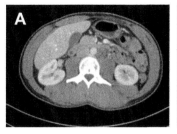 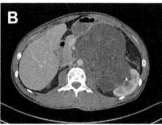

Fig. 2. (*A*) Abdominal computed tomography scan of a 29-year-old patient before chemotherapy. (*B*) Abdominal computed tomography scan after three cycles of chemotherapy with bleomycin/etoposide/cisplatin.

received complete resection and six patients had an incomplete resection. During follow-up, 3 of 24 (12%) patients undergoing complete resection presented with recurrent disease, whereas five of eight (83%) patients with incomplete resection experienced recurrence. Jeffery and colleagues[16] described a series of 13 patients (11 patients showing complete resection and two patients showing incomplete resection). Only the two patients with incomplete resection suffered from relapse. With a median follow-up of 28 months, one patient was still alive with a stable disease and one patient died after another retroperitoneal surgery during the postoperative setting.

A complete resection of the residual masses often requires multiple surgical procedures. Maroto and colleagues[49] described a series of 11 patients in whom altogether 24 surgical procedures had to be performed. Finally, six patients were rendered disease-free and five patients remained with stable disease.[49] The phenomenon of a stable, nonprogressive disease was also described by other working groups, most recently by André and colleagues[45] and Paffenholz and colleagues.[44]

For a complete resection, adjunctive procedures are necessary in 23% to 100%.[16,44,47–49] Most often vascular surgery, such as replacement of the vena cava or aorta, and nephrectomy are required.[44,47] This aspect has to be taken into consideration when planning surgical treatment of patients with GTS.

Despite the extent and numerous resections of patients with GTS, the morbidity of this surgery is acceptable, ranging from 18% to 44%.[16,44,47,48] Stella and colleagues[47] described surgery in 12 patients with GTS, all with the need of adjunctive procedures. Only 3 of 12 patients suffered from higher grade complications (Clavien Dindo ≥III). An additional for a complete resection in case of GTS is the higher rate of malignant disease recurrence, and therefore, the worse oncologic outcome in cases of incomplete resection. Rice and colleagues[50] and Giannatempo and colleagues[19] described a 5-year OS of only 50% in

patients with a recurrence of GTS including elements of malignant transformation.

The use of adjuvant chemotherapy in patients with GTS depends on the histopathologic findings. If only mature teratoma is found on histology, chemotherapy is not recommended because teratomas are not sensitive to chemotherapy. However, in cases of malignant transformation, especially in cases of recurrent disease, chemotherapy should be administered according to the histology of the recurrent disease.[19,20,50]

SUMMARY

GTS is a rare clinical phenomenon that is described with an incidence of up to 8%. The clinical appearance is characterized by growing metastatic nonseminomatous germ cell cancer masses while tumor markers are decreasing or normalizing during chemotherapy. The diagnosis is confirmed after resection by histologic presence of postpubertal teratoma only with the absence of vital, malignant tumor cells.

In this review, we have suggested a molecular model of how GTS might develop: embryonal carcinoma cells develop/differentiate into TAC under therapy, which are able to self-renew or differentiate further into cells of all three germ layers (mesoderm, ectoderm, endoderm), thereby fueling teratoma growth. We termed this special cell type TF-TAC.

After diagnosis and completion of chemotherapy a complete resection of all teratoma masses is mandatory. Because of the high incidence of adjunctive procedures in up to 23% to 100% of cases, treatment at a high-volume specialized center with access to multidisciplinary surgical care, such as vascular surgery, is recommended.

Improved oncologic outcomes are achieved by following three steps: (1) early recognition of the paradox development of tumor size and tumor markers during chemotherapy, (2) completion of initially stage-stratified numbers of chemotherapy courses under thorough monitoring of size and clinical appearance, and (3) complete surgical resection of residual masses.

REFERENCES

1. Shanmugalingam T, Soultati A, Chowdhury S, et al. Global incidence and outcome of testicular cancer. Clin Epidemiol 2013;5:417–27.

2. Siegel RL, Miller KD, Jemal A. Cancer statistics, 2018. CA Cancer J Clin 2018;68(1):7–30.

3. Le Cornet C, Lortet-Tieulent J, Forman D, et al. Testicular cancer incidence to rise by 25% by 2025 in Europe? Model-based predictions in 40 countries using population-based registry data. Eur J Cancer 2014;50(4):831–9.

4. Ghazarian AA, Trabert B, Devesa SS, et al. Recent trends in the incidence of testicular germ cell tumors in the United States. Andrology 2015;3(1):13–8.

5. Albers P, Albrecht W, Algaba F, et al. Guidelines on testicular cancer: 2015 update. Eur Urol 2015;68(6): 1054–68.

6. International germ cell consensus classification: a prognostic factor-based staging system for metastatic germ cell cancers. International Germ Cell Cancer Collaborative Group. J Clin Oncol 1997;15(2): 594–603.

7. Albany C, Adra N, Snavely AC, et al. Multidisciplinary clinic approach improves overall survival outcomes of patients with metastatic germ-cell tumors. Ann Oncol 2018;29(2):341–6.

8. Collette L, Sylvester RJ, Stenning SP, et al. Impact of the treating institution on survival of patients with "poor-prognosis" metastatic nonseminoma. European Organization for Research and Treatment of Cancer Genito-Urinary Tract Cancer Collaborative Group and the Medical Research Council Testicular Cancer Working Party. J Natl Cancer Inst 1999; 91(10):839–46.

9. Nayan M, Jewett MA, Anson-Cartwright L, et al. The association between institution at orchiectomy and outcomes on active surveillance for clinical stage I germ cell tumours. Can Urol Assoc J 2016;10(5–6): 204–9.

10. Adra N, Althouse SK, Liu H, et al. Prognostic factors in patients with poor-risk germ-cell tumors: a retrospective analysis of the Indiana University experience from 1990 to 2014. Ann Oncol 2016;27(5):875–9.

11. Lusch A, Albers P. Residual tumor resection (RTR). World J Urol 2017;35(8):1185–90.

12. Motzer RJ, Jonasch E, Agarwal N, et al. Testicular cancer, version 2.2015. J Natl Compr Canc Netw 2015;13(6):772–99.

13. Krege S, Beyer J, Souchon R, et al. European consensus conference on diagnosis and treatment of germ cell cancer: a report of the second meeting of the European Germ Cell Cancer Consensus group (EGCCCG): part I. Eur Urol 2008;53(3):478–96.

14. Logothetis CJ, Samuels ML, Trindade A, et al. The growing teratoma syndrome. Cancer 1982;50(8): 1629–35.

15. Tongaonkar HB, Deshmane VH, Dalal AV, et al. Growing teratoma syndrome. J Surg Oncol 1994; 55(1):56–60.

16. Jeffery GM, Theaker JM, Lee AHS, et al. The growing teratoma syndrome. Br J Urol 1991;67(2): 195–202.

17. Tonkin KS, Rustin GJ, Wignall B, et al. Successful treatment of patients in whom germ cell tumour masses enlarged on chemotherapy while their serum tumour markers decreased. Eur J Cancer Clin Oncol 1989;25(12):1739–43.

18. Motzer RJ, Amsterdam A, Prieto V, et al. Teratoma with malignant transformation: diverse malignant histologies arising in men with germ cell tumors. J Urol 1998;159(1):133–8.

19. Giannatempo P, Pond GR, Sonpavde G, et al. Treatment and clinical outcomes of patients with teratoma with somatic-type malignant transformation: an international collaboration. J Urol 2016;196(1):95–100.

20. Necchi A, Colecchia M, Nicolai N, et al. Towards the definition of the best management and prognostic factors of teratoma with malignant transformation: a single-institution case series and new proposal. BJU Int 2011;107(7):1088–94.

21. Oosterhuis JW, Looijenga LH. Testicular germ-cell tumours in a broader perspective. Nat Rev Cancer 2005;5(3):210–22.

22. Sonne SB, Almstrup K, Dalgaard M, et al. Analysis of gene expression profiles of microdissected cell populations indicates that testicular carcinoma in situ is an arrested gonocyte. Cancer Res 2009;69(12): 5241–50.

23. Biermann K, Heukamp LC, Nettersheim D, et al. Embryonal germ cells and germ cell tumors. Verh Dtsch Ges Pathol 2007;91:39–48 [in German].

24. Eckert D, Nettersheim D, Heukamp LC, et al. TCam-2 but not JKT-1 cells resemble seminoma in cell culture. Cell Tissue Res 2008;331(2):529–38.

25. Wermann H, Stoop H, Gillis AJ, et al. Global DNA methylation in fetal human germ cells and germ cell tumours: association with differentiation and cisplatin resistance. J Pathol 2010;221(4): 433–42.

26. Biermann K, Goke F, Nettersheim D, et al. c-KIT is frequently mutated in bilateral germ cell tumours and down-regulated during progression from intratubular germ cell neoplasia to seminoma. J Pathol 2007;213(3):311–8.

27. Eckert D, Biermann K, Nettersheim D, et al. Expression of BLIMP1/PRMT5 and concurrent histone H2A/H4 arginine 3 dimethylation in fetal germ cells, CIS/IGCNU and germ cell tumors. BMC Dev Biol 2008;8:106.

28. Nettersheim D, Heukamp LC, Fronhoffs F, et al. Analysis of TET expression/activity and 5mC oxidation during normal and malignant germ cell development. PLoS One 2013;8(12):e82881.

29. de Jong J, Stoop H, Gillis AJ, et al. Differential expression of SOX17 and SOX2 in germ cells and stem cells has biological and clinical implications. J Pathol 2008;215(1):21–30.

30. Godmann M, Gashaw I, Eildermann K, et al. The pluripotency transcription factor Kruppel-like factor 4 is strongly expressed in intratubular germ cell neoplasia unclassified and seminoma. Mol Hum Reprod 2009;15(8):479–88.

31. Nettersheim D, Jostes S, Sharma R, et al. BMP inhibition in seminomas initiates acquisition of pluripotency via NODAL signaling resulting in reprogramming to an embryonal carcinoma. PLoS Genet 2015; 11(7):e1005415.

32. Nettersheim D, Heimsoeth A, Jostes S, et al. SOX2 is essential for in vivo reprogramming of seminoma-like TCam-2 cells to an embryonal carcinoma-like fate. Oncotarget 2016;7(30):47095–110.

33. Milose JC, Filson CP, Weizer AZ, et al. Role of biochemical markers in testicular cancer: diagnosis, staging, and surveillance. Open Access J Urol 2011; 4:1–8.

34. Carl J, Christensen TB, von der Maase H. Cisplatinum dose dependent response in germ cell cancer evaluated by tumour marker modelling. Acta Oncol 1992;31(7):749–53.

35. Skinner DG, Scardino PT. Relevance of biochemical tumor markers and lymphadenectomy in management of non-seminomatous testis tumors: current perspective. J Urol 1980;123(3):378–82.

36. Kawasaki S, Tanioka H, Yamasaki K, et al. Expression and tissue distribution of p63 isoforms in human ocular surface epithelia. Exp Eye Res 2006;82(2): 293–9.

37. Farnie G, Clarke RB. Breast stem cells and cancer. Ernst Schering Found Symp Proc 2006;(5):141–53.

38. Petkova N, Hennenlotter J, Sobiesiak M, et al. Surface CD24 distinguishes between low differentiated and transit-amplifying cells in the basal layer of human prostate. Prostate 2013;73(14):1576–90.

39. Barrandon Y, Green H. Three clonal types of keratinocyte with different capacities for multiplication. Proc Natl Acad Sci U S A 1987;84(8):2302–6.

40. van der Flier LG, Clevers H. Stem cells, self-renewal, and differentiation in the intestinal epithelium. Annu Rev Physiol 2009;71:241–60.

41. Driskell RR, Giangreco A, Jensen KB, et al. Sox2-positive dermal papilla cells specify hair follicle type in mammalian epidermis. Development 2009; 136(16):2815–23.

42. Bak CW, Yoon TK, Choi Y. Functions of PIWI proteins in spermatogenesis. Clin Exp Reprod Med 2011; 38(2):61–7.

43. Green H. The birth of therapy with cultured cells. Bioessays 2008;30(9):897–903.

44. Paffenholz P, Pfister D, Matveev V, et al. Diagnosis and management of the growing teratoma syndrome: a single-center experience and review of the literature. Urol Oncol 2018;36(12):529.e23-30.

45. André F, Fizazi K, Culine S, et al. The growing teratoma syndrome: results of therapy and long-term follow-up of 33 patients. Eur J Cancer 2000;36(11): 1389–94.

46. Spiess PE, Kassouf W, Brown GA, et al. Surgical management of growing teratoma syndrome: the M. D. Anderson cancer center experience. J Urol 2007;177(4):1330–4 [discussion: 1334].

47. Stella M, Gandini A, Meeus P, et al. Retroperitoneal vascular surgery for the treatment of giant growing teratoma syndrome. Urology 2012;79(2):365–70.

48. Lee DJ, Djaladat H, Tadros NN, et al. Growing teratoma syndrome: clinical and radiographic characteristics. Int J Urol 2014;21(9):905–8.

49. Maroto P, Tabernero JM, Villavicencio H, et al. Growing teratoma syndrome: experience of a single institution. Eur Urol 1997;32(3):305–9.

50. Rice KR, Magers MJ, Beck SD, et al. Management of germ cell tumors with somatic type malignancy: pathological features, prognostic factors and survival outcomes. J Urol 2014;192(5):1403–9.

Complications of Retroperitoneal Lymph Node Dissection

Clint Cary, MD, MPH*, Richard S. Foster, MD,
Timothy A. Masterson, MD

KEYWORDS

- Retroperitoneal lymph node dissection • Germ cell tumors • Complications • Testicular cancer

KEY POINTS

- The overall incidence of complications during primary RPLND should be low and is reported to be less than 5% in high-volume centers, whereas the incidence is higher in the postchemotherapy setting, at approximately 10% to 15%, and may be higher depending on the necessity of concomitant procedures.
- Perioperative or postoperative complications in either the primary or postchemotherapy setting are directly correlated with surgeon and hospital volume and experience.
- Preservation of antegrade ejaculation, particularly in the primary RPLND setting, should approach 95% to 100% when performed by experienced surgeons.
- A significant component of this procedure requires the urologic surgeon to be well versed in vascular surgery techniques so as to minimize technical complications.

INTRODUCTION

Retroperitoneal lymph node dissection (RPLND) has long been integrated into the fabric of testicular cancer management strategies. The nuances and complexities of the operation are influenced by a variety of factors that modify the inherent risks of the procedure for patients. Some of these factors depend on patient characteristics such as body habitus, prior surgical interventions, and comorbid conditions. Disease-related factors such as histology of the primary tumor, staging/volume of primary or residual disease, and receipt of prior systemic or regional therapies also influence surgical difficulty. An important consideration lies in the fact that this is largely a vascular operation, and techniques of vascular control should be comfortable for the urologic surgeon performing the procedure. This article discusses the historical modifications of RPLND for the purpose of minimizing complications, discusses the known surgical complications inherent to RPLND, and reviews the relative incidence of surgical complications in the primary and postchemotherapy settings.

HISTORICAL PERSPECTIVES

Dating back to over 100 years ago, surgical removal of retroperitoneal (RP) lymph nodes had been successfully incorporated into the management of metastatic testicular germ cell tumor. In the absence of systemic therapies that are now readily available to patients with disseminated disease, surgical intervention with or without postoperative radiotherapy served as the only option to provide patients their best chance at long-term

Disclosure Statement: No author has any financial or commercial interests to disclose.
Department of Urology, Indiana University School of Medicine, 535 N Barnhill Drive, RT 420, Indianapolis, IN 46202, USA
* Corresponding author.
E-mail address: kcary@iupui.edu

Urol Clin N Am 46 (2019) 429–437
https://doi.org/10.1016/j.ucl.2019.04.012

survival. In 1914, Hinman[1] first published in *JAMA* his operative experience treating tumors of the testis. Surgical approaches at that time were largely performed through lower extraperitoneal, unilateral incisions, extending in a paramedian fashion from the tip of the 12th rib to the ipsilateral internal inguinal ring. Notable limitations included inadequate access to the ipsilateral renal pedicles and suprahilar (infradiaphragmatic) space that proved to represent potential sites for relapse and death.[2] Attempts at resection of these sites were associated with a higher risk of vascular accidents, thereby rendering a complete dissection impossible.

Incorporation of a thoracoabdominal approach extending from the posterior axillary line over the 10th rib and carrying this anteriorly/inferiorly into the peritoneal compartment allowed expansion of the surgical template to encompass all areas of disease, particularly the ipsilateral suprahilar region. This permitted a wider exposure of the involved region of lymphatic spread, facilitating a safer and more feasible resection of all sites of disease, including the contralateral retroperitoneum. Donohue[1] later published his anterior, transabdominal approach via a midline laparotomy incision that included further expansion of the surgical template with a bilateral suprarenal-hilar dissection,[3] touting more accurate staging of disease and the highest stage-for-stage survival outcomes for the time. However, with widening of the surgical template, major and minor surgical complications were noted to occur in 11.9% of patients,[4] comparing favorably with contemporary reports of the time.[5,6] These included greater risk for pancreatic injuries, vascular injuries, chylous ascites, and rendering patients anejaculatory.

With the introduction of platinum-based systemic chemotherapy in the 1970s, survival rates began to improve significantly.[7] However, negative consequences were noted with regard to the patient's nutritional reserve, pulmonary function, and hematologic status. Accordingly, higher rates of surgical complications were noted as surgical complexity increased in the postchemotherapy setting with reduced physiologic reserve.[4] Simultaneously in the setting of advanced-stage disease, reductions in bulk of residual disease after chemotherapy and higher rates of complete clinical response were noted, thus allowing for considerations to reduce the importance of radical resections to improve survival outcomes. With more effective chemotherapy, the focus on reducing the surgical morbidity became more relevant. Through a series of subsequent anatomic mapping studies, modifications in the surgical template were introduced, noting the predictable patterns of spread to the primary landing zones of the retroperitoneum in early and late staged metastatic disease.[8–10] This afforded the opportunity to omit the suprahilar and interiliac regions from routine dissection without jeopardizing the accuracy of staging or the therapeutic efficacy of RPLND, thus minimizing the risk of pancreatic fistulas and chyle leaks as well as reducing harm to the pelvic nerves responsible for ejaculation. Concomitantly, better anatomic understanding of the sympathetic neural pathways of the postganglionic fibers leading to the hypogastric plexus was realized.[11–14] Incorporation of nerve sparing through prospective identification and/or omission from the template via unilateral dissections in highly select patients have resulted in antegrade ejaculation rates in greater than 95% of patients in contemporary primary and postchemotherapy RPLND published series.[15,16]

CONTEMPORARY RISKS
Ejaculatory Function/Fertility

Until the anatomic characterization of the neural pathways responsible for seminal emission and antegrade ejaculation, it was largely accepted that a standard template to resect all lymphatic tissue in the retroperitoneum would result in the universal loss of ejaculatory function and its inherent negative impact on fertility. This side effect was the product of disruption to any component of the sympathetic innervation, including the postganglionic fibers of L1 through L4 extending from the sympathetic chain of ganglia along the posterior body wall, their coalescence as the right and left hypogastric plexus overlying the distal aorta anteriorly, or their course as the pelvic nerves to the seminal vesicles, ampulla of the vasa deferentia, vasa deferentia proper, bladder neck, and prostate.[12] As discussed previously, the preservation of the efferent postganglionic sympathetic fibers was feasible in select patients through incorporation of modified templates that reduced the surgical boundaries of dissection to avoid harm to the contralateral nerve branches[17,18] and/or prospective nerve-sparing techniques that allowed for prospective identification of these nerves within the template.[13]

In the primary setting, early studies looking at patients with clinical stage I or early stage II disease reported preservation rates in 75% to 87% of patients undergoing unilateral template modifications.[17–19] More contemporary reports have demonstrated further improvement in rates of antegrade ejaculation, attributable to experience and greater awareness of the path of the contralateral nerve fibers coursing caudal to the inferior mesenteric artery along the distal aorta. In the series published by Beck and colleagues,[15] 97% of patients undergoing a unilateral modified template without ipsilateral nerve sparing reported preservation of function.

Prospective nerve sparing within the template of dissection resulted in further improvement of antegrade ejaculation rates. Early experiences demonstrated success in 90% to 100% of patients.[12,15,20,21] In the study by Beck and colleagues,[15] the addition of ipsilateral nerve sparing to a unilateral template increased preservation rates from 97% to 99%. Investigators publishing on bilateral nerve-sparing approaches in the absence of template modifications have documented high rates of temporary loss of function in the immediate postoperative period,[20] owing to varying degrees of neuropraxia that recovers with time and nerve regeneration. In the setting of unilateral template modifications with or without ipsilateral nerve sparing, these periods of temporary anejaculation are largely avoided.[22] Similar outcomes can be achieved in the postchemotherapy setting. In a series by Pettus and colleagues,[23] 40% of consecutive patients undergoing a postchemotherapy resection were candidates for prospective nerve-sparing techniques. Among these, 79% were able to achieve successful antegrade emission after surgery, noting lower rates of functional recovery in right-sided tumors and larger volume disease. Among all of the aforementioned studies and others, no significant negative impact was noted on oncologic outcomes, providing evidence that these techniques can be safely incorporated among appropriately selected patients without compromising long-term survival.[12,21,24,25]

In the minimally invasive realm of surgical technique for RPLND, several investigators have demonstrated feasibility in preserving seminal emission and antegrade ejaculation. Most early studies accomplished this through the use of modified templates, with rates of preservation being noted in 85.7% to 100% of patients.[26–30] Limited data are available regarding the feasibility of prospective ipsilateral nerve sparing using the minimally invasive approach. In a series of 42 patients published by Steiner and colleagues,[31] successful recovery of function was noted in 85.7% of patients undergoing bilateral nerve sparing.

Ultimately, the goal of maintaining ejaculatory function is preservation of fertility. In the primary setting of RPLND, reports from the authors' institution demonstrated successful paternity in 76% of patients attempting pregnancy after undergoing nerve-sparing RPLND.[32] In the series by Beck and colleagues[15] similar success rates were reported, with 73% fathering children after nerve-sparing RPLND. Lower rates of paternity were noted among patients receiving chemotherapy for the management of relapse in this series. Similarly in the postchemotherapy setting for advanced disease, the negative impact of platinum-based regimens on spermatogenesis has been shown to persist for many years beyond treatment.[33] Therefore, given the well-documented oncologic effectiveness of surgery as a stand-alone treatment in the absence of adjuvant chemotherapy,[22,34–36] it remains the authors' disposition to avoid the routine use of adjuvant chemotherapy among patients in whom fertility remains an important consideration after primary RPLND.

Vascular (Venous Thromboembolism/ Pulmonary Embolism, Hemorrhage/Vascular Injury)

Venous thromboembolism

As with all major abdominal operations, the risk of venous thromboembolism (VTE) is inherent with primary and postchemotherapy RPLND. Fortunately, rates remain low for both populations of patients, with incidences of deep venous thrombosis (DVT) reported at less than 1%.[21,37] Similarly, the occurrence of pulmonary embolism (PE) is less than 1% in the primary setting,[21,37,38] and ranges from 0.1% to 3.1% in the postchemotherapy setting.[37,39] Although DVT remains an uncommon event, the low-risk, commonsense use of sequential compression devices before induction of anesthesia and maintenance when nonambulatory throughout hospitalization should be routinely incorporated. In addition, early mobilization and ambulation should be encouraged in essentially all patients when feasible.

The routine use of thromboprophylaxis remains more controversial. Pharmaceuticals such as subcutaneous low-dose unfractionated heparin and low molecular weight heparin have demonstrated efficacy in decreasing VTE rates in the postoperative period.[40] However, concerns regarding the increased risk of lymphocele and/or chylous ascites with their use in patients with prostate cancer have hampered their widespread use after RPLND.[41–43] Given the competing risks of VTE-related complications in comparison with lymphatic complications, consideration for chemical thromboprophylaxis should be made on a case-by-case basis, with prioritization of its use among high-risk patients because of known hypercoagulable states, anticipated vascular reconstruction, or personal histories of PE/DVT.

Hemorrhage and vascular injury

The potential for vascular injury intraoperatively and/or hemorrhage in the perioperative period remains a risk of any retroperitoneal operation. With RPLND, the volume of blood loss and number of transfusions correlates well with the complexity of the operation. In patients undergoing primary RPLND with or without nerve sparing, mean blood loss among contemporary studies ranged from 150 to 200 mL, with vascular injuries occurring in 0% to 2.5% of cases.[21,44] In a study by Baniel and colleagues,[45] 2 vascular complications were noted among unilateral or bilateral template procedures in the 478 patients evaluated (0.4%), including a scrotal hematoma requiring drainage and a rectus sheath hematoma in another. In a more recent report by Subramanian and colleagues[37] comparing primary and postchemotherapy complications, greater degrees of blood loss and transfusion rates were seem in the postchemotherapy RPLND setting. In addition, among 96 patients in the postchemotherapy group, 1 patient experienced delayed hemorrhage necessitating management. Delayed bleeding was also reported in the postchemotherapy RPLND setting by Baniel and colleagues[39] in 2 patients out of 603 reported cases (0.3%), both occurring in the setting of postoperative anticoagulation for VTE events. Comparisons have been made with regard to open versus laparoscopic approaches. In general, overall blood loss rates with minimally invasive techniques are touted to be less, although transfusion rates in the primary setting for either approach are similarly low. However, major vascular injuries are reported to occur at a higher frequency in the minimally invasive cohorts.[46,47]

Lymphatic (Lymphocele, Chylous Ascites)

Lymphocele

The development of localized lymphatic fluid accumulation in the surgical bed can occur in the presence or absence of symptoms. Subclinical lymphoceles are likely common after RPLND, although the true incidence has not been reliably evaluated and reported. Symptomatic lymphoceles are reported to occur in 0% to 1.7% of patients undergoing RPLND.[21,37,39,45] Patients may present clinically with symptoms caused by compression of adjacent structures, including the ureter causing obstruction and resultant colic, or venous compression leading to lower extremity swelling and edema. Further symptoms include abdominal distention, early satiety, nausea, and emesis when displacement of the stomach and proximal intestine occurs with larger volume collections. When colonized or seeded with bacteria, fever and regional pain may develop as infection sets in. Prevention remains paramount through the meticulous ligation of lymphatic channels

encountered and disrupted during RPLND. Observation of asymptomatic lymphoceles identified during routine imaging is acceptable, as most will reabsorb over the subsequent months. In the setting of symptoms, percutaneous aspiration and drainage is required. Systemic antibiotics should be administered when concerns for infection exist.

Chylous ascites

In contrast to a localized collection of lymphatic fluid in the retroperitoneum, chylous ascites represents a unique complication attributable to RPLND. This condition refers to the large-volume accumulation of chylomicron-containing lymphatic fluid that develops and is distributed throughout the retroperitoneal and peritoneal compartments. In the primary setting, it has been reported to occur in 0.2% to 2.1% of patients, with higher rates of 2% to 7% being noted in the postchemotherapy populations.[21,37,39,45,48] Though not typically present in the early postoperative period, chylous ascites tend to manifest in the second or third week after surgery with symptoms of massive abdominal distention, anorexia, nausea, emesis, and shortness of breath. Physical examination often demonstrates characteristic findings of an abdominal fluid wave and relative absence of tympany on percussion, helping to distinguish ascites from postoperative ileus. Imaging will reveal the diffuse presence of fluid throughout the abdominal cavity. Diagnosis is made on paracentesis, which reveals milky-colored fluid. Testing of the fluid will reveal alkaline, triglyceride-laden fluid that stains positive for Sudan black.

The etiology of chylous ascites is related to disruption of the cisterna chyli and its tributaries, located posterior to the medial surface of the aorta at the level of the L1/2 vertebral bodies and coursing to the retrocrural space. Dissections that incorporate the suprahilar area are at greater risk of this complication.[3] In addition, resection of the inferior vena cava has been associated with a higher incidence of this complication, attributable to higher venous pressures leading to increased capillary leak and secondary third spacing of lymphatic fluid in the retroperitoneum.[49] Others have reported increased rates of chylous ascites with increasing cycles of chemotherapy, greater volume of intraoperative blood loss, and longer operative times.[48]

Management strategies at the authors' institution have followed a graduated approach, with initial paracentesis as a first step for diagnostics and assessment of resolution of symptoms. Implementation of a low fat/medium-chain triglyceride diet is provided with help from nutritionists, as well as observation to determine the duration of the symptom-free interval, as many patients will require no further management. However, in the setting of prompt reaccumulation and development of recurrent symptoms, an indwelling tunneled drain is placed and initiation of total parenteral nutrition with restriction of oral intake recommended. Anecdotally the routine use of octreotide has not proved to be of great value in the authors' experience; however, it has demonstrated efficacy in minimizing chylous leaks after hepaticopancreaticobiliary surgery.[50,51]

With these modifications, persistence of high-volume chylous drainage (>100 mL/24 h) is exceedingly rare. In the circumstance of refractory or persistent large-volume ascites, placement of a peritoneovenous (LeVeen) shunt or surgical exploration with attempted ligation of the lymphatic leak remain options. These should be reserved as last resorts, as peritoneovenous shunts have been reported to be associated with a significant incidence of occlusion or malfunction, often requiring revision after placement, sepsis, and potentially fat embolization.[48]

Neurologic (Neuropraxia, Paralysis)

Temporary neuropraxia in the thigh can occur following either primary or postchemotherapy RPLND. This usually improves within 4 weeks but can persist for several months. In addition, numbness of the anterior and medial thigh will occur if the anterior femoral cutaneous, genitofemoral, and/or ilioinguinal nerve branches are resected during removal of the retroperitoneal nodes and/or masses. In the authors' experience, symptomatic management with narcotics and nerve pain medications, such as gabapentin and nonsteroidal anti-inflammatories, are of marginal benefit with most improvement seen simply with additional convalescence. The incidence of spinal cord ischemia with subsequent lower extremity paralysis is one of the most devastating neurologic complications that can occur. In a report by Leibovitch and colleagues,[52] this occurred in only 4 of 712 (0.56%) postchemotherapy RPLND cases and no primary RPLND cases. Contributing factors in the 4 cases were extensive residual masses, combined retroperitoneal and mediastinal dissection with division of lumbar and intercostal arteries, and previous abdominal irradiation. In a review of 268 patients undergoing postchemotherapy resection of mediastinal disease for testicular or primary retroperitoneal germ cell tumor, Kesler and colleagues[53] reported 6 patients (2.2%) with paraplegia. Patients with bulky mediastinal and retroperitoneal disease are at an increased risk of

developing paraplegia. The likelihood of neurologic complications increases with the scale of para-aortic resection.

Pulmonary

Major pulmonary complications are rare but occur more commonly in the postchemotherapy setting in 1% to 8% of postchemotherapy RPLND cases.[37,54] These complications can include PE, pneumonia, and acute respiratory distress syndrome with mechanical ventilation. Historically, patients treated with bleomycin regimens were at risk of acute respiratory distress syndrome requiring prolonged ventilator support. With improvements in supportive care intraoperatively and postoperatively, and surgical efficiency, the incidence of respiratory complications has declined over the years. In a contemporary report of 234 good-risk postchemotherapy RPLND patients treated initially with either 3 cycles of bleomycin/etoposide/cisplatin or 4 cycles of etoposide/cisplatin, there was no increase in pulmonary complications postoperatively in patients treated with bleomycin.[55] Indeed, no patient required intensive care unit admission for ventilation, all patients were extubated at the end of the surgical procedure, and duration of supplemental oxygen was less than 48 hours regardless of the use of bleomycin. The role of an experienced anesthesiologist should not be understated regarding intraoperative and postoperative pulmonary issues. Typically the fraction of inspired oxygen intraoperatively is kept between 30% and 40% for most of the operation. Intraoperative fluid resuscitation is minimized and not driven by intraoperative urine output. Additional fluid is not given to compensate for nothing-by-mouth status. Patients typically are given 4 mL/kg/h lactated Ringer solution and 2 mL/kg/h albumin for the first 2 hours of the operation. Volume and vital status are then reassessed at that point to dictate additional resuscitation. Blood transfusions are administered only if clinically indicated.

Gastrointestinal

Ileus and small bowel obstruction

One of the more common complications reported after either primary or postchemotherapy RPLND is postoperative paralytic ileus. Incidence of this varies in the literature largely because of diverse definitions of ileus. One study reported that ileus accounted for 63% and 45% of all complications in primary and postchemotherapy RPLND patients, respectively.[37] In recent studies, significant ileus has occurred in 0% to 12% of cases.[16,21,37,54,56] A 2017 study of 68 patients reported no cases of ileus using a midline extraperitoneal approach.[16] Most cases do not require routine postoperative nasogastric tubes. However, if duodenal resection or primary repair are required, the authors would recommend a nasogastric tube in the immediate postoperative period. The reported incidence of small bowel obstruction requiring operative intervention is less than 1% of cases. This has been reported to occur early within 30 days of RPLND and also years following RPLND.

Mortality

Mortality in the primary RPLND setting should generally be zero.[21,22,37] In more advanced disease, the risk of postoperative mortality following postchemotherapy RPLND remains low but is related to surgical volume. Capitanio and colleagues[57] used the Surveillance, Epidemiology, and End Results (SEER) database to compare the incidence of perioperative mortality in the community with reports from centers of excellence with significant surgical experience. The incidence of mortality in the community was 6% versus 0.8% in the center of excellence for patients with advanced disease. The Indiana group has updated their experience using a more contemporary cohort, whereby the risk of perioperative mortality was 0.26% in 755 patients who underwent postchemotherapy RPLND.[54]

INCIDENCE OF COMPLICATIONS

The overall incidence of complications from retroperitoneal lymph node dissection varies between the primary and postchemotherapy setting. This is largely due to the desmoplastic reaction following chemotherapy and variable residual mass sizes around the great vessels.

Primary Retroperitoneal Lymph Node Dissection

As detailed in the previous sections, several types of complications may occur following primary RPLND. The incidence of these complications is lower in the primary setting compared with after chemotherapy. The incidence also varies depending on surgeon and hospital volume. For example, overall postoperative complications in the primary setting range from 1.3% to 24%.[21,37,38,44] The proportion of complications is directly correlated with surgical experience, as demonstrated in the German series that explored this question in 7 centers (**Fig. 1**).[21] In this study, the highest volume surgeons/centers had the lowest incidence of complications (12%) compared with lowest

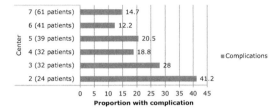

Fig. 1. Minor and major complications. (*Data from* Heidenreich A, Albers P, Hartmann M, et al. Complications of primary nerve sparing retroperitoneal lymph node dissection for clinical stage I nonseminomatous germ cell tumors of the testis: experience of the German Testicular Cancer Study Group. J Urol 2003;169(5):1710–4. https://doi.org/10.1097/01.ju. 0000060960.18092.54.)

volumes surgeons/centers (41%). This volume relationship has also been shown using the Nationwide Inpatient Sample in the United States. Higher hospital volume was associated with fewer respiratory, miscellaneous medical complications and overall complications, $P<.047$.[58] Beck and colleagues[44] also demonstrated a low incidence (1.3%) of complications in a more contemporary cohort at a high-volume single center.

Intraoperative complications during primary procedures should be minimal and mostly have been reported to involve vascular structures.[21,38] Reports of renal artery, superior mesenteric artery, and inferior vena cava injury occurred in 2.5% of the multicenter German study, of which all but one were surgically repaired. One patient with a renal artery injury required nephrectomy.[21] Other potential injuries include accidental ureteral injury and inadvertent enterotomy.

Postchemotherapy Retroperitoneal Lymph Node Dissection

Surgery following chemotherapy for metastatic disease is technically a more demanding operation when compared with primary RPLND. Owing to the desmoplastic reaction created following chemotherapy, natural tissue planes around the great vessels are most often obliterated. As such, the number of complications is greater than in the primary setting. Depending on the years of study, postoperative complications range from 3.7% to 32%.[16,37,54,59] In a study over time from Indiana University, a decreased risk in postoperative complications was noted from the 1990s (13.9%) to early 2000s (6.7%).[59] The likelihood of complications is directly related to the complexity of the surgery represented by size of the retroperitoneal mass at the time of surgery. In addition, postchemotherapy seminoma surgeries are also known to result in a more difficult dissection.

Heidenreich and colleagues[60] recently reported on a group of 25 "complex" patients who required additional procedures such as vascular grafting or resection of vertebral bodies. The median mass size was 18 cm and all patients had either intermediate-risk or poor-risk disease. In this group of 25 patients the incidence of complications was 41%, representing the challenging nature of this patient population. Regarding seminoma patients, Mosharafa and colleagues[61] demonstrated the risk of complications to be 24% in the seminoma group compared with 20% in the group without seminoma, $P = .29$. However, the need for additional procedures such as nephrectomy or vascular procedures was significantly higher in the seminoma group than in the nonseminoma group, 38% versus 26%, respectively ($P = .02$). The association of surgical volume with postoperative outcome also holds true in the postchemotherapy setting, including the risk of perioperative death. As already mentioned, this was demonstrated by Capitanio and colleagues[57] with a higher risk of perioperative mortality of 6% in SEER data versus 0.8% at higher-volume centers, suggesting that these complex patients should be managed at centers of excellence when possible.

Intraoperative complications are also largely vascular in nature in the postchemotherapy setting. This is explained by the increased need for vascular grafting procedures and nephrectomies. Subramanian and colleagues[37] reported an 11% intraoperative complication risk, all of which were vascular in nature, compared with 5% overall complication risk in the primary RPLND setting. Furthermore, in a study of 755 postchemotherapy patients, the incidence of additional intraoperative procedures was 22% with nephrectomy being the most common. Significant risk factors for additional procedures were preoperative mass size, elevated markers at the time of surgery, and retroperitoneal pathology, all $P<.05$.[54]

REFERENCES

1. Hinman F. The operative treatment of tumors of the testicle: with the report of thirty cases treated by orchidectomy. JAMA 1914;LXIII(23):2009–15.

2. Chevassu M. Tumeurs de la glande sous-maxillaire. Rev Chir 1910;41:145–70.

3. Donohue JP. Retroperitoneal lymphadenectomy: the anterior approach including bilateral suprarenal-hilar dissection. Urol Clin North Am 1977;4(3):509–21.

4. Donohue JP, Rowland RG. Complications of retroperitoneal lymph node dissection. J Urol 1981;125(3):338–40.

5. Sago AL, Ball TP, Novicki DE. Complications of retroperitoneal lymphadenectomy. Urology 1979;13(3):241–3.

6. Staubitz WJ, Early KS, Magoss IV, et al. Surgical management of testis tumor. J Urol 1974;111(2):205–9.

7. Einhorn LH, Donohue JP. Improved chemotherapy in disseminated testicular cancer. J Urol 1977;117(1):65–9.

8. Donohue JP, Zachary JM, Maynard BR. Distribution of nodal metastases in nonseminomatous testis cancer. J Urol 1982;128(2):315–20.

9. Ray B, Hajdu SI, Whitmore WF. Distribution of retroperitoneal lymph node metastases in testicular germinal tumors. Cancer 1974;33(2):340–8.

10. Weissbach L, Boedefeld EA. Localization of solitary and multiple metastases in stage II nonseminomatous testis tumor as basis for a modified staging lymph node dissection in stage I. J Urol 1987;138(1):77–82.

11. Narayan P, Lange PH, Fraley EE. Ejaculation and fertility after extended retroperitoneal lymph node dissection for testicular cancer. J Urol 1982;127(4):685–8.

12. Donohue JP, Foster RS, Rowland RG, et al. Nerve-sparing retroperitoneal lymphadenectomy with preservation of ejaculation. J Urol 1990;144(2 Pt 1):287–91 [discussion: 291–2].

13. Jewett MAS, Kong YS, Goldberg SD, et al. Retroperitoneal lymphadenectomy for testis tumor with nerve sparing for ejaculation. J Urol 1988;139(6):1220–4.

14. Colleselli K, Poisel S, Schachtner W, et al. Nerve-preserving bilateral retroperitoneal lymphadenectomy: anatomical study and operative approach. J Urol 1990;144(2 Pt 1):293–7 [discussion: 297–8].

15. Beck SDW, Bey AL, Bihrle R, et al. Ejaculatory status and fertility rates after primary retroperitoneal lymph node dissection. J Urol 2010;184(5):2078–80.

16. Syan-Bhanvadia S, Bazargani ST, Clifford TG, et al. Midline extraperitoneal approach to retroperitoneal lymph node dissection in testicular cancer: minimizing surgical morbidity. Eur Urol 2017;72(5):814–20.

17. Pizzocaro G, Salvioni R, Zanoni F. Unilateral lymphadenectomy in intraoperative stage I nonseminomatous germinal testis cancer. J Urol 1985;134(3):485–9.

18. Weissbach L, Boedefeld EA, Oberdörster W. Modified RLND as a means to preserve ejaculation. Prog Clin Biol Res 1985;203:323–34.

19. Fossa SD, Ous S. Primary unilateral retroperitoneal lymph node dissection (RLND) in nonseminomatous testicular cancer. Prog Clin Biol Res 1985;203:319.

20. Jewett MAS, Torbey C. Nerve-sparing techniques in retroperitoneal lymphadenectomy in patients with

low-stage testicular cancer. Semin Urol 1988;6(3): 233–7.

21. Heidenreich A, Albers P, Hartmann M, et al. Complications of primary nerve sparing retroperitoneal lymph node dissection for clinical stage I nonseminomatous germ cell tumors of the testis: experience of the German Testicular Cancer Study Group. J Urol 2003;169(5):1710–4.

22. Donohue JP, Thornhill JA, Foster RS, et al. Retroperitoneal lymphadenectomy for clinical stage A testis cancer (1965 to 1989): modifications of technique and impact on ejaculation. J Urol 1993;149(2): 237–43.

23. Pettus JA, Carver BS, Masterson T, et al. Preservation of ejaculation in patients undergoing nerve-sparing postchemotherapy retroperitoneal lymph node dissection for metastatic testicular cancer. Urology 2009;73(2):328–31 [discussion: 331–2].

24. Babaian RJ, Bracken RB, Johnson DE. Complications of transabdominal retroperitoneal lymphadenectomy. Urology 1981;17(2):126–8.

25. Skinner DG, Melamud A, Lieskovsky G. Complications of thoracoabdominal retroperitoneal lymph node dissection. J Urol 1982;127(6):1107–10.

26. Cheney SM, Andrews PE, Leibovich BC, et al. Robot-assisted retroperitoneal lymph node dissection: technique and initial case series of 18 patients. BJU Int 2015;115(1):114–20.

27. Hyams ES, Pierorazio P, Proteek O, et al. Laparoscopic retroperitoneal lymph node dissection for clinical stage I nonseminomatous germ cell tumor: a large single institution experience. J Urol 2012; 187(2):487–92.

28. Skolarus TA, Bhayani SB, Chiang HC, et al. Laparoscopic retroperitoneal lymph node dissection for low-stage testicular cancer. J Endourol 2008;22(7): 1485–9.

29. Cresswell J, Scheitlin W, Gozen A, et al. Laparoscopic retroperitoneal lymph node dissection combined with adjuvant chemotherapy for pathological stage II disease in nonseminomatous germ cell tumours: a 15-year experience. BJU Int 2008;102(7): 844–8.

30. Bhayani SB, Ong A, Oh WK, et al. Laparoscopic retroperitoneal lymph node dissection for clinical stage I nonseminomatous germ cell testicular cancer: a long-term update. Urology 2003;62(2): 324–7.

31. Steiner H, Zangerl F, Stöhr B, et al. Results of bilateral nerve sparing laparoscopic retroperitoneal lymph node dissection for testicular cancer. J Urol 2008;180(4):1348–52 [discussion: 1352–3].

32. Foster RS, McNulty A, Rubin LR, et al. The fertility of patients with clinical stage I testis cancer managed by nerve sparing retroperitoneal lymph node dissection. J Urol 1994;152(4):1139–42 [discussion: 1142–3].

33. Lampe H, Horwich A, Norman A, et al. Fertility after chemotherapy for testicular germ cell cancers. J Clin Oncol 1997;15(1):239–45.

34. Richie JP, Kantoff PW. Is adjuvant chemotherapy necessary for patients with stage B1 testicular cancer? J Clin Oncol 1991;9(8):1393–6.

35. Hermans BP, Sweeney CJ, Foster RS, et al. Risk of systemic metastases in clinical stage I nonseminoma germ cell testis tumor managed by retroperitoneal lymph node dissection. J Urol 2000;163(6): 1721–4.

36. Nicolai N, Miceli R, Artusi R, et al. A simple model for predicting nodal metastasis in patients with clinical stage I nonseminomatous germ cell testicular tumors undergoing retroperitoneal lymph node dissection only. J Urol 2004;171(1):172–6.

37. Subramanian VS, Nguyen CT, Stephenson AJ, et al. Complications of open primary and post-chemotherapy retroperitoneal lymph node dissection for testicular cancer. Urol Oncol 2010;28(5): 504–9.

38. Baniel J, Foster RS, Rowland RG, et al. Complications of primary retroperitoneal lymph-node dissection for low-stage testicular cancer. World J Urol 1994;12(3):139–42.

39. Baniel J, Foster RS, Rowland RG, et al. Complications of post-chemotherapy retroperitoneal lymph node dissection. J Urol 1995;153(3 Pt 2): 976–80.

40. Collins R, Scrimgeour A, Yusuf S, et al. Reduction in fatal pulmonary embolism and venous thrombosis by perioperative administration of subcutaneous heparin. Overview of results of randomized trials in general, orthopedic, and urologic surgery. N Engl J Med 1988;318(18):1162–73.

41. Bigg SW, Catalona WJ. Prophylactic mini-dose heparin in patients undergoing radical retropubic prostatectomy. A prospective trial. Urology 1992;39(4): 309–13.

42. Koch MO, Smith JA. Low molecular weight heparin and radical prostatectomy: a prospective analysis of safety and side effects. Prostate Cancer Prostatic Dis 1997;1(2):101–4.

43. Schmitges J, Trinh QD, Jonas L, et al. Influence of low-molecular-weight heparin dosage on red blood cell transfusion, lymphocele rate and drainage duration after open radical prostatectomy. Eur J Surg Oncol 2012;38(11):1082–8.

44. Beck SDW, Peterson MD, Bihrle R, et al. Short-term morbidity of primary retroperitoneal lymph node dissection in a contemporary group of patients. J Urol 2007;178(2):504–6 [discussion: 506].

45. Baniel J, Foster RS, Rowland RG, et al. Complications of primary retroperitoneal lymph node dissection. J Urol 1994;152(2 Pt 1):424–7.

46. Pearce SM, Golan S, Gorin MA, et al. Safety and early oncologic effectiveness of primary robotic

retroperitoneal lymph node dissection for nonseminomatous germ cell testicular cancer. Eur Urol 2017;71(3):476–82.

47. Harris KT, Gorin MA, Ball MW, et al. A comparative analysis of robotic vs laparoscopic retroperitoneal lymph node dissection for testicular cancer. BJU Int 2015;116(6):920–3.

48. Evans JG, Spiess PE, Kamat AM, et al. Chylous ascites after post-chemotherapy retroperitoneal lymph node dissection: review of the M. D. Anderson experience. J Urol 2006;176(4):1463–7.

49. Baniel J, Foster RS, Rowland RG, et al. Management of chylous ascites after retroperitoneal lymph node dissection for testicular cancer. J Urol 1993;150(5): 1422–4.

50. Shapiro AM, Bain VG, Sigalet DL, et al. Rapid resolution of chylous ascites after liver transplantation using somatostatin analog and total parenteral nutrition. Transplantation 1996;61(9):1410–1.

51. Kuboki S, Shimizu H, Yoshidome H, et al. Chylous ascites after hepatopancreatobiliary surgery. Br J Surg 2013;100(4):522–7.

52. Leibovitch I, Nash PA, Little JS, et al. Spinal cord ischemia after post-chemotherapy retroperitoneal lymph node dissection for nonseminomatous germ cell cancer. J Urol 1996;155(3):947–51.

53. Kesler KA, Brooks JA, Rieger KM, et al. Mediastinal metastases from testicular nonseminomatous germ cell tumors: patterns of dissemination and predictors of long-term survival with surgery. J Thorac Cardiovasc Surg 2003;125(4):913–23.

54. Cary C, Masterson TA, Bihrle R, et al. Contemporary trends in postchemotherapy retroperitoneal lymph node dissection: additional procedures and perioperative complications. Urol Oncol 2015;33(9):389.e15-21.

55. Calaway AC, Foster RS, Adra N, et al. Risk of bleomycin-related pulmonary toxicities and operative morbidity after postchemotherapy retroperitoneal lymph node dissection in patients with good-risk germ cell tumors. J Clin Oncol 2018;36(29): 2950–4.

56. Spiess PE, Brown GA, Liu P, et al. Predictors of outcome in patients undergoing postchemotherapy retroperitoneal lymph node dissection for testicular cancer. Cancer 2006;107(7):1483–90.

57. Capitanio U, Jeldres C, Perrotte P, et al. Population-based study of perioperative mortality after retroperitoneal lymphadenectomy for nonseminomatous testicular germ cell tumors. Urology 2009;74(2): 373–7.

58. Yu H-Y, Hevelone ND, Patel S, et al. Hospital surgical volume, utilization, costs and outcomes of retroperitoneal lymph node dissection for testis cancer. Adv Urol 2012;2012(2):1–8.

59. Mosharafa AA, Foster RS, Koch MO, et al. Complications of post-chemotherapy retroperitoneal lymph node dissection for testis cancer. J Urol 2004; 171(5):1839–41.

60. Heidenreich A, Haidl F, Paffenholz P, et al. Surgical management of complex residual masses following systemic chemotherapy for metastatic testicular germ cell tumours. Ann Oncol 2017;28(2):362–7.

61. Mosharafa AA, Foster RS, Leibovich BC, et al. Is post-chemotherapy resection of seminomatous elements associated with higher acute morbidity? J Urol 2003;169(6):2126–8.

High-Dose Chemotherapy and Autologous Stem Cell Transplant

Nabil Adra, MD, MSc*, Rafat Abonour, MD

KEYWORDS

- Testicular cancer • Germ cell tumor • High-dose chemotherapy • Salvage chemotherapy
- Stem cell transplant

KEY POINTS

- First-line cisplatin-based chemotherapy will cure about 80% of patients with metastatic germ cell tumors.
- Despite the substantial advances in germ cell tumors, 20% to 30% of patients will relapse after first-line chemotherapy and will require additional salvage therapies.
- High-dose chemotherapy followed by bone marrow transplant was first investigated for relapsed metastatic germ cell tumors at Indiana University in 1986.
- In 1996, bone marrow transplant was replaced by peripheral blood stem cell transplant allowing for more rapid engraftment and fewer delays in delivering a second cycle of high-dose chemotherapy.
- Using high-dose chemotherapy and peripheral blood stem cell transplant along with modern supportive care measures, cures are achieved in up to 60% of patients with relapsed germ cell tumor.

INTRODUCTION

Germ cell tumors (GCT) are the most common cancer in men between 15 and 35 years of age and the incidence has increased during the past several decades.[1] The International Germ Cell Cancer Collaborative Group (IGCCCG) classified patients with metastatic GCT into good-, intermediate-, and poor-risk disease based on specified prognostic criteria.[2] Per the IGCCCG, the good-risk category represents 60%, intermediate-risk 26%, and poor-risk 14% of patients with metastatic GCT. Patients with metastatic GCT are curable even in the presence of metastatic disease.[3] Using contemporary cisplatin-based frontline combination chemotherapy, cure rates at the authors' institution for good, intermediate, and poor risk disease are 90%, 84%, and 54% respectively.[4] Salvage surgery is appropriate for patients who relapse with anatomically confined disease after initial chemotherapy.[5] The vast majority of patients, however, will be treated with salvage chemotherapy; the most effective regimen for these patients remains unsettled. Second-line standard dose chemotherapy options include etoposide plus ifosfamide plus cisplatin (VIP), vinblastine plus ifosfamide plus cisplatin, or paclitaxel plus ifosfamide plus cisplatin (TIP).[6–8]

High-dose chemotherapy (HDCT) followed by bone marrow transplant was first investigated at Indiana University in 1986.[9] Bone marrow transplantation was replaced by peripheral blood stem cell transplant (PBSCT) in 1996. This allowed for more rapid engraftment and hence fewer delays in delivering a second course of HDCT.

This article reviews the current knowledge on HDCT and stem cell transplant for salvage treatment of patients with relapsed metastatic GCT.

Disclosure Statement: The authors have no conflict of interests to disclose.
Division of Hematology & Medical Oncology, Melvin & Bren Simon Cancer Center, Indiana University School of Medicine, 535 Barnhill Drive, RT 400, Indianapolis, IN 46202, USA
* Corresponding author.
E-mail address: nadra@iu.edu

Urol Clin N Am 46 (2019) 439–448
https://doi.org/10.1016/j.ucl.2019.04.007
0094-0143/19/© 2019 Elsevier Inc. All rights reserved.

Furthermore, the authors attempt to dissect the controversy of using standard-dose versus high-dose therapy as initial salvage and identify patients who are most likely to benefit from HDCT and PBSCT.

HISTORY OF HIGH-DOSE CHEMOTHERAPY FOR METASTATIC GERM CELL TUMORS

Metastatic testicular cancer has always been sensitive to chemotherapy. When HDCT and autologous stem cell transplant were first introduced in the 1970s and after successful testing in patients with multiple myeloma and lymphoma, this strategy was further tested in a variety of solid tumors. Patients with relapsed GCT were of particular interest, given the known chemosensitivity of these tumors, young age at diagnosis, minimal comorbid conditions, and ability to escalate the doses of active drugs such as carboplatin and etoposide with main toxicity being myelosuppression, which can be overcome with stem cell transplant.

Initial studies of HDCT in the 1980s evaluated dose escalation of single-agent etoposide or carboplatin followed by autologous stem cell transplant in patients with previously treated GCT.[10,11] These studies established that dose escalation of single-agent chemotherapy has clinical activity with a tolerable toxicity profile. Initial studies evaluating high-dose cyclophosphamide were unsuccessful.[12] A landmark phase I/II study initiated in 1986 at Indiana University investigated the combination of high-dose carboplatin and etoposide followed by bone marrow transplant in 33 patients with relapsed refractory GCT.[9] Patients were treated with a fixed total dose of etoposide 1200 mg/m^2 divided over 3 days with each cycle. The carboplatin dose ranged from 900 mg/m^2 to 2000 mg/m^2 with a maximal tolerated dose identified to be 1500 mg/m^2. The most common nonhematologic toxicity was moderate enterocolitis. In this study, 2 cycles of HDCT were administered. Although 21% of patients had treatment-related deaths, substantial responses were observed with 8 out of 33 patients achieving complete remissions. Most patients on this study were treated in the third-line or later setting.

A multicenter Eastern Cooperative Oncology Group study was able to reproduce these results with 40 patients with relapsed refractory GCT enrolled.[13] Forty-five percent of patients achieved objective responses, including 8 partial and 9 complete remissions. Five patients suffered treatment-related mortality. This trial further established the potentially curative role of high-dose carboplatin and etoposide followed by autologous bone marrow transplantation in patients with relapsed GCT.

TRANSITION FROM BONE MARROW TO PERIPHERAL BLOOD STEM CELL TRANSPLANT

Encouraging results with bone marrow transplant were offset by delays in engraftment and hematologic recovery. In February 1996, Indiana University shifted from using bone marrow stem cells to peripheral blood stem cells after the introduction of granulocyte colony-stimulating factor in the mid-1990s allowing for easier harvest of peripheral blood stem cells. This allowed more rapid engraftment and delivering the second course of HDCT with fewer delays. With the introduction of peripheral blood stem cells, patients with rapidly progressive disease, such as progressive brain metastases or primary mediastinal nonseminoma, who previously were not amenable to cures were now offered a curative chance with HDCT and PBSCT. Up until this day, PBSCT remains standard for patients with relapsed GCT undergoing HDCT.

IMPROVED EFFICACY WITH DECREASED TOXICITY

Given promising results in initial studies, further efforts focused on improving efficacy while decreasing short-term toxicity of HDCT. The transition to peripheral blood stem cells allowed for shorter duration of neutropenia and transfusion dependence and therefore shorter delays in delivering the subsequent cycle of HDCT. In addition, the addition of granulocyte colony-stimulating factor plus supportive care including appropriate administration of antibiotics has decreased treatment-related mortality from 21% in the initial studies to about 2% to 3% in the modern era.[14–16] The earlier administration of HDCT and PBSCT in the course of the disease has had a substantial impact on decreasing morbidity and improving cure rates. **Table 1** highlights landmark prospective and retrospective studies evaluating salvage HDCT in patients with relapsed GCT.

Among the first 184 patients treated with high-dose carboplatin (2100 mg/m^2 per cycle) and etoposide (2250 mg/m^2 per cycle) with PBSCT at Indiana University, cures were achieved in 70% of patients in the second-line setting and in 45% of patients who were treated in the third-line or subsequent setting.[15] One hundred seventy-three patents received both planned cycles of HDCT. Only 3 acute drug-related deaths occurred, and secondary acute leukemia developed in 3 additional patients. Patients with primary mediastinal

Table 1
Landmark studies evaluating high-dose chemotherapy in germ cell tumors

Study	Regimen	N	Years	Results	Toxicity	Comments/Conclusions
Lorch et al,[20] 2012	VIPx1 + HD carboplatin + etoposide x3 vs VIPx3 + HD carboplatin + etoposide + cyclophosphamide x1	211	1999–2004	5-y OS 49% vs 5-y OS 39%	4% TRM vs 16% TRM	More toxicity and no survival advantage of single-cycle HDCT, which incorporates cyclophosphamide compared with 3 cycles of HDCT with carboplatin plus etoposide
Lorch et al,[29] 2011	HDCT vs standard-dose chemotherapy	1594	1990–2008	5-y OS 53% vs 5-y OS 41%	Not reported	HDCT was superior to standard-dose chemotherapy with respect to PFS and OS. These results were consistent within almost every prognostic subgroup evaluated except among the low-risk category
Pico et al,[28] 2005	VIP/VeIP x3 + HD carboplatin + etoposide + cyclophosphamidex1 vs VIP/VeIP x4	263	1994–2001	42% EFS vs 35% EFS	7% TRM vs 3% TRM	No survival benefit for single cycle of HDCT that incorporates cyclophosphamide over standard-dose chemotherapy
Einhorn et al,[15] 2007	HD carboplatin + etoposide x2	184	1996–2004	63% DFS 2nd line: 70% DFS 3rd line: 45% DFS	2% TRM	Patients with relapsed refractory GCT are curable by HDCT and PBSCT Poor prognostic features include • Using HDCT as ≥3rd-line therapy • Platinum-refractory disease (progression within 4 wk of standard-dose chemotherapy) • IGCCCG poor-risk disease

(continued on next page)

Table 1
(continued)

Study	Regimen	N	Years	Results	Toxicity	Comments/Conclusions
Feldman et al,[16] 2010	Paclitaxel + Ifosfamide x2 → HD carboplatin + etoposide x3 (TI-CE)	107	1993–2006	47% DFS 52% OS	2% TRM	Relapsed refractory GCT patients with poor prognostic features are curable with HDCT Most notable poor prognostic features: primary mediastinal nonseminoma and ≥2 prior lines of standard-dose chemotherapy
Adra et al,[31] 2016	HD carboplatin + etoposide x2	364	2004–2014	2-y PFS 60% 2-y OS 66% 2nd line: 63% PFS 3rd line: 49% PFS	2% TRM	Relapsed refractory GCT patients are curable with HDCT and PBSCT using HD carboplatin + etoposide x2 even when used in ≥3rd-line therapy Cures achieved in patients with primary mediastinal nonseminoma (23% PFS), platinum-refractory disease (33% PFS), progressive brain metastases (40% PFS), and ≥3rd-line or further therapy (49% PFS)

Abbreviations: EFS, event-free survival; HD, high-dose; PFS, progression-free survival; TRM, treatment-related mortality; VeIP, vinblastine-ifosfamide-cisplatin; VIP, etoposide-ifosfamide-cisplatin.

nonseminomatous GCT and late relapse were excluded from this study. This was a landmark study highlighting that optimal patient selection, earlier administration of HDCT in the disease course, switching to peripheral blood stem cells, further escalation of carboplatin and etoposide doses, and improved supportive care were all key to achieving higher number of cures with less toxicity.

Several studies attempted to capitulate on these successes by adding a third drug to the carboplatin-etoposide backbone. At Indiana University, a study evaluating the combination of ifosfamide, carboplatin, and etoposide was closed early due to nephrotoxicity experienced by the 4 of the first 7 patients treated at the lowest dose level.[17] A study from Germany evaluating the combination of ifosfamide, carboplatin, and etoposide in relapsed or refractory GCT did not show excess toxicity in 74 patients treated, albeit with lower carboplatin doses used.[18] Two-year overall survival (OS) was 44%, 2-year event-free survival (EFS) was 35%, and 2-year relapse-free survival was 67%. Treatment-related mortality was 3%.

Investigators at Memorial Sloan Kettering Cancer Center (MSKCC) evaluated a regimen incorporating cyclophosphamide to high-dose carboplatin and etoposide in 58 patients with GCT progressing after incomplete response to first-line chemotherapy or after salvage standard-dose chemotherapy.[19] Forty percent of patients achieved a complete response and 21% achieved a durable remission at 28 months. Myelosuppression was severe and there were 7 (12%) treatment-related deaths. A randomized phase III study comparing sequential with a single course of high-dose chemotherapy showed superior OS in the arm receiving sequential high-dose chemotherapy.[20] Between 1999 and 2004, 211 patients with relapsed or refractory GCT were randomized to 1 cycle of cisplatin, 100 mg/m^2; etoposide, 375 mg/m^2; and ifosfamide, 6 g/m^2, (VIP) plus 3 cycles of high-dose carboplatin, 1500 mg/m^2; and etoposide, 1500 mg/m^2, or 3 cycles of VIP plus 1 cycle of high-dose carboplatin, 2200 mg/m^2; etoposide, 1800 mg/m^2; and cyclophosphamide, 6400 mg/m^2. followed by autologous stem cell reinfusion. More patients experienced early treatment-related death with the single HDCT compared with the sequential HDCT regimen highlighting the additional toxicity and limited further therapeutic benefit of cyclophosphamide in this setting.

The incorporation of paclitaxel and ifosfamide to HDCT regimens was a novel approach pioneered by investigators at MSKCC. This regimen incorporates paclitaxel and ifosfamide as induction

chemotherapy and stem cell mobilization followed by high-dose carboplatin area under the curve 24 and etoposide, 1200 mg/m^2, each divided over 3 days followed by PBSCT for 3 cycles (TI-CE regimen).[16] In a phase I/II trial that enrolled 107 patients with unfavorable features such as extragonadal primary site, incomplete response to first-line chemotherapy, short duration of complete or partial response, or progressive disease after salvage standard-dose chemotherapy, the reported 5-year disease-free survival was 47% and OS was 52%. Mediastinal primary site and having received 2 or more prior lines of therapy predict poor disease-free survival. In this study, 5 of 21 patients with primary mediastinal nonseminoma and 2 of 7 patients with late relapse achieved long-term remissions with TI-CE.[16]

The combination of high-dose paclitaxel, ifosfamide, and carboplatin (TIC) has also been investigated. At MSKCC, this combination led to progressive renal insufficiency in 3 out of 23 patients treated with this regimen; significant acute and chronic renal toxicity was reported.[21] Investigators at City of Hope evaluated 1 cycle of high-dose paclitaxel in combination with carboplatin and etoposide followed by 1 cycle of high-dose TIC.[22,23] This study reported durable remissions with acceptable quality of life in long-term survivors.

Other regimens incorporating thiotepa, epirubicin, gemcitabine, docetaxel, melphalan, or bevacizumab have failed to show an additive survival advantage to standard HDCT regimens with carboplatin and etoposide.[24–27] Therefore, high-dose carboplatin and etoposide followed by PBSCT continues to be the backbone of almost all HDCT regimens used as salvage therapy in relapsed GCT. The most commonly used regimens for HDCT and PBSCT are listed in **Table 2**.

INITIAL SALVAGE REGIMEN AND NUMBER OF HIGH-DOSE CHEMOTHERAPY CYCLES

The choice of initial salvage chemotherapy for relapsed testicular cancer remains controversial. One of the challenges is determining which patients should be treated with salvage standard-dose chemotherapy versus high-dose chemotherapy. A randomized phase III study comparing sequential versus a single course of HDCT showed superior OS in the arm receiving sequential HDC.[20] A prospective phase III trial did not show a difference in survival when comparing VIP for 4 cycles versus VIP for 3 cycles followed by HDCT with carboplatin and etoposide plus cyclophosphamide for one cycle.[28] In 2011, Lorch and colleagues[29] reported outcomes from a large multiinstitutional

Table 2
Established high-dose chemotherapy regimens for relapsed germ cell tumor

Regimen	Dose	Days	Reference
Indiana University—Double Tandem Approach[a]			
Carboplatin	700 mg/m^2	1–3	Einhorn et al,[15] 2007
Etoposide	750 mg/m^2	1–3	Adra et al,[31] 2016
MSKCC—TIGER trial—Triple Sequential Approach[b]			
Carboplatin	AUC 8 mg/mL/min	1–3	Feldman et al,[16] 2010
Etoposide	400 mg/m^2	1–3	

Abbreviations: AUC, area under the curve; MSKCC, Memorial Sloan Kettering Cancer Center.
[a] Repeated every 21 to 28 days after hematologic recovery x2.
[b] Repeated every 21 to 28 days after hematologic recovery x3.

database evaluating 1594 patients with relapsed GCT. This retrospective study included a diverse patient population stratified to prognostic subgroups according to the International Prognostic Factors Study Group.[30] Patients were treated with heterogeneous salvage chemotherapy regimens between 1990 and 2008. In this study, HDCT achieved superior outcomes compared with standard-dose chemotherapy and there was an overall 56% decrease in the risk of progression after first salvage treatment, favoring HDCT. This translated into statistically significant improvement in OS with HDCT in all prognostic subgroups except the low-risk group. The superior outcomes with HDCT were more pronounced in patients with intermediate-, high-, or very high-risk disease.

Prospective and retrospective studies have demonstrated good outcomes with either 2 or 3 cycles of high-dose carboplatin and etoposide with no formal comparison to suggest the optimal number of cycles.[15,16]

In an updated analysis from Indiana University, 364 consecutive patients with relapsed GCT were treated with HDCT and autologous PBSCT between 2004 and 2014.[31] With a median follow-up of 3.3 years, the 2-year progression-free survival (PFS) was 60% and the 2-year OS was 66%. Three hundred three patients received HDCT as second-line therapy with a 2-year PFS of 63% and 61 patients received HDCT as third-line or later therapy with a 2-year PFS of 49%. There were 122 patients with platinum refractory disease, defined as tumor progression within 4 weeks of platinum-based chemotherapy, with a 2-year PFS of 33%. Five of 20 patients with primary mediastinal nonseminoma were disease-free after HDCT. Eight of 20 patients with progressive brain metastases at initiation of HDCT achieved remission and were disease-free after HDCT. There were 90 patients with seminoma on

this study with a 2-year PFS of 90%. Treatment-related death rate was 2.5%.

The role of HDCT and stem cell transplant in first-line therapy for patients with IGCCCG intermediate or poor-risk GCT was investigated in a randomized phase III trial where patients received bleomycin-etoposide-cisplatin (BEP) x4 versus BEPx2 followed by HDCTx2.[32] Two-hundred nineteen patients enrolled, and this study failed to show any survival advantage with incorporating HDCT to the first-line setting in high-risk patients.

Based on compelling clinical trial and large retrospective observational data, the preferred initial salvage regimen at Indiana University remains HDCT with carboplatin and etoposide followed by PBSCT for 2 cycles. Other investigators advocate the use of HDCT only in high-risk patients, those who have had a relapse after receiving ifosfamide-based chemotherapy or those who have had a relapse after 2 lines of standard salvage therapy. Optimal patient selection for HDCT versus standard-dose chemotherapy as initial salvage is currently being studied in a randomized phase III trial as part of an international collaboration (ClinicalTrials.gov identifier, NCT02375204). This trial (TIGER or a Randomized Phase III Trial of Initial Salvage Chemotherapy for Patients with Germ Cell Tumors) randomizes patients to receive TIP for 4 cycles or ifosfamide plus paclitaxel followed by high-dose carboplatin and etoposide and PBSCT for 3 cycles.

PROGNOSTIC FACTORS IN RELAPSED GERM CELL TUMORS

Patients who experience treatment failure after first-line cisplatin-based combination chemotherapy and thus require salvage therapies represent a heterogeneous group. Factors consistently associated with favorable outcome with salvage therapies include gonadal primary tumor site, complete response to first-line chemotherapy, and normal or low serum tumor markers (including alpha-fetoprotein [AFP] and human chorionic gonadotropin [hCG]) at time of initiation of salvage therapy.[33]

Beyer and colleagues[34] were the first to report a prognostic model for patients with relapsed GCT undergoing HDCT regimens at 4 different centers in Europe and the United States. This study included 310 patients and multivariate analysis identified the following adverse prognostic features: progressive disease before HDCT, mediastinal nonseminomatous primary tumor, refractory or absolute refractory disease to conventional-dose cisplatin, and hCG greater than 1000 mIU/mL before HDCT.

Single institution studies from Indiana University and MSKCC have identified several prognostic factors predicting inferior outcomes with HDCT and PBSCT. The initial Indiana University study with HDCT and PBSCT identified the following adverse prognostic features: treatment with HDCT as greater than or equal to third-line therapy, platinum refractory disease, and IGCCCG poor-risk category at time of initiation of first-line chemotherapy.[15] Feldman and colleagues[16] reported the following adverse prognostic features in 107 patients treated with salvage TI-CE and PBSCT: primary mediastinal nonseminoma, presence of lung metastases, hCG greater than or equal to 1000 mIU/mL, greater than or equal to 3 metastatic sites, and IGCCCG intermediate- or poor-risk classification at first-line chemotherapy. A second study from Indiana University evaluating 364 patients with relapsed GCT treated with HDCT and PBSCT identified the following poor prognostic features: treatment with HDCT as greater than or equal to third-line or subsequent therapy, platinum refractory disease, primary mediastinal primary site, nonseminoma histology, IGCCCG intermediate- or poor-risk disease, and hCG greater than or equal to 1000 mIU/mL.[31]

The International Prognostic Factor Study Group was formed to develop a prognostic model for patients who relapse and will be treated with standard-dose chemotherapy or HDCT. Data from 1984 patients with relapsed GCT who progressed after first-line chemotherapy and were treated with cisplatin-based conventional-dose or carboplatin-based HDCT were used to build the prognostic model.[30] The risk factors included the following:

- Primary tumor site,
- Prior response to first-line chemotherapy,
- Progression-free interval after first-line chemotherapy,
- AFP level at salvage therapy,
- hCG level at salvage therapy, and
- The presence of liver, brain, or bone metastases.

Each risk factor was assigned a numerical value based on its prognostic significance with the sum. Total score was used to classify patients into 5 risk groups: very low, low, intermediate, high, and very high risk. These prognostic categories differed significantly with regard to 2-year PFS: 75% in very low-risk, 51% in low-risk, 40% in intermediate-risk, 26% in high-risk, and 6% in the very high-risk category.

TUMOR MARKER DECLINE DURING HIGH-DOSE CHEMOTHERAPY AND PERIPHERAL-BLOOD STEM CELL TRANSPLANT

Adequate serum tumor marker decline, including AFP and hCG, during first-line standard-dose chemotherapy predicts outcome and chance of achieving cures.[35] Moreover, adequate serum tumor marker decline also predicts outcomes in patients receiving salvage chemotherapy.[36,37] The importance of serum tumor marker decline during HDCT and PBSCT was studied by investigators at MSKCC using the TI-CE regimen. Adequate serum tumor marker decline during HDCT predicted favorable PFS and OS, mostly driven by hCG. However, unsatisfactory declines did not exclude long-term PFS/OS.[38] A series of 25 patients reported from Indiana University with increasing tumor markers at the start of the second cycle of HDCT showed that increasing markers represented an adverse prognostic sign; however, cure was still possible in a small subset of these patients.[39]

ROLE OF RESIDUAL TUMOR RESECTION AFTER HIGH-DOSE CHEMOTHERAPY AND PERIPHERAL-BLOOD STEM CELL TRANSPLANT

Complete resection of all detectable residual masses after HDCT and PBSCT, if feasible, is of clinical importance to achieve long-term remissions. In reported retrospective series, the proportion of patients with viable cancer, with or without necrosis or teratoma, in resected specimens after HDCT was as high as 46%.[40,41] In a series of patients undergoing retroperitoneal lymph-node dissection post-HDCT, 72% of patients harbored teratoma or active cancer in the retroperitoneal specimen underscoring the importance of resection of all residual masses to render patients free of disease and providing optimal chance for long-term remissions.[40]

SURVIVORSHIP IN TESTICULAR CANCER SURVIVORS CURED WITH HIGH-DOSE CHEMOTHERAPY AND PERIPHERAL-BLOOD STEM CELL TRANSPLANT

Testicular cancer survivors are at risk for multiple late consequences of therapy contributing to cumulative burden of morbidity including metabolic syndrome, cardiovascular disease, hypertension, infertility, neurotoxicity, nephrotoxicity, pulmonary toxicity, hypogonadism, psychosocial disorders, and secondary malignancies.[42,43] In testicular cancer survivors, cumulative doses of etoposide have been associated with an increased risk of developing secondary leukemia that typically exhibits a short latency period, a chromosomal translocation (11q23 and 21q22), and rearrangement of the mixed-lineage leukemia gene.[44] Published data suggest that the risk of secondary leukemia is dose related and that the risk of treatment with etoposide totaling more than 2 g/m^2, almost always encountered in relapsed patients treated with HDCT, is approximately 2% to 3%.[45,46] Therefore, careful follow-up with routine hematological evaluation is important in survivors cured with HDCT and PBSCT.

A multiinstitutional study evaluating the genetic predisposition of long-term cisplatin toxicities, identifying single nucleotide polymorphisms associated with these toxicities, and collecting data regarding various cardiovascular risk factors in testicular cancer survivors is currently underway. Data regarding the long-term adverse health outcomes in testicular cancer survivors cured with HDCT are lacking. Future investigation in this patient population is of utmost importance.

SUMMARY

The modern history of testicular cancer is that of an oncological success story. The advances made in the diagnosis, prognostication, and treatment of patients with relapsed disease have resulted from collaborations among investigators across the globe. HDCT followed by PBSCT is an effective salvage therapy for relapsed GCT delineating the remarkable chemosensitivity of this disease. However, there remains a proportion of patients who are incurable despite intensification of therapy with HDCT and PBSCT. Further investigation will need to evaluate the biology and identify biomarkers of disease response/early resistance and introduce novel agents into the treatment paradigm.

REFERENCES

1. Nigam M, Aschebrook-Kilfoy B, Shikanov S, et al. Increasing incidence of testicular cancer in the United States and Europe between 1992 and 2009. World J Urol 2015;33(5):623–31.
2. International Germ Cell Consensus Classification: a prognostic factor-based staging system for metastatic germ cell cancers. International Germ Cell Cancer Collaborative Group. J Clin Oncol 1997;15(2):594–603.
3. Hanna NH, Einhorn LH. Testicular cancer–discoveries and updates. N Engl J Med 2014;371(21):2005–16.
4. Albany C, Adra N, Snavely A, et al. Multidisciplinary clinic approach improves overall survival outcomes of patients with metastatic germ-cell tumors. Ann Oncol 2017;29(2):341–6.
5. Murphy BR, Breeden ES, Donohue JP, et al. Surgical salvage of chemorefractory germ cell tumors. J Clin Oncol 1993;11(2):324–9.
6. Loehrer PJ Sr, Einhorn LH, Williams SD. VP-16 plus ifosfamide plus cisplatin as salvage therapy in refractory germ cell cancer. J Clin Oncol 1986;4(4):528–36.
7. Loehrer PJ Sr, Gonin R, Nichols CR, et al. Vinblastine plus ifosfamide plus cisplatin as initial salvage therapy in recurrent germ cell tumor. J Clin Oncol 1998;16(7):2500–4.
8. Kondagunta GV, Bacik J, Donadio A, et al. Combination of paclitaxel, ifosfamide, and cisplatin is an effective second-line therapy for patients with relapsed testicular germ cell tumors. J Clin Oncol 2005;23(27):6549–55.
9. Nichols CR, Tricot G, Williams SD, et al. Dose-intensive chemotherapy in refractory germ cell cancer–a phase I/II trial of high-dose carboplatin and etoposide with autologous bone marrow transplantation. J Clin Oncol 1989;7(7):932–9.
10. Shea TC, Flaherty M, Elias A, et al. A phase I clinical and pharmacokinetic study of carboplatin and autologous bone marrow support. J Clin Oncol 1989;7(8):1177.
11. Wolff SN, Johnson DH, Hainsworth J, et al. High-dose VP-16-213 monotherapy for refractory germinal malignancies: a phase II study. J Clin Oncol 1984;2(4):271–4.
12. Buckner C, Clift R, Fefer A, et al. High dose cyclophosphamide (NSC 26271) for the treatment of metastatic testicular neoplasms. Cancer Chemother Rep 1974;58(5 Pt 1):709–14.
13. Nichols CR, Andersen J, Lazarus HM, et al. High-dose carboplatin and etoposide with autologous bone marrow transplantation in refractory germ cell cancer: an Eastern Cooperative Oncology Group protocol. J Clin Oncol 1992;10(4):558–63.
14. Adra N, Althouse SK, Liu H, et al. Prognostic factors in patients with poor-risk germ-cell tumors: a retrospective analysis of the Indiana University experience from 1990 to 2014. Ann Oncol 2016;27(5):875–9.

15. Einhorn LH, Williams SD, Chamness A, et al. High-dose chemotherapy and stem-cell rescue for metastatic germ-cell tumors. N Engl J Med 2007;357(4): 340–8.

16. Feldman DR, Sheinfeld J, Bajorin DF, et al. TI-CE high-dose chemotherapy for patients with previously treated germ cell tumors: results and prognostic factor analysis. J Clin Oncol 2010;28(10):1706–13.

17. Broun E, Nichols C, Tricot G, et al. High dose carboplatin/VP-16 plus ifosfamide with autologous bone marrow support in the treatment of refractory germ cell tumors. Bone Marrow Transplant 1991; 7(1):53–6.

18. Siegert W, Beyer J, Strohscheer I, et al. High-dose treatment with carboplatin, etoposide, and ifosfamide followed by autologous stem-cell transplantation in relapsed or refractory germ cell cancer: a phase I/II study. The German Testicular Cancer Cooperative Study Group. J Clin Oncol 1994;12(6): 1223–31.

19. Motzer RJ, Mazumdar M, Bosl GJ, et al. High-dose carboplatin, etoposide, and cyclophosphamide for patients with refractory germ cell tumors: treatment results and prognostic factors for survival and toxicity. J Clin Oncol 1996;14(4):1098–105.

20. Lorch A, Kleinhans A, Kramar A, et al. Sequential versus single high-dose chemotherapy in patients with relapsed or refractory germ cell tumors: long-term results of a prospective randomized trial. J Clin Oncol 2012;30(8):800–5.

21. Feldman DR, Glezerman I, Patil S, et al. Phase I/II study of paclitaxel plus ifosfamide followed by high-dose paclitaxel, ifosfamide, and carboplatin with autologous stem cell reinfusion for salvage treatment of germ cell tumors. Biol Blood Marrow Transplant 2014;20(2):S90.

22. Margolin KA, Doroshow JH, Frankel P, et al. Paclitaxel-based high-dose chemotherapy with autologous stem cell rescue for relapsed germ cell cancer. Biol Blood Marrow Transplant 2005;11(11): 903–11.

23. Pal SK, Yamzon J, Sun V, et al. Paclitaxel-based high-dose chemotherapy with autologous stem cell rescue for relapsed germ cell tumor: clinical outcome and quality of life in long-term survivors. Clin Genitourin Cancer 2013;11(2):121–7.

24. Lotz J-P, Bui B, Gomez F, et al. Sequential high-dose chemotherapy protocol for relapsed poor prognosis germ cell tumors combining two mobilization and cytoreductive treatments followed by three high-dose chemotherapy regimens supported by autologous stem cell transplantation. Results of the phase II multicentric TAXIF trial. Ann Oncol 2005;16(3): 411–8.

25. Selle F, Fizazi K, Biron P, et al. The taxif ii protocol final results: a phase ii trial of high-dose chemotherapy supported by haematopoietic stem cell transplantation in patients with disseminated germ-cell tumors failing chemotherapy and with adverse prognostic factors. Paper presented at: European Society of Medical Oncology, 2012.

26. Nieto Y, Tannir NM, Tu S-M, et al. Phase II trial of bevacizumab (BEV)/high-dose chemotherapy (HDC) for refractory germ-cell tumors (GCT). Journal of Clinical Oncology; 2012.

27. Nieto Y, Tu SM, Bassett R, et al. Bevacizumab/high-dose chemotherapy with autologous stem-cell transplant for poor-risk relapsed or refractory germ-cell tumors. Ann Oncol 2015;26(10):2125–32.

28. Pico JL, Rosti G, Kramar A, et al. A randomised trial of high-dose chemotherapy in the salvage treatment of patients failing first-line platinum chemotherapy for advanced germ cell tumours. Ann Oncol 2005; 16(7):1152–9.

29. Lorch A, Bascoul-Mollevi C, Kramar A, et al. Conventional-dose versus high-dose chemotherapy as first salvage treatment in male patients with metastatic germ cell tumors: evidence from a large international database. J Clin Oncol 2011;29(16):2178–84.

30. Lorch A, Beyer J, Bascoul-Mollevi C, et al. Prognostic factors in patients with metastatic germ cell tumors who experienced treatment failure with cisplatin-based first-line chemotherapy. J Clin Oncol 2010;28(33):4906–11.

31. Adra N, Abonour R, Althouse SK, et al. High-dose chemotherapy and autologous peripheral-blood stem-cell transplantation for relapsed metastatic germ cell tumors: the Indiana University experience. J Clin Oncol 2016;35(10):1096–102.

32. Motzer RJ, Nichols CJ, Margolin KA, et al. Phase III randomized trial of conventional-dose chemotherapy with or without high-dose chemotherapy and autologous hematopoietic stem-cell rescue as first-line treatment for patients with poor-prognosis metastatic germ cell tumors. J Clin Oncol 2007; 25(3):247–56.

33. Fosså SD, Stenning SP, Gerl A, et al. Prognostic factors in patients progressing after cisplatin-based chemotherapy for malignant non-seminomatous germ cell tumours. Br J Cancer 1999;80(9):1392.

34. Beyer J, Kramar A, Mandanas R, et al. High-dose chemotherapy as salvage treatment in germ cell tumors: a multivariate analysis of prognostic variables. J Clin Oncol 1996;14(10):2638–45.

35. Fizazi K, Culine S, Kramar A, et al. Early predicted time to normalization of tumor markers predicts outcome in poor-prognosis nonseminomatous germ cell tumors. J Clin Oncol 2004;22(19): 3868–76.

36. Murphy BA, Motzer RJ, Mazumdar M, et al. Serum tumor marker decline is an early predictor of treatment outcome in germ cell tumor patients treated with cisplatin and ifosfamide salvage chemotherapy. Cancer 1994;73(10):2520–6.

37. Massard C, Kramar A, Beyer J, et al. Tumor marker kinetics predict outcome in patients with relapsed disseminated non-seminomatous germ-cell tumors. Ann Oncol 2013;24(2):322–8.

38. Feldman DR, Voss MH, Jia X, et al. Serum tumor marker (STM) decline rates during high-dose chemotherapy (HDCT) to predict outcome for germ cell tumor (GCT) patients (pts). Journal of Clinical Oncology; 2012.

39. Pant-Purohit M, Brames MJ, Abonour R, et al. Tumor marker rise during second course high-dose chemotherapy in recurrent testicular cancer: Outcome analysis. J Clin Oncol 2011;29(15_suppl): 4612.

40. Cary C, Pedrosa JA, Jacob J, et al. Outcomes of postchemotherapy retroperitoneal lymph node dissection following high-dose chemotherapy with stem cell transplantation. Cancer 2015;121(24): 4369–75.

41. Rick O, Bokemeyer C, Weinknecht S, et al. Residual tumor resection after high-dose chemotherapy in patients with relapsed or refractory germ cell cancer. J Clin Oncol 2004;22(18):3713–9.

42. Fung C, Sesso HD, Williams AM, et al. Multi-institutional assessment of adverse health outcomes among north american testicular cancer survivors after modern cisplatin-based chemotherapy. J Clin Oncol 2017;35(11):1211–22.

43. Kerns SL, Fung C, Monahan PO, et al. Cumulative burden of morbidity among testicular cancer survivors after standard cisplatin-based chemotherapy: a multi-institutional study. J Clin Oncol 2018;36(15): 1505–12.

44. Travis LB, Fossa SD, Schonfeld SJ, et al. Second cancers among 40,576 testicular cancer patients: focus on long-term survivors. J Natl Cancer Inst 2005;97(18):1354–65.

45. Houck W, Abonour R, Vance G, et al. Secondary leukemias in refractory germ cell tumor patients undergoing autologous stem-cell transplantation using high-dose etoposide. J Clin Oncol 2004;22(11): 2155–8.

46. Kollmannsberger C, Hartmann JT, Kanz L, et al. Risk of secondary myeloid leukemia and myelodysplastic syndrome following standard-dose chemotherapy or high-dose chemotherapy with stem cell support in patients with potentially curable malignancies. J Cancer Res Clin Oncol 1998;124(3–4): 207–14.

MicroRNAs as Biomarkers for Germ Cell Tumors

Lucia Nappi, MD, PhD[a,b], Craig Nichols, MD[c,d],*

KEYWORDS

- Testicular cancer • Germ cell tumor • Management of testis cancer • MicroRNAs • Biomarkers

KEY POINTS

- Germ cell testicular cancer is curable with cisplatin-based chemotherapy and represents one of the successes of the medical oncology in the past 40 years.
- Some clinical scenarios, including clinical stage I, tumor marker negative stage IIA, and postchemotherapy residual disease, still are equivocal because of the lack of sensitivity and specificity of the current imaging and tumor markers.
- Circulating microRNAs are specifically expressed by germ cell tumors, both seminoma and noseminoma, and can be detected in the blood of patients with germ cell tumors.
- Large prospective trials to validate the clinical utility of those circulating microRNAs have been planned.
- If their high sensitivity and specificity are confirmed prospectively, those microRNAs will become clinical biomarkers to overcome the uncertainty of equivocal clinical settings and ultimately improve the quality of the care of patients with germ cell tumors.

INTRODUCTION

The treatment of testicular cancer is one of the top 5 successes of the modern medical oncology.[1] Cisplatin-based chemotherapy has dramatically changed the prognosis of patients with germ cell testicular cancer (GCT),[2] and over the past 40 years there has been a continuous dynamic process to learn how to maximize the positive effects of chemotherapy and reduce the negative long-term effects deriving from it.[3–5] The authors also observed a switch of the priority in this curable disease: from cure to cure plus preservation of quality of life of survivors.[6,7] The high survival rate, however, is related to some variables and to the delivery of the care by expert centers. The differences in the outcomes of the patients treated in high volume compared with the centers with minimal exposure to GCTs have an impact on the quality of the care that the patients receive.[8] This is true particularly for patients who need surgical treatments (retroperitoneal lymph node dissection [RPLND]) but also for chemotherapy.[9,10] Emerging evidences suggest that both under-treatments and over-treatments may have an impact on quality of life and life expectancy and should be avoided to ensure the best quality of care.[11] There are some clinical settings in GCTs where the degree of uncertainty is still high and the experience of the care providers makes a huge difference. The risk of overtreatment is particularly high in some equivocal scenarios, such as clinical stage I (CSI),[12] tumor marker negative stage IIA,[13] and patients with postchemotherapy residual disease.[14] The use of biomarkers able to predict with high fidelity the presence of viable GCT can significantly contribute to clarifying the disease and guiding the selection of the patients who need treatments.

Disclosure Statement: The authors have nothing to disclose.
[a] Department of Medicine, Medical Oncology Division, BC Cancer Agency, University of British Columbia, 600 West 10th Avenue, Vancouver, British Columbia V5Z 4E6, Canada; [b] Department of Urologic Sciences, Vancouver Prostate Centre, University of British Columbia, Vancouver, British Columbia, Canada; [c] Testicular Cancer Commons, Vancouver, WA, USA; [d] SWOG Group Chairs Office, 2611 Southwest 3rd Avenue MQ280, Portland, OR 97201, USA
* Corresponding author. 2611 Southwest 3rd Avenue MQ280, Portland, OR 97201.
E-mail address: craig@tccommons.org

urologic.theclinics.com

MANAGEMENT OF EQUIVOCAL CLINICAL SCENARIOS

Clinical Stage I Seminoma

CSI represents the most frequent presentation of GCTs. It is defined as the absence of detectable metastatic deposits outside the testis and normal tumor markers. Although the survival of CSI patients is almost 100%, there are still open controversies about the beneficial role of adjuvant treatments to reduce the risk of relapse. Approximately 75% to 80% of seminoma patients present CSI at diagnosis. Among those patients, approximately 15% have a relapse. The size of the primary testicular tumor is associated with the risk of relapse.[15] As demonstrated by Chung and colleagues,[16] however, the tumor size is a continuous variable and, even in presence of a primary tumor greater than 7 cm, the risk of relapse is less than 30%. The cutoff of 4 cm has been abandoned as main factor to select patients for adjuvant chemotherapy. Carboplatin has demonstrated equivalent to radiation therapy to reduce the risk of relapse in patients with CSI seminoma.[17] The modern approach shared by both European and Canadian–American experts is to manage all patients with CSI seminoma with active surveillance.[18,19] As demonstrated by large retrospective analysis, the 5-year survival of patients with CSI seminoma on surveillance is 99%.[20] There are pockets primarily in Europe that favor adjuvant carboplatin, but this management strategy is uncommon. Patients experiencing a relapse on surveillance are cured with chemotherapy or radiotherapy, and this strategy can spare long-term toxicity in 85% of patients.[20]

Clinical stage I nonseminoma

The most common presentation of nonseminoma is also CSI. The risk of relapse postorchiectomy is estimated at approximately 15% to 50%. The presence of lymphovascular invasion (LVI) assessed pathologically in the primary tumor predicts a 50% risk of relapse.[21] Other risk factors (ie, percentage of embryonal carcinoma component, expression of chemokine (C-X-C motif) ligand 2 (CXCL2),[22] and craniocaudal diameter of suspicious lymph nodes[23]) have been associated with a higher risk of relapse, but they have not been validated. Although primary RPLND has been abandoned in most of these cases,[24] the role of adjuvant chemotherapy in the LVI positive patients is still controversial.

Two cycles of bleomycin, etoposide, and platinum (BEP) have been demonstrated to reduce the risk of relapse from 50% to 2% to 4%[25] and, most recently, phase II experiences and a phase III clinical trial have demonstrated that 1 cycle of BEP has comparable outcomes.[26,27] The presence of LVI, however, predicts 50% of risk of relapse, and the treatment of all those patients consists of overtreatment of 50% of patients who are cured by orchiectomy alone. Because of the high effectiveness of BEP chemotherapy in the metastatic setting[20] and the long life expectancy of those patients, many experts favor active surveillance even in high-risk patients because adjuvant BEP still unnecessarily exposes half of those patients to potential harmful long-term side effects.[28] BEP × 1 cycle remains the preferred option only in selected situations and certain geographies.

Stage IIA tumor marker negative germ cell testicular cancer

The management of small, less than 2 cm, enlarging retroperitoneal masses in absence of elevated tumor markers is challenging. The risk of overtreatment is high in absence of a clear evidence of tumor growth. As demonstrated by retrospective surgical series, in this clinical stage, 40% to 50% of patients have no tumor.[13,14] The commonly used conservative approach in those cases characterized by a high uncertainty is to repeat a CT scan to assess the growth of the suspicious nodes and defer the treatment until there is evidence of tumor growth. This situation is particularly common in seminoma patients, often presenting with normal tumor markers. Once the tumor growth has been established, the treatment consists of either BEP × 3 cycles (seminoma and nonseminoma) or radiation therapy (seminoma).[18,19] The risk of second malignancies, however, is high in the long term with RT[29] and chemotherapy is the preferred option, unless clearly contraindicated.

Postchemotherapy residual disease

Management of postchemotherapy residual disease in patients with normal tumor markers is controversial and depends on the histology.

The management of postchemotherapy nonseminoma consists of surgical removal of residual retroperitoneal lesions larger than 1 cm. This is related mainly to the risk of teratoma, present in almost 40% of the residual tumors, and viable GCTs, identified in 10% to 15% of the patients. Therefore, 40% to 50% of patients have no teratoma or viable GCTs and are exposed to unnecessary surgeries.[30] In seminoma, the PET-CT scan has been shown to have a high negative predictive value with a greater than 3-cm residual disease[31] but its positive predictive value is low because of the high rate of false-positive results related to inflammatory or granulomatous reaction associated to seminomas.[32]

POTENTIAL CHANGE IN THE MANAGEMENT OF GERM CELL TESTICULAR CANCER PATIENTS WITH THE INTRODUCTION OF MicroRNAs
Biology of MicroRNAs in Germ Cell Testicular Cancers

MicroRNAs (miRNAs) are small (approximately 22 nucleotides) noncoding RNAs involved in the regulation of mRNA transcription and translation.[33] miRNA expression studies have shown specific patterns of expression in different solid tumors.[34] Although the human genome expresses greater than 900 miRNAs,[35] only 31 miRNAs are expressed by stem cells.[36] This finding has narrowed down the search for aberrant expression of the miRNAs in GCTs.

In 2006, Voorhoeve and colleagues[37] performed the first miRNA expression study of GCT tissue, observing that 2 miRNAs (miR), miR372a-3p and miR373a-3p, were particularly abundant in GCT tissue and cell lines. Subsequently the same group published the data of RNome of GCTs, describing that miR372 and miR373 are part of 2 similar clusters of miRNAs that are overexpressed in GCTs: cluster miR302a to miR302d and miR371 to miR373.[38] Those 8 miRNAs are part of the 31 miRNAs overexpressed in stem cells. Palmer and colleagues[39] confirmed the very high expression of those 8 miRNAs in GCTs tissue and human GCT cell lines compared with the normal peritumoral tissue and teratoma in both pediatric and adult GCTs. Overall, these 3 independent studies demonstrated for the first time that GCTs are characterized by a miRNA expression signature characteristic of stem cells and very specific for this type of malignancy.

Voorhoeve and colleagues[37] also explored the biological functions of those miRNAs. With the limitation of few data in this regard, LATS2 seems the most likely target. LATS2 is a negative regulator of the cell cycle, and preclinical evidence suggests that those miRNAs are able to induce tumor proliferation by promoting the transition from phase G1 to phase S of the cell cycle. The inhibition of those miRNAs by antisense oligonucleotides resulted in the arrest of the cell cycle. In cells, however, this led to a reduction of the response to cisplatin, probably because of the block of cell cycle in G1 phase.[36]

Those data support the use of miRNAs as tumor biomarkers rather than therapeutic targets.

Circulating MicroRNAs in Germ Cell Testicular Cancers

Compared with the circulating tumor DNA, miRNAs have demonstrated to be stable and to resist to the degradation of serum RNAses.[40]

MiRNAs 371 to 373 and 302 clusters were detected for the first time in the serum of a pediatric GCT patient by Murray and colleagues[41] in 2011. Since then, several groups have been working on the optimization of the method to extract, quantify, and analyze those circulating miRNAs.

METHODS

Three different methodologies[42–44] have been used to evaluate circulating miRNAs in GCTS. The technique to assess the expression is the same consisting of a real-time (RT)–polymerase chain reaction (PCR) of the target miRNAs after normalization for some reference miRNAs.

The methods differ for collection tubes, types of blood samples, miRNA extractions, normalization, and establishment of the cutoff to assess the performance of the test.

Collection Tubes

Most of the studies conducted to evaluate miRNA expression in the blood of GCTs patients are retrospective and have been conducted using frozen serum collected in serum separator tubes.[42,45,46] More recently, Streck tubes have been used to collect blood for cell-free DNA and circulating tumor DNA analysis. Those tubes have the advantage of being stored at room temperature up until 1 week with stabilizing the cell-free DNA, a characteristic particularly relevant in the context of samples collection to establish a biobank.

Blood Samples

Most of the miRNA studies in GCTs have demonstrated that miRNAs can be efficiently extracted from the peripheral blood. Nappi and colleagues[44] recently reported that miR371a-3p can be extracted from plasma collected with Streck tubes with comparable results in terms of sensitivity and slightly better specificity. Compared with serum, the plasma obtained from the Streck tubes have lower expression of miR23a-3p, a miRNA proposed for evaluating hemolysis.[43] Because of this variability in plasma compared with serum, the use of miR23a-3p is not recommended as reference miRNA when plasma is used.[47]

MicroRNA Extraction

- Magnetic beads–conjugated miRNAs: Gillis and colleagues[42] have developed a targeted miRNA extraction (TSmiR) based on magnetic beads conjugated to 389 antisense oligonucleotides complementary to the targeted ones, including the reference miRNAs. The volume of serum used with this method is

50 μL (lower than the one used in other methods) and no preamplification was used. After the incubation, the magnetic beads are pulled down using a magnetic separator and the miRNAs are isolated using an elution solution and then quantified by RT-PCR.

- Direct miRNAs extraction: the extraction from serum or plasma can be done directly by using a serum/plasma extraction kit (Qiagen, Germany or mirVana [Life Technologies, California, US]).[41,48] With this method, a slightly higher sample volume (200–400 μL) is needed and preamplification has been used to increase the sensitivity of detecting miRNAs amplification.

MicroRNA Expression

RT-PCR has been used to assess targeted miRNA amplification, regardless of the method chosen to extract the miRNAs. As for other biomarker panels, this technique is based on multiple steps. The RNA is reverse transcribed to produce clonal DNA. In this phase, a multiplexed RT is performed and the probes of the miRNAs of interest are used. One preamplification of the RT products has been used by most of the groups. The preamplified clonal DNA then is used to assess the targeted miRNA expression by single-plexed quantitative PCR.

Normalization

To reduce this variability of the miRNAs expression, the cycle threshold (Ct) of the targeted miR-NAs is normalized to reference miRNAs.[49] The reference miRNA expression does not change based on tumor characteristics. Usually an external spike-in miRNA also is added to the blood samples before the extraction to evaluate the extraction efficiency. To reduce the variability of the results, several references miRNAs are chosen. In GCTs, miR30b-5p was selected as the best reference miRNAs among a pool of 10 miRNAs because of its lowest variability in expression.[50] Moreover, miR451a and miR23a-3p,

indicators of hemolysis, have been selected to reduce the effect of hemolysis on the targeted miRNAs.[43] Although some studies have used 1 reference miRNA,[48] the authors' recommendation is to use several reference miRNAs to reduce the variability of expression (miR30b-5p, miR39-3p, miR451a, and miR23a-3p).

CLINICAL VALIDITY OF MicroRNAs IN GERM CELL TESTICULAR CANCERS
Obvious Germ Cell Testicular Cancers: Primary in Situ and Metastatic Germ Cell Testicular Cancers

MiRNAs have demonstrated to have a very high sensitivity and specificity to detect viable GCTs. As proof of feasibility, most of the available data have been collected in patients with primary testicular cancer prior to and after to orchiectomy (**Table 1**).

The half-life of miR371 after the orchiectomy was evaluated in 24 patients with CSI GCT prior to and for 3 days after the surgery. The serum levels of miR371 decreased to 2.6%, 1.2%, and 0.47% of the preorchiectomy levels at day 1, 2, and 3, respectively. The calculated half-life was 7 hours to 12 hours, which is shorter than the classic tumor markers, β–human chorionic gonadotropin and α-fetoprotein.[51]

Using the TSmiR test, Gillis and colleagues[42] demonstrated that miR371 to miR373 and 302 clusters can be detectable in the serum of most patients with GCTs, seminoma and nonseminoma. Most of the patients had miRNAs evaluated prior to orchiectomy and postorchiectomy, and the expression of miRNAs was compared with normal healthy volunteers (n = 47) or to patients with non-GCT testicular masses (n = 12). Combining the results of miRNAs 371 to 372 with miRNAs 373 and 367, sensitivity was 98% and specificity was 48.3%, whereas the specificity was 60% to 91% and sensitivity was 90% when those miRNAs were analyzed individually.

The results of TSmiR test were confirmed in a larger cohort (n = 250) of patients with CSI GCTs

Table 1
Serum microRNA 367, microRNA 371, microRNA 372, and microRNA 373 accuracy

	Dieckmann et al,[48] 2017		Gillis et al,[42] 2013		van Agthoven et al,[52] 2016	
	Area Under the Curve	P Value	Area Under the Curve	P Value	Area Under the Curve	P Value
miR371	0.9432	.001	0.89	<.0001	0.951	.000
miR367	0.8173	.006	0.94	<.0001	0.861	.034
miR372	0.7875	>.05	0.91	<.0001	NA	NA
miR373	0.7697	>.05	0.96	<.0001	0.888	.003

prior orchiectomy. In this study, the levels of miR371, miR372 and miR373 were compared with 60 non-GCT patients and 104 male healthy volunteers. The area under the curve (AUC) of the receiver operating characteristic (ROC) curve for miR371 was higher than the AUC of miR372 and miR373 and was comparable to the AUC of the 3 miRNAs combined (0.951 vs 0.962), with a sensitivity of 90% and a specificity of 86% to 91%. The quantification of the expression was compared with the raw Ct data and similar results were obtained. Dieckmann and colleagues[48] published the largest series of serum miRNA in patients with GCTs, prior to and after orchiectomy and in patients with stage II and stage III GCTs prior to, during, and after chemotherapy. In the development cohort, 50 patients were evaluated for miR371, miR372, miR373, and miR367 and the sensitivity of miR371 was comparable to the combined miRNAs (**Table 2**). miR371 was demonstrated to be highly expressed prior to orchiectomy and to decrease after surgery. Overall, 160 patients were analyzed and compared with healthy male volunteers. This study demonstrated that miR371 was able to predict the presence of viable GCTs with a sensitivity of 92% and a specificity of 80%. The levels of serum miRNAs were related to tumor burden; however, no patients in this study presented with a tumor volume less than 1.5 cm. The levels of miR371 decreased during chemotherapy in patients with metastatic disease. Only 18 patients of the 166 analyzed had relapsed disease and miR371 was overexpressed in all those patients. The cutoff for sensitivity was set up at a relative expression (RQ) of 5. Although a significant reduction of the serum levels was observed after treatments, no data about the post-treatment follow-up were reported and more specifically no data were available about post-treatment residual or relapsed disease.[48] Both those studies[48,52] used only miR93 as reference miRNA for normalization and no control for hemolysis was adopted.

In March 2019, Dieckman and colleagues[53] published the first prospective study of serum miR371 in patients with GCT. The serum expression of miR371 in patients with testicular GCT (n = 616) was compared with 258 male controls.

Most of the patients enrolled had the miR371 assessed prior to the orchiectomy and presented with CSI disease, 201 patients had metastatic disease and 46 were evaluated at the time of tumor relapse. The sensitivity of miR371 in detecting GCT prior to the orchiectomy was 90.1%, specificity 94.0%, positive predictive value 97.2%, and AUC 0.966. The investigators confirmed that miR371 expression levels were associated with clinical stage, primary tumor size, and response to treatment. MiR371 also was overexpressed in patients who presented with GCT relapse and normalized to normal levels on remission.

Equivocal Germ Cell Testicular Cancers

Postchemotherapy residual disease
MiRNAs 371, 373, and 367 were analyzed using the TSmiR technique in 82 patients postchemotherapy and prior to RPLND. Only 12 patients had residual viable GCTs and serum miR371 predicted viable GCTs, with specificity of 50% and sensitivity of 100%, in cases of a residual disease greater than 3 cm. Residual postchemotherapy teratoma and fibrosis did not present high levels of serum miRNAs. The AUC of miR371 alone was 0.874, comparable to the combined miRNAs 371 and 373 (AUC 0.885).[46]

Germ cell neoplasia in situ
Germ cell neoplasia in situ (GCNIS) is considered a preinvasive stage of GCTs. Although a group from the Netherlands using TSmiR test did not reveal miRNA in 6 patients with GCNIS,[52] a recent publication from the Dieckmann group demonstrated that serum miR371 was overexpressed in 50% of the 27 patients with GCNIS analyzed.[54] Although preliminary and involving small number of patients, these results are encouraging to support the use of circulating miRNAs to identify microscopic GCTs in early stages of disease.

FUTURE CLINICAL IMPLICATIONS OF MicroRNAs

Promising results showing consistent high sensitivity and specificity in identifying GCTs from

Table 2
Sensitivity and specificity of serum miR371 compared with microRNA 367, microRNA 371, microRNA 372, and microRNA 373 tested together

	Dieckmann et al,[48] 2017		van Agthoven et al,[52] 2016	
	Sensitivity (%)	Specificity (%)	Sensitivity (%)	Specificity (%)
miR371	92	84	90	86
miR371, miR372, miR373, and miR367 (all 4 together)	92	80	90	91

Table 3
Differences in the extraction and analysis of microRNAs across the different studies

	Targeted MicroRNA Extraction[42]	Targeted MicroRNA Extraction[42]	Serum MicroRNA Extraction[48]	Serum MicroRNA Extraction[50]	Plasma MicroRNA Extraction[44]
Blood collection tubes	Not specified	Not specified	Serum separator	Serum separator	Streck
Extraction method	Magnetic beads	Magnetic beads	Serum with extraction kit	Serum with extraction kit	Plasma with extraction kit
Preamplification	none	10 min at 95°C, 12 cycles at 95°C for 15 s, and 60°C for 1 min	10 min at 95°C, 14 cycles at 95°C for 15 s, and 60°C for 1 min	10 min at 95°C, 14 cycles at 95°C for 15 s, and 60°C for 4 min	10 min at 95°C, 14 cycles at 95°C for 15 s, and 60°C for 1 min
Normalization	miR20a miR93-5p	miR30b-5p	miR93-5p	miR30b-5p cel–miR39-3p	miR30b-5p cel–miR39-3p miR451a
Quantification	RQ	RQ	RQ	RQ	RQ and qualitative
Spike in miRNAs	Cel–miR39-3p Ath–miR159a	Cel–miR39-3p Ath–miR159a	Cel–miR39-3p	Cel–miR39-3p	Cel–miR39-3p
Quality control	Intraplates and interplates variability	Hemolysis	NA	Ct values of miR30b-5p cel–miR39-3p miR451a miR23a-3p hemolysis	Ct values of miR30b-5p cel–miR39-3p miR451a miR23a-3p hemolysis
Serum volume	50 µL	50 µL	200 µL	200 µL	200 µL
Data analysis	No pre-established cutoffs Cutoffs of RQ adjusted to reach a certain sensitivity	No pre-established cutoffs Cutoffs of RQ adjusted to reach a certain sensitivity	Cutoff: RQ ≥5 to evaluate sensitivity and specificity	Cutoff: RQ ≥2 to define miRNA overexpression	Quantitative and qualitative analysis The definition of +ve or −ve miR371-based on cT value ≤40 assuming acceptable values of miR30b-5p, miR39-3p, and miR451a

several groups around the world have encouraged further prospective studies to validate circulating miRNAs analysis in several clinical settings.

MiRNAs will be evaluated as an optional translational component of the Children's Oncology Group (COG) study AGCT1531 that is randomizing pediatric and adult patients with germ cell malignancy to surveillance or specific treatments. This phase III multicenter study randomizes pediatric and adult patients to 5 arms based on the clinical stage at presentation and the risk factors of relapse in patients with CSI. Patients with low risk CSI are followed with surveillance, and blood is optionally collected during the follow-up. Patients with high-risk CSI GCT and metastatic GCT are randomized to chemotherapy regimens with either carboplatin or cisplatin. The primary endpoints of the study are overall survival and event-free survival. The utility of the 4-miRNA panel (miR371, miR372, miR373, and miR367) is one of the secondary endpoints of the study. Although informative for the pediatric GCT population, the COG AGCT1531 study will add few data about adult GCT, especially for seminoma, considering that this group is under-represented in the pediatric population of GCTs.

Considering the outstanding performance of miRNA detection, its use may be extremely informative in equivocal clinical situations characterized by high uncertainty and that are prone to mistakes, which lead to either over-treatment or under-treatment in these patients.

If circulating miRNAs are confirmed to have the same sensitivity demonstrated in advanced disease, this test will solve the clinical dilemma of management of patients with tumor marker negative stage IIA, avoiding repeated imaging and unnecessary invasive procedures or unnecessary treatments.

CSI is the most frequent presentation of GCTs and a good predictive biomarker of relapse to select patients for adjuvant treatments is an unmet clinical need. If their sensitivity also is confirmed in this early stage of disease, miRNAs may contribute to solving the unavailability of a good biomarker of relapse in clinical stage I. In this regard and to answer the clinical utility of miRNAs in predicting relapse in patients with clinical stage I, a large cohort prospective trial (SWOG S1823) enrolling more than 1000 patients with CSI seminoma and nonseminoma is planned.

CRITICISMS AND CHALLENGES

The cutoff to assign the significance to the (over) expression of the miRNAs has been established on the post-hoc sensitivity to identify viable GCTs, and none of the studies has proposed a standard cutoff that can be used prospectively (**Table 3**). The inconsistency among the studies may be reduced by a standard method that to uniform the extraction method, protocol of preamplifications, type and number of reference miRNAs, and blood samples/collecting tubes. To reduce the interexperiment variability, the significance of the overexpression should be assessed based on a cutoff established on the sensitivity of the technique to detect the lowest tumor volume possible (ie, microscopic disease in patients with CSI tumor).

A possible solution to obtaining a standard method may be to use a qualitative rather quantitative method based on the analysis of the raw Ct of the targeted miRNA, once normalized for the reference miRNAs.[44]

Although miRNAs have demonstrated as expressed and detectable in the blood of patients with viable GCTs, it is known that they are not expressed by teratoma. A negative miRNA result in patients with GCT and radiologic evidence of metastatic disease is suspicious for the presence of disseminated teratoma or for non-GCT conditions. Especially in the postchemotherapy setting of nonseminoma patients with residual disease, however, a negative miRNA cannot rule out the presence of teratoma and, therefore, cannot be used to inform clinical decisions. Promising data for the identification of teratoma-specific biomarkers have demonstrated that miR375 is overexpressed in teratoma tissue[55] but no data about the detection of this miRNA in the blood of patients with teratoma are available.

SUMMARY

The results obtained in several independent laboratories around the world confirming the high sensitivity and specificity are reassuring of the biological value of miRNAs as biomarkers of viable GCTs. Conjunct efforts are needed to standardize the methods and obtain more uniform results. Prospective trials planned will be valuable to definitely validate the use of those circulating miRNAs, especially in early-stage GCTs and in other equivocal scenarios where the rate of uncertainty is concerning.

REFERENCES

1. Goldberg K: ASCO50th anniversary poll names the top 5 advances from the past 50 years, 2014.
2. Einhorn LH. Testicular cancer as a model for a curable neoplasm: the Richard and Hinda Rosenthal Foundation Award Lecture. Cancer Res 1981;41:3275–80.

3. Kollmannsberger C, Tyldesley S, Moore C, et al. Evolution in management of testicular seminoma: population-based outcomes with selective utilization of active therapies. Ann Oncol 2011;22:808–14.

4. Nichols C, Kollmannsberger C. Alternatives to standard BEP x 3 in good-prognosis germ cell tumors–you bet your life. J Natl Cancer Inst 2010;102:1214–5.

5. Fein DE, Paulus JK, Mathew P. Reassessment of 4-cycle etoposide and cisplatin as the standard of care for good-risk metastatic germ cell tumors. JAMA Oncol 2018;4(12):1661–2.

6. Fung C, Sesso HD, Williams AM, et al. Multi-institutional assessment of adverse health outcomes among North American testicular cancer survivors after modern cisplatin-based chemotherapy. J Clin Oncol 2017;35:1211–22.

7. Kerns SL, Fung C, Monahan PO, et al. Cumulative burden of morbidity among testicular cancer survivors after standard cisplatin-based chemotherapy: a multi-institutional study. J Clin Oncol 2018;36:1505–12.

8. Jeldres C, Pham KN, Daneshmand S, et al. Association of higher institutional volume with improved overall survival in clinical stage III testicular cancer: Results from the National Cancer Data Base (1998-2011). J Clin Oncol 2014;32(Suppl 15):4519.

9. Flum AS, Bachrach L, Jovanovic BD, et al. Patterns of performance of retroperitoneal lymph node dissections by American urologists: most retroperitoneal lymph node dissections in the United States are performed by low-volume surgeons. Urology 2014;84:1325–8.

10. Feuer EJ, Sheinfeld J, Bosl GJ. Does size matter? Association between number of patients treated and patient outcome in metastatic testicular cancer. J Natl Cancer Inst 1999;91:816–8.

11. Tandstad T, Kollmannsberger CK, Roth BJ, et al. Practice makes perfect: the rest of the story in testicular cancer as a model curable neoplasm. J Clin Oncol 2017;35:3525–8.

12. Nappi L, Nichols CR, Kollmannsberger CK. New treatments for stage I testicular cancer. Clin Adv Hematol Oncol 2017;15:626–31.

13. Stephenson AJ, Bosl GJ, Motzer RJ, et al. Retroperitoneal lymph node dissection for nonseminomatous germ cell testicular cancer: impact of patient selection factors on outcome. J Clin Oncol 2005;23:2781–8.

14. Daneshmand S, Albers P, Fossa SD, et al. Contemporary management of postchemotherapy testis cancer. Eur Urol 2012;62:867–76.

15. Warde P, Specht L, Horwich A, et al. Prognostic factors for relapse in stage I seminoma managed by surveillance: a pooled analysis. J Clin Oncol 2002;20:4448–52.

16. Chung P, Daugaard G, Tyldesley S, et al. Evaluation of a prognostic model for risk of relapse in stage I seminoma surveillance. Cancer Med 2015;4:155–60.

17. Oliver RT, Mead GM, Rustin GJ, et al. Randomized trial of carboplatin versus radiotherapy for stage I seminoma: mature results on relapse and contralateral testis cancer rates in MRC TE19/EORTC 30982 study (ISRCTN27163214). J Clin Oncol 2011;29:957–62.

18. Albers P, Albrecht W, Algaba F, et al. Guidelines on testicular cancer: 2015 update. Eur Urol 2015;68:1054–68.

19. Motzer RJ, Jonasch E, Agarwal N, et al. Testicular cancer, version 2.2015. J Natl Compr Canc Netw 2015;13:772–99.

20. Kollmannsberger C, Tandstad T, Bedard PL, et al. Patterns of relapse in patients with clinical stage I testicular cancer managed with active surveillance. J Clin Oncol 2015;33:51–7.

21. Albers P, Siener R, Kliesch S, et al. Risk factors for relapse in clinical stage I nonseminomatous testicular germ cell tumors: results of the German Testicular Cancer Study Group Trial. J Clin Oncol 2003;21:1505–12.

22. Gilbert DC, Al-Saadi R, Thway K, et al. Defining a new prognostic index for stage I nonseminomatous germ cell tumors using CXCL12 expression and proportion of embryonal carcinoma. Clin Cancer Res 2016;22:1265–73.

23. Howard SA, Gray KP, O'Donnell EK, et al. Craniocaudal retroperitoneal node length as a risk factor for relapse from clinical stage I testicular germ cell tumor. AJR Am J Roentgenol 2014;203:W415–20.

24. Nicolai N, Miceli R, Necchi A, et al. Retroperitoneal lymph node dissection with no adjuvant chemotherapy in clinical stage I nonseminomatous germ cell tumours: long-term outcome and analysis of risk factors of recurrence. Eur Urol 2010;58:912–8.

25. Tandstad T, Cohn-Cedermark G, Dahl O, et al. Long-term follow-up after risk-adapted treatment in clinical stage 1 (CS1) nonseminomatous germ-cell testicular cancer (NSGCT) implementing adjuvant CVB chemotherapy. A SWENOTECA study. Ann Oncol 2010;21:1858–63.

26. Huddart RA, Joffe JK, White JD, et al. 111: A single-arm trial evaluating one cycle of BEP as adjuvant chemotherapy in high-risk, stage 1 nonseminomatous or combined germ cell tumors of the testis (NSGCTT). J Clin Oncol 2017;35(Suppl 6):400.

27. Tandstad T, Stahl O, Hakansson U, et al. One course of adjuvant BEP in clinical stage I nonseminoma mature and expanded results from the SWENOTECA group. Ann Oncol 2014;25:2167–72.

28. Nichols CR, Roth B, Albers P, et al. Active surveillance is the preferred approach to clinical stage I testicular cancer. J Clin Oncol 2013;31:3490–3.

29. Travis LB, Ng AK, Allan JM, et al. Second malignant neoplasms and cardiovascular disease following radiotherapy. J Natl Cancer Inst 2012; 104:357–70.

30. Steyerberg EW, Keizer HJ, Fossa SD, et al. Prediction of residual retroperitoneal mass histology after chemotherapy for metastatic nonseminomatous germ cell tumor: multivariate analysis of individual patient data from six study groups. J Clin Oncol 1995;13:1177–87.

31. De Santis M, Becherer A, Bokemeyer C, et al. 2-18fluoro-deoxy-D-glucose positron emission tomography is a reliable predictor for viable tumor in post-chemotherapy seminoma: an update of the prospective multicentric SEMPET trial. J Clin Oncol 2004;22:1034–9.

32. Cathomas R, Klingbiel D, Bernard B, et al. Questioning the value of fluorodeoxyglucose positron emission tomography for residual lesions after chemotherapy for metastatic seminoma: results of an international global germ cell cancer group registry. J Clin Oncol 2018. [Epub ahead of print].

33. Zamore PD, Haley B. Ribo-gnome: the big world of small RNAs. Science 2005;309:1519–24.

34. Catto JWF, Alcaraz A, Bjartell AS, et al. MicroRNA in prostate, bladder, and kidney cancer: a systematic review. Eur Urol 2011;59:671–81.

35. Winter J, Jung S, Keller S, et al. Many roads to maturity: microRNA biogenesis pathways and their regulation. Nat Cell Biol 2009;11:228–34.

36. Eini R, Dorssers LC, Looijenga LH. Role of stem cell proteins and microRNAs in embryogenesis and germ cell cancer. Int J Dev Biol 2013;57:319–32.

37. Voorhoeve PM, le Sage C, Schrier M, et al. A genetic screen implicates miRNA-372 and miRNA-373 as oncogenes in testicular germ cell tumors. Cell 2006;124:1169–81.

38. Gillis AJM, Stoop HJ, Hersmus R, et al. High-throughput microRNAome analysis in human germ cell tumours. J Pathol 2007;213:319–28.

39. Palmer RD, Murray MJ, Saini HK, et al. Malignant germ cell tumors display common microRNA profiles resulting in global changes in expression of messenger RNA targets. Cancer Res 2010;70: 2911–23.

40. Mitchell PS, Parkin RK, Kroh EM, et al. Circulating microRNAs as stable blood-based markers for cancer detection. Proc Natl Acad Sci U S A 2008;105: 10513–8.

41. Murray MJ, Halsall DJ, Hook CE, et al. Identification of microRNAs From the miR-371~373 and miR-302 clusters as potential serum biomarkers of malignant germ cell tumors. Am J Clin Pathol 2011;135: 119–25.

42. Gillis AJ, Rijlaarsdam MA, Eini R, et al. Targeted serum miRNA (TSmiR) test for diagnosis and follow-up of (testicular) germ cell cancer patients: a proof of principle. Mol Oncol 2013;7:1083–92.

43. Murray MJ, Huddart RA, Coleman N. The present and future of serum diagnostic tests for testicular germ cell tumours. Nat Rev Urol 2016;13:715–25.

44. Nappi L, Neil BO, Daneshmand S, et al. Circulating miR-371a-3p for the detection of low volume viable germ cell tumor: Expanded pilot data, clinical implications and future study. J Clin Oncol 2018; 36(Suppl 15):4549.

45. Murray MJ, Raby KL, Saini HK, et al. Solid tumors of childhood display specific serum microRNA profiles. Cancer Epidemiol Biomarkers Prev 2015;24:350–60.

46. Leao R, van Agthoven T, Figueiredo A, et al. Serum miRNA predicts viable disease after chemotherapy in patients with testicular nonseminoma germ cell tumor. J Urol 2018;200:126–35.

47. Murray MJ, Watson HL, Ward D, et al. "Future-proofing" blood processing for measurement of circulating miRNAs in samples from biobanks and prospective clinical trials. Cancer Epidemiol Biomarkers Prev 2018;27:208–18.

48. Dieckmann KP, Radtke A, Spiekermann M, et al. Serum levels of MicroRNA miR-371a-3p: a sensitive and specific new biomarker for germ cell tumours. Eur Urol 2017;71:213–20.

49. Lohmann S, Herold A, Bergauer T, et al. Gene expression analysis in biomarker research and early drug development using function tested reverse transcription quantitative real-time PCR assays. Methods 2013;59:10–9.

50. Murray MJ, Bell E, Raby KL, et al. A pipeline to quantify serum and cerebrospinal fluid microRNAs for diagnosis and detection of relapse in paediatric malignant germ-cell tumours. Br J Cancer 2016; 114:151–62.

51. Radtke A, Hennig F, Ikogho R, et al. The novel biomarker of germ cell tumours, Micro-RNA-371a-3p, has a very rapid decay in patients with clinical stage 1. Urologia Internationalis 2018;100:470–5.

52. van Agthoven T, Looijenga LHJ. Accurate primary germ cell cancer diagnosis using serum based microRNA detection (ampTSmiR test). Oncotarget 2017;8:58037–49.

53. Dieckmann KP, Radtke A, Geczi L, et al. Serum levels of MicroRNA-371a-3p (M371 Test) as a new biomarker of testicular germ cell tumors: results of a prospective multicentric study. J Clin Oncol 2019. [Epub ahead of print].

54. Radtke A, Cremers JF, Kliesch S, et al. Can germ cell neoplasia in situ be diagnosed by measuring serum levels of microRNA371a-3p? J Cancer Res Clin Oncol 2017;143:2383–92.

55. Shen H, Shih J, Hollern DP, et al. Integrated molecular characterization of testicular germ cell tumors. Cell Rep 2018;23:3392–406.

Moving?

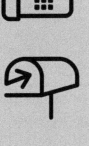

Printed and bound by CPI Group (UK) Ltd, Croydon, CR0 4YY

03/10/2024

01040371-0013